Outdoor and Mountain Medicine

Kindly supported by MAMMUT
Absolute alpine.

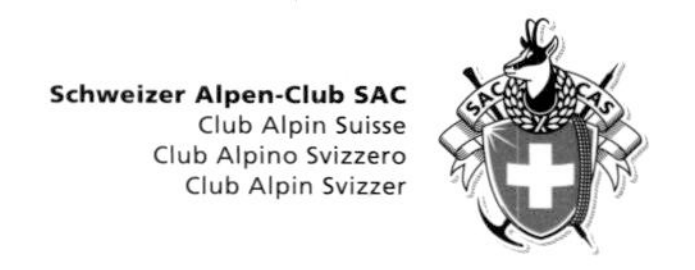

A.G. Brunello / M. Walliser / U. Hefti

Outdoor and Mountain Medicine

Mountaineering Rescue and First Aid Care

Education

1st English edition
edited by «Language 4u» and Martin Walliser

SAC Verlag

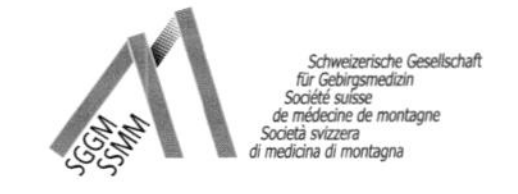

Graphics and typesetting: Egger AG, Frutigen
Lithos: Egger AG, Frutigen
Printed and bound in Italy by Printer Trento S.r.l.
Cover design: Buch & Grafik, Barbara Willi-Halter, Zurich
Cover illustrations: Swiss Exped research expedition 2009/ Tommy Dätwyler (front), Urs Wiget (back)

ISBN 978-3-85902-394-9

Index of Contents

Preface

What counts in life is not the number of breaths you take but the moments that take your breath away. Such moments may be of a positive or negative nature. Understandably, it is everyone's hope that they will only experience the positive ones. If you are keen to experience those wonderful exhilarating moments for yourself, you could do worse than to consult the program offered by a "Bergschule" run by people who are familiar with all the different aspects of mountaineering activity. In order to ensure that you avoid any encounters with those negative moments of breathlessness, the authors have taken time out to write the chapters of this book which you now hold in your hands. Studying its contents will help you to minimize the likelihood of falling victim to ailments and accidents.

Venturing into the mountains is by no means the same as embarking on a trip to the seaside. Even with the most meticulous of preparations it is still possible to encounter rockfalls, it is easy to put a foot wrong and slip and predicting altitude sickness is like trying to forecast the weather. What risks a tour of the mountains, a trekking trip or even staying out in the open air may involve, what preparations we can make and what we need to do should an accident happen are all set out in the pages of this enthralling book. Its handy format means that you can also take it along in your rucksack and use it as a guidebook, something to read in your hut or as a companion on an expedition. This, the first issue, represents a pooling in compressed format of current knowledge on all matters related to mountain and outdoor medicine. The authors include distinguished Swiss experts in high-altitude medicine. I would like to take the opportunity of congratulating authors Brunello, Walliser and Hefti on their work and assure them of the support of the Swiss Society of Mountain Medicine not only now but also in the future, in their efforts by to make our mountains safer, to optimize the treatment of victims of sickness or accidents and to implement the best possible emergency treatment.

Walo Pfeifhofer
President SGGM

May 2010

We are happy and proud to be able to present the second book in our series "Education" in collaboration with the Swiss Society of Mountain Medicine (SGGM). What has emerged is a straightforward and articulate work of nonfiction clearly geared to the requirements of Alpinists and instructors alike. We would also like to express our thanks to the team of authors under the direction of Anna Brunello and the SGGM for a fruitful collaboration.

Meyrin – Geneva, June 2010
President of the Publishing Committee of the Swiss Alpine Club (SAC)

Hans Bräm

After this extensive work has been published already in its second edition in the German language and also successful in the French language, the SAC (Swiss Alpine Club) is very pleased to offer now also the Italian and English first edition. The SAC endeavors whenever possible to publish in Italian as the third national language. The English edition is a further step to gain international attention and recognition. We thank the author team led by Anna Brunello and the SGGM (Swiss Society of Mountain Medicine) for their support.

Hünibach/Thun, April 2014
President of the Publishing Committee of the Swiss Alpine Club (SAC)

Peter Hubacher

Foreword

Medical experts specializing in mountain medicine have always aspired to ensuring that the emergency patient in the mountains has approximately the same chances of survival as would be expected in a lowland environment. Unfortunately, in addition to the subjective principles, there are also objective circumstances as well which further jeopardize the sick person's or accident victim's chances of survival. Rescuing a patient in the mountains is a more complicated and protracted procedure than at low levels; consequently the time taken to reach hospital tends to be longer. In the mountains there are medical problems that are practically unknown in lowland areas. Rescuing an avalanche victim or treating a patient with suspension trauma are problems specifically encountered in relation to mountain medicine. All these factors demonstrate the need for a training manual in mountain medicine.

It was some years ago that Bruno Durrer, Urs Wiget and I first gave some thought to writing a book on mountain medicine. The idea came about during the first of the summer courses in mountain medicine on the Furka Pass and in the winter on the Oberalp Pass. Our thoughts centered on a small booklet on First Aid that could be easily packed in a rucksack and a larger work on mountain medicine to keep at home. Based on various documents relating to courses for SAC rescue teams, mountain guides, avalanche dog handlers and piste patrollers, the book "First Aid for Hikers and Mountaineers" (Durrer, Jacomet, Wiget, 3rd edition, SAC Publishing, Berne) was born. The work on the book on mountain medicine was plagued by delays until a new group of young and enthusiastic medical experts specializing in mountain medicine got to work and made the original idea a reality.
Today the work – drafted by doctors involved in mountain medicine, mountain rescue and high altitude mountaineering – is at last available. The fact that the authors all have such relevant experience can only be of benefit as far as the present volume is concerned – the people who have worked on it are not mere theorists, they are all practitioners and members of the SGGM. The experience of the older generation coupled with the medical knowledge of younger colleagues is what makes the book so interesting and valuable.
The various topics in relation to mountain medicine are clearly dealt with, the reader can find the answer to the vast majority of questions he may have in relation to the sector. The book represents a valuable medical companion to learning for anyone involved with First Aid in the mountains, either on a professional or voluntary basis.

I would like, on behalf of all users, to thank my colleagues, the authors, most sincerely for the work they have done. The successful outcome of their work will undoubtedly be more than gratifying recompense for all those hours spent in the mountains. SAC Publishing can be proud of having a work of this nature on its library shelves. I wish all readers every enjoyment when it comes to immersing themselves in topics relating to mountain medicine.

Hans Jacomet

On behalf of all the authors (for contact details see under "Authorship," Page 313) I would like to take this opportunity of extending my sincere thanks for all the comments and suggestions for improvements that have already been received and any that are still to be received and which will be used to advantage in the next edition.

In this first English edition, there is particular focus on the topic of resuscitation in accordance with the 2010 guidelines. In conjunction with this the subject of artificial respiration has assumed new importance in the resuscitation guidelines. Special thanks to our english friends Dr. Parminder Chaggar, Dr. Gareth James and Dr. Mike Wilde for their tremendous support in reviewing the chapters.

Particular thanks also to Urs and Walli for their fantastic ongoing support, to Andrea and Steffi for compiling the lexicon so quickly, to the "old guys" for their many contributions and the lively discussions, to René Wellig (Egger AG) and Hans Ott (SAC Publishers) for their patience and help.
And, of course, to all participants in the SAC "First Aid" courses who inspired the project and to the Swiss Society of Mountain Medicine who made it possible.

And we extend our special thoughts to Willi Kuhn (1961–2011), long-term SAC mountain rescuer, trainer and emergency medical technician. With his extensive knowledge of mountain rescue and what it has to teach us, Willi supported and enriched this book with valuable tips conveyed by way of content as well as through the medium of illustrations.

Anna G. Brunello, Martin Walliser
March 2014

Introduction

Hints

 Important aspects for the implementation of learned concepts into practice.

 Important additional information, please note.

 Didactic advice

Safety in the Mountains

Regardless of how difficult the tour is and how familiar you are with the route, it is essential that you keep to the following rules:

- Find out about conditions and the weather!
- Leave nothing to chance! Any good tour or any variation on it needs to be planned. You always need a good Plan B.
- Keep your strength up! When on a mountain you are well-advised to maintain a stock of reserves. It is only in this way that you will be in a position to respond to unpleasant surprises.
- Don't stint! Basic equipment like good footwear, safety equipment appropriate to the particular season and the tour are things that you must have with you at all costs.
- Watch out for slippery surfaces! Snow, ice and wet grass call for experience and skill. Give some thought to whether you are up to coping with the difficulties.
- Don't keep it to yourself! Doubts, aspirations, decisions, they all have a place on the discussion table when you are in the mountains! Thinking in unison helps keep everyone's spirits up and paves the way for good decisions.
- Take a good look at yourself! Observe the way you behave. When are you open-minded, at what point do you become stubborn, where do you feel secure, where do you not feel secure? Learn the art of self-esteem as well as how to assess your own capabilities.

Alpine Hazards

The easiest way to prevent a mountaineering accident is to be cautious when planning a tour, to consistently review your plans while on the tour, to ensure that no member of the group is overstretched and that everyone is alert and aware of the risks. Some possible hazards are listed below and strategies for dealing with them explained.

Falling: Go slowly and concentrate when on exposed paths and difficult terrain. Help weaker members of the group along (rope?). If in an area where there is a potential risk of falling and an accumulation of unfavorable factors such as poor going underfoot, wet, snow, time pressures and fatigue, extreme caution should be exercised and consideration given to possibly even abandoning the attempt.

Bad weather: In bad weather the difficulty and risk associated with a tour is intensified. If you are still determined to proceed, you should adopt an extremely defensive approach. This will ensure an intense experience even on a fairly short and simple tour. Take special care in the case of cold fronts and thunderstorms. If there is lightning retreat from exposed areas, belay yourself and sit on your rucksack!

Avalanches: The main source of danger on tours that take place in the winter. Observe and assess are the keywords, both when planning the tour (Avalanche Report) and while you are actually on the tour. Even in the summer, avalanches present a threat which needs to be taken seriously. The risk increases with each new fall of snow and/or significant degree of warming. Even a small quantity of snow slipping down can lead to a fall.

Fall into a crevasse: Make sure that you are always roped up when walking on snowbound glaciers, except you can completely exclude the risk of crevasses. Your map or markings on alpine hiking routes will not be sufficient to cover this eventuality. If you are on skis you should rope up in areas where there are crevasses if the visibility is poor or where there are crevasses which have an insufficient covering of snow. Corresponding equipment (rope, harness, crevasse rescue materials) should always be carried. Do not linger on snowbound glaciers; retreat before the bridges over the crevasses become soft.

Rockfalls: In steep terrain, in particular when snow and rock alternate, there is a risk of rockfall. In warm weather this risk increases. Wear a helmet, make sure you get back early, avoid gullies and slopes and instead keep to ridges and edges. Rockfalls may also be caused by other mountaineers, animals or the onset of rain.

Ice falls: Unstable areas of an ice collapse, e.g. ice blocks (seracs) may topple at any time (no increase of risk during the course of the day). Avoid discharge area (often very extensive) or pass by quickly. Keep a watch on seracs and give some thought to an escape route.

Cornice collapse: Even for specialists, it is practically impossible to identify the threat of a cornice collapse. Ascertain the size of the cornice and give the edge a wide berth. Be very critical when assessing tracks.

Risk Factors

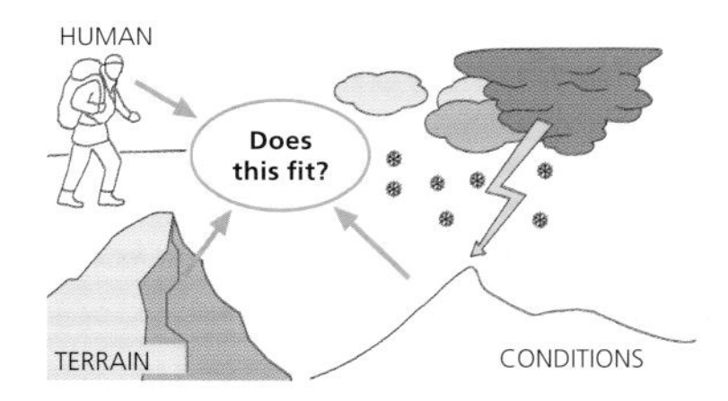

Whether you are at risk from a specific hazard depends on three risk factors, that is, the conditions, the terrain and the person themselves. These factors are individually assessed during pre-tour planning, at the start of the tour (in the region), immediately before a specific stage and with hindsight once home again. You should constantly question the fit of these three factors.

Conditions

What are the challenges currently being presented to you by the natural environment and is your plan still reasonable, bearing in mind the prevailing conditions? What sort of condition is the route in, how is the weather likely to turn out? Is the route snowy or dry? In the winter the focus is estimating the risk of avalanche. See section: Dealing with conditions and terrain in winter.

Terrain

What is the physical composition of the terrain in which the tour is to take place (steepness–gentleness, scree, rock or ice…)? What are the factors characterizing the main difficulties and risks? Steep grassy slope with risk of falling, narrow gully, rock passageway?

Person

In the majority of cases it is we who must accept liability for placing ourselves in a dangerous situation. The ability to adopt a critical view of one's own behavior is consequently of importance in the mountains.

The way a person behaves in a situation where a decision is called for is governed by a number of different behavioral patterns. Courage, detachment, determination, ambition and the will to succeed are qualities that we find tend to accumulate in men. Emotions, intuition, striving after security and social exchange are often to be seen in women. Of course, each human being has his own mix of characteristics of this nature. In order to be able to make the best possible decision in risk situations, this mix needs to be made up of characteristics from both categories. Otherwise one is inclined to assume increased risks. When it comes to making a decision within a group this effect undergoes additional reinforcement. The following recommendations are pertinent here:

- Get to know your own behavioural patterns and scrutinize them critically. Discuss your observations with your partners on the tour too. This will generate an open, judicial atmosphere, leading to an optimum basis for good decisions.
- **When it comes to a particular point for decision, adopt a different stance to the one you would usually take:**
  - What is my gut feeling when I contemplate this key passage? If you identify a vaguely negative feeling, try and figure out where it comes from. What exactly is it that you find disturbing at this point?

- What is the very worst thing that could happen to us at this place (i.e. what is the "worst case scenario"?) Think about how you can prevent this or what the odds are that it will not happen.
- How does the member of the group with the least experience feel about this passage (before others have voiced their own feelings on the matter)?
- How important is it for me that we get past this key passage? If the answer is "It is very important, giving up now would not be the right thing to do," the chances are that you will be more prepared to take on increased risks.

Preparing for the tour

Good tour planning is the key to safe and successful mountaineering. It saves us from many a dangerous situation and a lot of hard grind. It is worth investing sufficient time for it. The aim is to find a tour that corresponds to the predominant conditions and skills of the group in the best possible way. With this in mind, proceed as follows:

Collect information: Sketch the tour, including possible variations, into your map, read the guide to the area. Find out about the weather and the conditions relating to the tour and ask experts for the most up to date information. Ask yourself whether all the participants will be up to coping with the difficulties and whether your material is right for the tour.

Key passages: Trace the route of the tour on your map and think about where you are likely to encounter difficult stages. How can these be made easier, how will you proceed and at what point could it be sensible to abandon the attempt? What alternatives will you have up your sleeve should you find you are not able to get past a particular stage? Ask yourself again whether your group's abilities actually meet the requirements at the key passages.

Tour Plan and Timetable: How long will the tour take going by the guidebook and in your estimation? Plan so that you have some time in reserve. Are all participants up to coping with the length of the tour?

Checks: Go over the tour once again in your mind and think about all the things that can go wrong. What can you do to prevent them? Do you get a good feeling when you think about the tour? If not, why not? What is there about the plan that you can change in order to improve your feelings about it?

Once you have finished planning your tour you should be able to endorse the following statements:

- I have found out about the weather and conditions.
- The current conditions allow us to anticipate the tour and I have a good feeling about it. I have contemplated the conditions under which I would abandon any further thoughts of embarking on the tour.
- I am clear about the course of the route. I have outlined it on the map and memorised it.
- I have looked for the key passages, am familiar with their characteristics and have developed some sound basic tactics for tackling the route.
- My tour plan is realistic (timetable, personal ability, equipment etc.).
- I have given consideration to alternatives and all participants know about them.
- Clear arrangements are in place as regards the leadership of the group. All members of the group are fully informed and motivated.

Possible conclusions if you are not able to tick all the boxes:

- Maybe you have not thought the tour through wherever possible. Take the time to do this – it's important.
- At best there may be a contradiction in the Conditions-Terrain-Person framework. Go into this in depth otherwise you will be lacking in a solid basis for the tour. Should the doubt refuse to go away, look around for a different tour.
- At most you may have doubts because the conditions or the terrain are not sufficiently clearly defined. Plan decision points and determine decision criteria in case you need to give up. Communicate alternatives (including giving up).

Local Assessment

During the planning phase you made some assumptions. As soon as you arrive in the region, you should check these against the conditions you encounter and draw the necessary conclusions.

At a local level, you should be able to endorse the following statements:

- The current conditions concur with the assumptions made when planning the tour.
- I have still not found any factors that argue against the tour and my gut feeling about it is good.
- My timetable would appear to be realistic and we are not behind.
- Out of the various options that I had allowed for we are on the one that is most suitable for today's excursion.

- The participants are just as experienced and fit as I had assumed they would be when planning the tour. They are able to cope with what we have in mind for today.
- The equipment is complete, suitable for the undertaking and in working order. I have everything with me that I needed to pack.

Possible conclusions if you are not able to tick all the boxes:

- Careful, you have uncovered a factor that places a question mark over the tour. Define and communicate your misgivings. Set yourself a binding time for making a decision. Up to that point you should collect up further information as regards your doubts and contemplate some decision criteria. If, by the time the point for a decision arrives, you have not managed to dispel your misgivings, go around or give up.

Evaluating a key passage

At each imminent stage, you should pause to once again identify possible risks and check whether Conditions, Terrain and Person square with one another at this point or not.

Immediately before any key passage you should be able to endorse the following statements:

- The terrain meets my expectations. All participants are now able to cope with the demands of transiting this section.
- The conditions (snow, ice, wet, weather) at this point meet my expectations from the planning stage. They permit us all to ascend.
- All participants are confident and motivated as regards transiting this section. The leaders of the group can offer assistance as to ensure that everyone feels happy about passing this site.
- Our tactics as regards this passage are ideally suited to the conditions and the group. All are informed about the procedure.

Possible conclusions if you are not able to tick all the boxes:

- Be careful! There is a key passage in front of you and you have doubts! Why have you got them and how serious are they? Talk this over between yourselves. Can you eliminate the doubts by means of enhanced safety measures or by a change in tactics? If not, adapt or abandon.

- Consider what the worst case scenario at this key passage would mean. How serious are the consequences? If they are serious, there is a very high probability that this worst case scenario will need to be excluded. Everything should indicate that it will not happen. Otherwise adapt or abandon.

One principle that extends life and makes it easier: mountain tours are fraught with hazards. If you don't feel that you are able to cope with them, don't go! For future preparation, take advice from specialists, **learn more about strategies when dealing with risk, develop your abilities on the mountain.** You will then be able to come back to the same place and have the satisfaction of mastering it. The experience of success will be significantly greater than it would have been with an angst-ridden knee-jerk action.

Safer Touring in Winter

Ski tours call for a knowledge of how to deal with the risk of avalanche. At this point we would like to bring in the most important tools for assessing this hazard. **NB: this in no way replaces a solid basic training.** Regardless of how high the risk of avalanche is and how well acquainted you are with the tour, ensure that you keep to the following rules:

- **Be well-informed.** Make a prior study of the conditions and the weather. The Avalanche Bulletin is especially important.
- **Assess and decide.** During and in the course of the tour you should constantly check the conditions (see typical avalanche problems), the terrain (my mental picture and reality), the people involved (take doubts seriously!). Do they all square with one another?
- **Check** that all search devices for people buried by avalanches are in transmit mode and are checked at the start of the tour. Always keep a shovel and a probe to hand.
- **Give a wide berth to wind-driven accumulations of fresh snow** (see typical avalanche problems).
- **Conduct yourself with caution.** Negotiate key passages and precipices one at a time.
- **Be aware of warming.** In the spring the risk of avalanche increases as the day goes on (see typical avalanche problems).

	CHARACTERISTICS (RELEASE PROBABILITY, DISTRIBUTION AND FREQUENCY OF DANGEROUS SLOPES, TYPE OF AVALANCHES)	CONSEQUENCES AND RECOMMENDATIONS FOR RECREATIONISTS OUTSIDE OF CONTROLLED SKI AREAS
1 **LOW** GERING, FAIBLE, DEBOLE	Triggering is generally possible only with high additional loads (e.g. groups without intervals) and on very few locations in steep extreme terrain. Only a few sluffs and small natural avalanches are possible. Forecasted for about 20% of the winter season. About 7% of the recreational fatalities.	**Generally favourable conditions.** Ski one by one on extremely steep slopes. If possible avoid recent accumulations of wind-driven snow on extreme slopes. Beware of the danger of falling and of possibly unfavourable conditions in high alpine terrain.
2 **MODERATE** MÄSSIG, LIMITÉ, MODERATO	Triggering possible in particular with high additional loads, particularly on the steep slopes indicated in the bulletin. Large natural avalanches not likely. Forecasted for nearly 50% of the winter season. About 34% of the recreational fatalities.	**Favourable conditions, for the most part.** Routes should be selected with care, in particular on steep slopes of the aspect and altitude indicated in the bulletin. Avoid all extremely steep slopes of the aspect and altitude indicated in the bulletin and recent accumulations of wind-driven snow. Ski one by one and with caution on very steep slopes.
3 **CONSIDERABLE** ERHEBLICH, MARQUÉ, MARCATO	Triggering possible even with low additional loads (e.g. single person), particularly on the steep slopes indicated in the bulletin. In some conditions, medium and occasionally large natural avalanches may occur. Frequently alarm signals exist (whumpfs, natural releases). Forecasted for nearly 33% of the winter season. About 47% of the recreational fatalities.	**Partly unfavourable conditions. Critical situation.** Experience in avalanche hazard assessment and in selecting good routes required. Avoid very steep slopes of the aspect and altitude indicated in the bulletin if possible. Pay attention to remotely triggered avalanches. Proceed with caution on traverses or when travelling into unknown terrain.
4 **HIGH** GROSS, FORT, FORTE	Triggering probable even with low additional loads on many steep slopes of all aspect. In some conditions, many medium and several large natural avalanches are likely. Forecasted for a few days only of the winter season. About 12% of the recreational fatalities.	**Unfavourable conditions. Acute Situation.** Lines of transport might be endangered. Sound experience in avalanche hazard assessment required. Stay in moderately steep terrain; beware of runout zones. Remotely triggered avalanches are typical, even over large distances.
5 **VERY HIGH** SEHR GROSS TRÈS FORT, MOLTO FORTE	Numerous large natural avalanches are likely, even in moderately steep terrain. Avalanches run to the valley bottom. Rarely forecasted, on average for one day of the winter season. No recreational fatalities.	**Very unfavourable conditions. Catastrophic situation.** Parts of villages endangered, evacuations might be necessary. Travel in avalanche terrain not recommended.

Slope Angle Classifications: **moderately steep terrain:** slopes flatter than about 30° **very steep slopes:** slopes steeper than 35°
steep slopes: slopes with an angle of more than about 30° **extreme slopes:** steeper than 40° and slopes that are inherently dangerous due to terrain profile or close proximity to ridges.

The risk of avalanche is estimated by the SLF on a 5-level scale (in the winter at 17.00 hrs each day for the following day). This information forms the basis for all decisions.

Critical quantity of new snow: The following quantities of new snow are a sure sign of risk stage "Considerable," regardless of what the Avalanche Bulletin says! Further signs of this are also whumpf! sounds and spontaneous avalanche discharges.

10–20 cm under unfavorable conditions. These include: strong winds, low temperatures (colder than -5° C), unfavorable topping of old snow (surface frost, frozen snow or ice, very old surface).

20–30 cm under moderate conditions and 30–50 cm under favorable conditions. These include: hardly any to moderate wind or temperatures only slightly below 0° C, favorable topping of old snow (which means highly irregular surface). Regular skiing activities in the slope throughout the skiing season.

Reduction Method

By way of a further central aid to assessment of the avalanche risk the **Reduction Method** may be used. It takes into account the risk level, inclination of slope and aspect. In the case of unfavorable aspect, the avalanche risk is as follows:

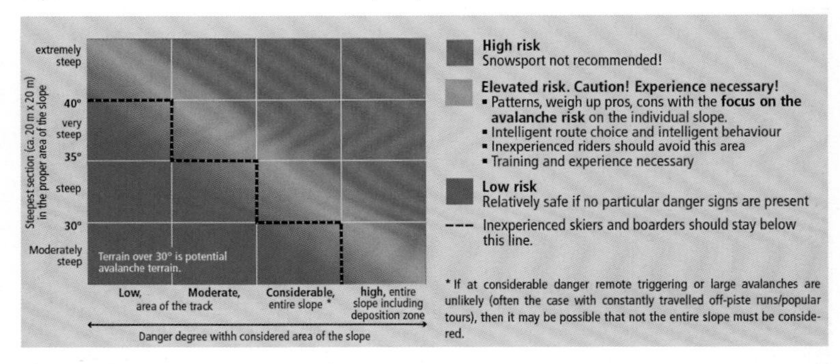

The following are regarded as unfavorable aspects: shady slopes, wind-loaded slopes, steep hillsides and high altitudes, slopes we know nothing about. For favorable slopes (sunny slope without wind loading and not in the core area of the Avalanche Bulletin) one may assume the next risk level down.

Typical avalanche problems (principal risk)

It makes sense, before and during the tour, to identify the principal risk emanating from the current conditions. One of the following four situations may typically represent this principal risk:

«Neuschnee.» During snowfall and 1–3 days afterward. Typically considerable risk of avalanche. Often critical quantity of new snow and alarm signs. The places at risk are spread over a wide area; there may be very few possibilities to circumvent. Observe Reduction Method!

«Triebschnee» (snow transported in windy conditions). During and for 1–2 days after snowfall and/or strong winds. Invariably wind signs and once in a while alarm signs may be evident. The hazard points are irregularly distributed. Avoid accumulations of snow. Fresh driving snow steeper than 30° tricky, circumvent!

«Nassschnee.» On days featuring appreciable warming. Can be recognized by the fact that the snow cover has become sodden. The hazardous locations are frequently situated on sunny slopes and in deeper locations. Be careful of spontaneous avalanches, terminate tour early!

«Altschnee.» Weak layers within the snow cover. Typically moderate risk of avalanche, difficult to identify. Note information in Bulletin, stick to Reduction Method!

Points to note as regards terrain evaluation in winter

- Steepness: Increasing steepness means increasing risk. Measure with slope inclination gauge on 1:25000 map. When in the terrain, use poles or other aids to measure. Estimate: hairpin turn terrain begins at around 30°, scree below a rock face is around 35° steep, steep, rocky terrain is more than approx. 40° steep
- Hillside location: avoid very steep and shaded ridges wherever possible.
- Sparse woods do not protect from avalanches.
- Relief/terrain: avoid troughs and walk on ridges.
- Slope aspect: shady slopes are often more risky than sunny ones. Where significant warming is a factor and where there is a risk of wet snow, sunny slopes are trickier.
- Size of slope: in the case of large slopes or those that are located above trenches or ditches, there is a risk of being buried deep by an avalanche.
- Prominent slope: slopes that are located above rocky terrain may bear a greater risk for falls.

Avalanche–Rescue

If buried. Try to get out of the area of the avalanche, otherwise let go of poles, undo bindings if you can (rarely possible). In an avalanche pull knees toward your chest and hold your arms in front of your face. Fight like hell!

If not buried

- Precisely monitor avalanche flow and persons caught in it (point of disappearance) Gain an overview–think–act, assess your own safety, avoid any further accidents
- Raise the alarm: be aware of time factor! The main thing is that the victim should still be able to breathe so the most important thing is the rescue! If there are a number of victims, there may be reason to suspect that they are buried deep, so ensure there are enough helpers and alert rescue service straight away.
- Determine primary search area (in the direction of flow below the point of disappearance).

- Switch off any transceivers that are not in use. Begin searching immediately with eyes and ears at the same time deploying an avalanche transceiver (*search band width for all devices with analogue sound signal min. 40 m. For digital devices note manufacturer's instructions).
- Pinpoint search with avalanche probe (finding the precise position with avalanche transceiver unlikely).
- Methodical digging over large area, dig in a V-shape.
- Uncover head and chest as quickly as possible, clear the breathing passages, check if there is a breathing cavity in the snow (snow-filled airways = no breathing cavity).
- Start artificial respiration (mouth to nose), if circulation has stopped start cardio-pulmonary resuscitation simultaneously.
- Carry out resuscitation measures on the casualty until a doctor is available to take over.
- Protect from further cooling, position accordingly if unconscious. Concentrate on monitoring and taking care of patient.
- Careful evacuation by helicopter.

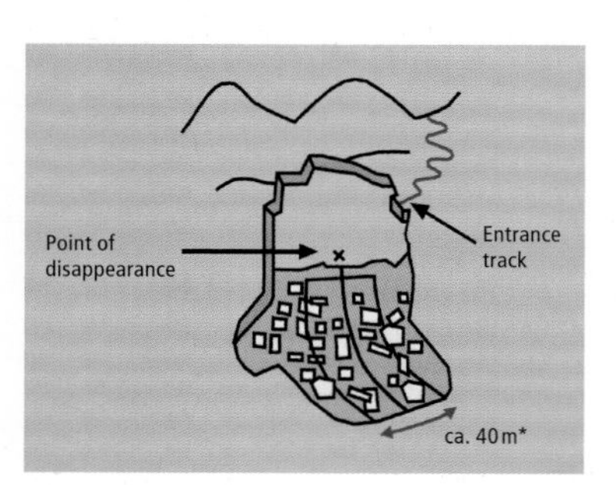

Air Rescue

Only approach helicopter once the rotor is standing still. If the rotor is operating, only embark and disembark if accompanied by a member of the crew and always maintain eye contact with the pilot.

Hazards in the Landing Area

Do not leave any loose objects lying about. Be careful with skis, avalanche probes etc.

Safer in Rocky Terrain

Regardless of how well you know the area or how much experience you may have, it is essential to adhere to the following rules when rock climbing:

- **Partnercheck.** Check on your partners before each route. Carry out a mutual check on harness fasteners, roping-up knots, safety equipment, belaying device, carabiner safety locks, knots in the end of the rope. See illustration.
- **Warm up before climbing.** Gymnastics and warm-up pre-climbing exercises will protect your joints, tendons and muscles from injury and increase your performance.
- **Correct behaviour during belaying.** Operate belaying device properly and assume correct position, be alert, make sure rope is not slack, maintain control when lowering.
- **Correct behaviour when climbing.** Fit intermediate fixing points from stable position and close to roping-up point. Pay attention to rope guidance.
- **Clear communication.** Clarity of communication avoids misunderstandings. Inform the person doing the belaying before you hang on the rope. Address faults in your own team or where other climbers are concerned.
- **Never rope on rope.** Only use metal bolts (deflections). Never fit two ropes in the same carabiner.
- **No unsecured bolts (deflections).** The bolt for top rope climbing should consist of a carabiner with a safety lock or two normal carabiners.
- **Protect your head.** When climbing out of doors always wear a helmet; it will protect you from head injuries in the event of a fall as well as from rock falls.
- **Behave with consideration.** Respect other climbers and draw their attention to any faults or hazards; in addition be aware of their fall zone. Find out about the "local rules." Observe any existing climbing restrictions.
- **Don't expect too much of children.** Be aware of difference in weight, less strength in the hands and limited concentration capability.
- **Carry out critical check on hook material.** A hook breaking away can have fatal consequences, especially at a stance. Caution is advisable in the case of old material. Conduct a critical check on the material; in cases of doubt, it may be advisable to retreat. Additional strengthening of the stance should be provided by means of mobile safety equipment (wedges, friends).

Safer on "Via Ferratas"

Regardless of how familiar you are with the "via ferrata," or however much experience you have, ensure compliance with the following rules:

- **Partnercheck.** Check on your partners before each start. Carry out a mutual check as regards fastenings on harnesses and correct securing of the "via ferrata" set. Ensure that the brake cable can run unimpeded into the brake but that it does not restrict continuous movement.
- **"Via ferrata" brake.** Only brakes in Y-form conforming to UIAA should be used. A home-made "via ferrata" set offers no protection if you fall. The impact force (= braking force) is too high for man and material.
- **Protect your head.** When climbing out of doors always wear a helmet; it will protect you from head injuries should you fall as well as from any from rock falls.
- **Correct behaviour during climbing.** One carabiner after the other is arranged at the intermediate bolt points. The openings of the carabiners face in opposite directions. Pay attention to the previous person's fall zone. In the majority of cases overtaking manoeuvres are dangerous. Discuss with others on the "via ferrata."
- **Behave with consideration.** Respect other climbers and draw their attention to any faults or hazards as applicable. Adopt a fair and clear approach to communication.
- **Keep an eye on the weather.** A "via ferrata" is a major conductor of lightning! If there is a risk of thunderstorms do not ascend! Turning back from a "via ferrata" is difficult and time consuming. Particularly when other people are following behind.
- **Complete equipment.** In addition to a helmet, a "via ferrata" set and a harness you will need gloves, good footwear (think about coming down), suitable clothes and a small First Aid kit. Belaying with a length of rope can also be used to secure weaker participants, particularly children. An additional sling with a carabiner on the climbing belt can be attached when it comes to resting.

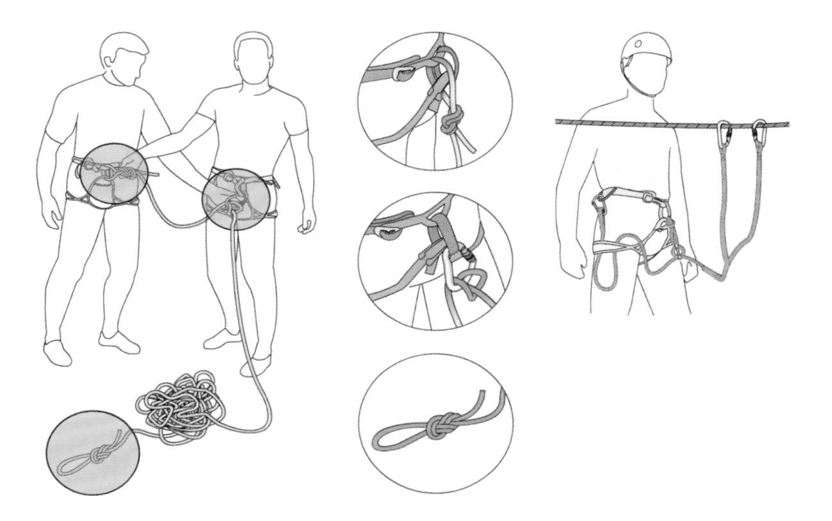

Information/Emergency

Weather

General overview:	www.meteoschweiz.ch, Tel. 162
Alternative, especially precipitation:	www.meteoblue.ch
Webcams:	www.swisswebcams.ch
Smartphone App:	MeteoSwiss
Swiss alpine weather report:	Tel. 0900 162 138
Personal weather information:	Tel. 0900 162 333

Winter conditions

Snow and avalanche information:	www.slf.ch
Smartphone App:	White Risk

(The forecast issued at 17.00 hrs gives the avalanche risk for the following 24 hours. At 08.00 hrs a new report is issued and this is valid until 17.00 hrs.)

Huts, Routes, Ideas

Huts, ascents, routes:	www.sac-cas.ch
Up to date tour reports:	www.gipfelbuch.ch, www.camptocamp.org
Tours by public transport:	www.oev-touren.ch
Alpine taxi:	www.alpentaxi.ch

Emergencies

Rega:	Tel. 1414 (in CH GSM network and with CH SIM card)
Rega:	Tel. 0041 333 333 333 (from abroad or with foreign SIM card in Switzerland)
Emergency ambulance service:	Tel. 144 (use this number in Wallis)
International emergency number:	Tel. 112

Sources:
Realisation: Markus Müller, Bruno Hasler, Swiss Alpine Club SAC (2010)
Illustrations: Swiss Alpine Club SAC (www.sac-cas.ch)

Additional Literature:

1) Winkler, K., Brehm, H.-P., Haltmeier, J. Bergsport Winter; Technik, Taktik, Sicherheit. SAC-Verlag (2008). ISBN 3-85902-241-5. (Order under www.sac-verlag.ch)
2) Winkler, K., Brehm, H.-P., Haltmeier, J. Bergsport Sommer; Technik, Taktik, Sicherheit. SAC-Verlag. (2008). ISBN 3-85902-247-4. (Order under www.sac-verlag.ch)
3) Wassermann, E., Wicky, M. Lawinen und Risikomanagement. Edition Filidor (2006). ISBN 3-906087-22-1. (Order under www.bergpunkt.ch)
4) Wassermann, E., Wicky, M. Technik und Taktik Plaisir Klettern. Edition Filidor (2007). ISBN 3-906087-29-8. (Order under www.bergpunkt.ch)
5) Wassermann, E., Wicky, M. Technik und Taktik für leichte Hochtouren. Edition Filidor (2005). ISBN 3-906087-25-5. (Order under www.bergpunkt.ch)

1. Training

D. Walter

Per aspera ad astra
(Through difficulties to the stars)
Seneca

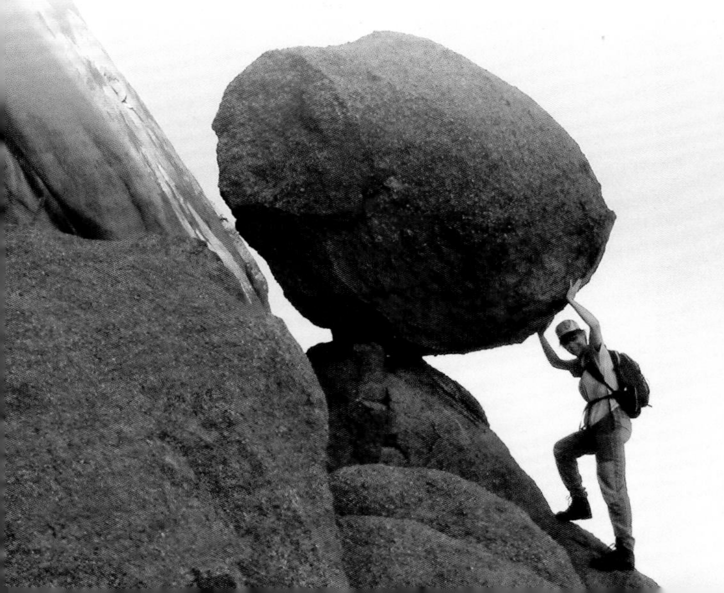

1.1 Theoretical Principles

Training in any sports discipline is a targeted process of activity aimed at improving a specific ability or performance. The training stimulus triggers an adaptive response at the structural, cellular or molecular level, something which, assuming the choice of training momentum at the right time and the right intensity, will lead to an improvement in performance ("super-compensation") where the system achieves an enhanced level of performance. Basic considerations relevant for mountain sports and/or trekking activities and expeditions are discussed in the following. For further, general or more detailed information, please refer to the relevant specific literature.[1) 2) 8)]

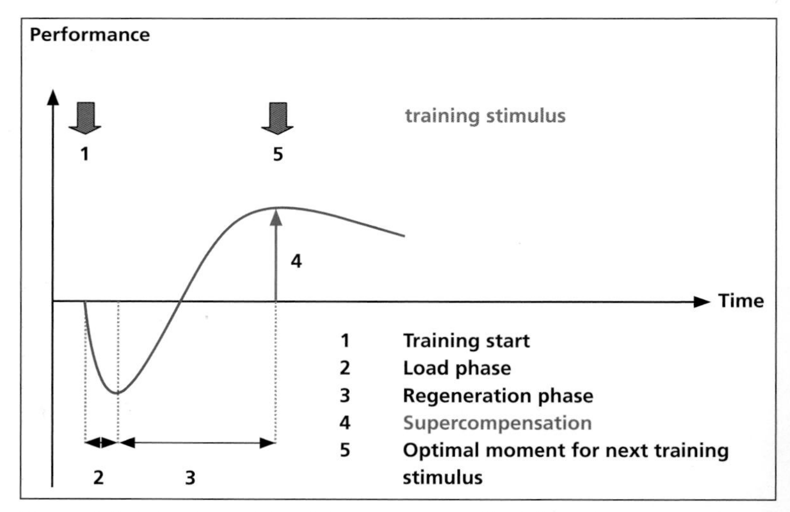

Figure 1.1: *Achieving a state of "super-compensation" through optimal timing of the next training stimulus.*

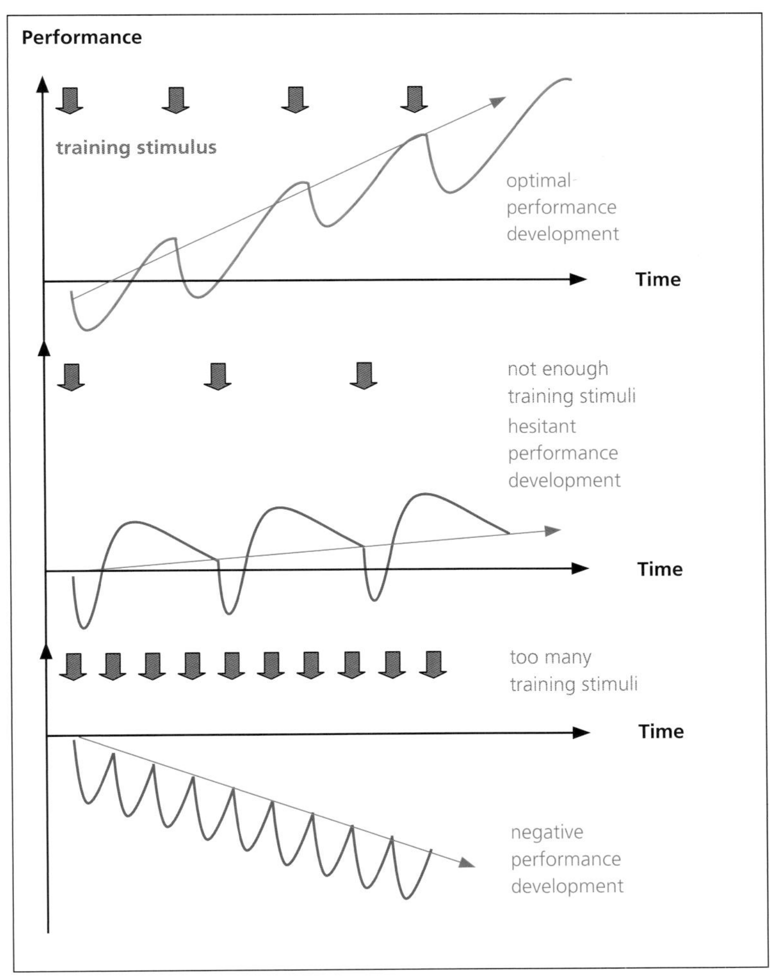

Figure 1.2: *Top: Time-optimised training intervals will lead to an improvement in performance. Centre: Stringing training stimuli together with insufficient frequency of stimulus will result in only a slow improvement in performance. Below: Too many training units will lead to a fall in performance (this is also known as overtraining or "overreaching."*

1.2 Training for Specific Activities

A broad range of well-developed constitutional factors is necessary to be able to cope with long-term exercise, which may involve carrying a heavy rucksack uphill and downhill and over rough terrain. Duration, strength and proprioception (perception, direction of movement, coordination) are all needed to some extent and play a major part in ensuring maximum possible safety on the mountain, on treks and expeditions. The principle of endurance training is the basis for any ongoing form of physical training. Especially the extensive continuous method, that is, exercise as applied to the whole of the body (e.g. Nordic Walking, swimming, running, hiking in the mountains etc.) on an continuous basis leads, through economization of cardiovascular activity, to an increase in the formation of capillaries (the smallest vessels) in the muscle and optimization of the lipometabolism resulting in greater tolerance of exercise. In addition, training of this kind also contributes to preventing ailments associated with lack of exercise and diseases of modern society. The level of intensity is low (in accordance with the so-called "speaking rule"), although the overall spread is high (several hours a week).

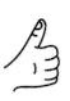

The **"speaking rule"** states that it should be possible to converse in continuous sentences within a group, for example, during an endurance run. As soon as the pace of running hots up, this will get more and more difficult.

On the other hand it is possible, by focusing on general strength-building exercises alongside energy-based adaptations (optimization of energy metabolism), to achieve effects that are predominantly positive. By means of powerfully developed musculature, the passive structures (cartilage, bones, ligaments, tendons, intervertebral discs) can be actively protected/controlled. Let's look, for example, at the immense forces that occur when you are walking downhill carrying a heavy rucksack ... Strength-building is possible by simply relying on your own body weight, in- or outdoor, with only basic additional equipment (e.g. Thera Band, PET bottles filled with water) or in the studio (on power equipment). Before embarking on your first session of strength-building, you should first get into training. By making use of very high quality exercises you prepare your body for the new forms of exertion and stresses using low weights (or even dispensing with weights completely) and repeating up to 20 times. A training session involving a cross-section of muscles will help with bodybuilding. This involves 3 sets of exercises repeated 10–12 times. Repeating the last set of exercises should have the effect of exhausting the muscles. It is only after this that you can even start to think about power training at greater intensity for better control/economization of the muscular system (so-called neuromuscular adaptation for intra- and

inter-muscular coordination). You will find that, with a clear reduction in the rate of repeats, the weights will go up, the movements will get faster or may even be carried out moving in the negative direction ("plyometric" training, as it is known).
In general, preference should be given to training that involves entire chains of muscles. Ultimately those muscles that have become weaker, mostly the phasic muscles (muscles of the torso with vertical and diagonal stomach muscles as well as back and/or intervertebral muscles, together with the musculature of the shoulder blades) need to undergo special training in order to counteract any muscular dysbalance. The latter has, taking into account the avoidance of injuries due to overexertion as well as bad posture, seen a massive increase in importance in the last few years.
Proprioception, i.e. the overall complement of systems that are responsible for balance, is of major importance as far as walking in open country is concerned, particularly where the terrain underfoot is uneven or incorporates ridges. Proprioceptives, which are also referred to as "sensorimotor training," can also be easily incorporated in strength-building activities (e.g. knee bends, barbell or dumbbell training on an unstable surface) or endurance training (consciously selected hikes without resorting to the use of poles). In addition, skills exercises can also be integrated into everyday living (e.g. brushing the teeth on one leg, maybe hopping with eyes closed; balancing across stones).

You don't need any elaborate infrastructure for strength-building. Physio- and sports therapists are familiar with a broad range of meaningful exercises aimed at strength-building which can, for example, also be practised in the natural environment. By contrast, exercises that are carried out thoughtlessly – in particular those involving heavy additional weights – can sometimes lead to over-exertion or even to injuries.

1.3 Training and Age

The ability to undergo training in a complex sequence of activities is not suppressed even as we age, although coordinative capabilities are certainly easier to acquire during childhood when the neuromuscular system is still developing. Indeed, it is never wrong to embark on a course of training – regardless of what kind of training it is. On the other hand, there is no storage facility for any ability once we have undergone training in it: training is a lifetime business (remember, "A rolling stone gathers no moss")! There is no exact definition as to when "old age" begins. The loss of muscle mass, strength, tolerance of injury and performance capability, all of which appear to be factors contingent on old age, are as a rule due to a lack of movement and exercise.[1)] Repeated opportunities have arisen for showing that a strength workout or training aimed at building up strength (here used as synonyms)[3) 9)] as well as training in *proprioception*[4)] have decidedly positive effects on the options available in old age. If sporting activities are to be resumed either from around the age of 35 or after a long abstinence from sport or renewed consideration is being given to performance-orientated training, then it is certainly advisable to book in for a sports medical examination and benefit from the support of a professional in this particular discipline.

Doctors with qualifications relating to **"Sports Medicine"** can be found at "www.sgsm.ch"

1.4 Training the Altitude

Tolerance of altitude is not basically something in which it is possible to undergo training. In the final analysis, it is always the speed of ascent and the individual's personal compatibility with altitude that are responsible for whether a period spent at high altitude will be tolerated or not. Consideration may be given to pre-acclimatisation if the destination altitude is to be attained in no more than 10 days, even better in no more than a week. In principle, it is possible to simulate altitude on the flat by reducing the concentration of oxygen over a number of hours or intermittently in the surrounding air (this is known as normobaric hypoxia) e.g. in a tent with reduced-oxygen ambient air. However, this form of "altitude training" is probably best described as monotonous and expensive … There are indications that pre-acclimatisation efforts of this kind undertaken over a period of 1–5 weeks for 1–4 hours daily at a simulated height of 4000 m are capable of reducing the incidence of acute mountain sickness (or AMS) see Chapter 17.3, Page 213.[10)]
Scientifically not proven but nevertheless frequently reported by mountaineers who routinely find themselves at great heights is the fact that repeated exposure to altitude may generate a certain "memory effect". The period spent at high altitude is, subjectively-speaking, better tolerated.

High-altitude tours with overnight stays in huts situated at high altitudes are an excellent way of preparing for an expedition or a trek. These should be deferred wherever possible until shortly before departure and definitely have their advantages. However, under no circumstances do they provide a replacement for common-sense acclimatisation tactics on the mountain itself!

1.5 Principles of Practical Training

Analogous to the findings in the previous chapter, training specific to mountain sports should, as far as possible, be practiced in a way that is varied and consistent yet administered in correct doses, not forgetting the importance of the fun factor. The more sports genre-specific the preparations are, the more those muscles that will be used for trekking or an expedition will be trained. Correspondingly, long mountain tours, represent an excellent opportunity for training. But, even on the flat, there are a number of options when it comes to individual preparation. In many places extended walks can be taken in hilly country, maybe with heavy boots and a rucksack. In urban areas there is always the possibility offered by flights of stairs in high rise buildings or training on the stepper in a fitness center.

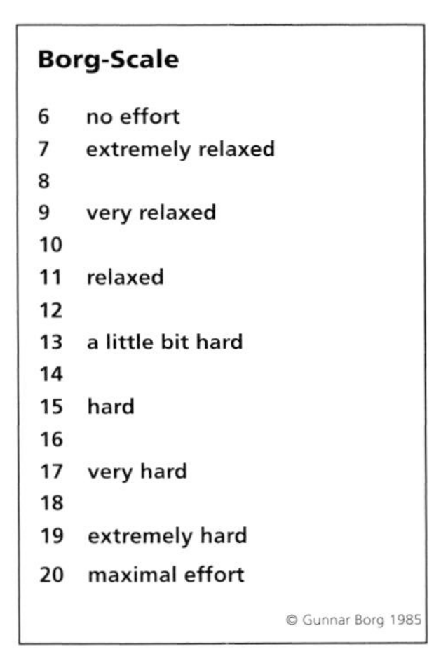

Borg-Scale

6	no effort
7	extremely relaxed
8	
9	very relaxed
10	
11	relaxed
12	
13	a little bit hard
14	
15	hard
16	
17	very hard
18	
19	extremely hard
20	maximal effort

© Gunnar Borg 1985

Figure 1.3: *So called "Borg-Scale": Gradation of the subjective sensation of effort/load.*

A performance test (4 x 1000 m running test, 12-minute running test as per Cooper, Conconi running test) can provide a snapshot of an individual's possible performance potential at a given moment, even though the training recommendations, especially when it comes to training on the mountain with the pulse monitor, should only be applied with some reservations (increase in pulse rate relatively speaking too high). A more mountain-specific test is a test of climbing performance or, if necessary, a step test on the treadmill at an inclined angle. Valuable recommendations as regards training management can be derived from a performance test. The maximum oxygen absorption capacity *(VO_2max)* determined bears no direct relationship to altitude performance–a number of well-known altitude pioneers (among them Reinhold Messner and Sir Edmund Hilary) have a "proven" excellent head for heights, despite only moderately good rates of VO_2max.[5) 6)]

A subjective perception of exertion can be described by recourse to the so-called **"Borg Scale."** If identical Borg values are obtained during training on the flat and on the mountain (i.e. with the same physical sensation) only the velocity of movement will be different. Correspondingly, a training instruction manual may, for example, read as follows: "Train for an hour three times a week at a Borg Value of 13–15 (regardless of terrain)."

1.6 Training Mistakes

When people are striving to achieve high aims, the outcome can sometimes be negative due to the fact that they have been overambitious or are in poor training. If the intensity or density of stimulus is too high (e.g. too many rapid training sessions in running) can lead to a state of overtraining and this may manifest itself in the form of exhaustion or increased susceptibility to infection. One-sided training can lead to overload injuries to the locomotor system. When it comes to treks and expeditions in particular, "high levels of psychological motivation, persistence, patience, teamwork capability, experience, technical skills, capacity for self-esteem and enjoyment of this specific form of physical activity"[7] are all crucial factors in addition to the purely physical components. This means that the training targets must also be realistically formulated. By contrast to this, an endurance run may also be made in driving snow or rain and wind ("overcoming one's own internal resistance and vanquishing the demons within!").
In summary, maximum priority should be assigned to training in basic endurance and economy of movement, followed by a general training session in strength-building (if possible incorporating sensorimotoric exercises). Highly intensive training or training units staged at intervals are, on the other hand, only of subordinate importance as far as mountain sport is concerned as an improvement in VO_2max at high altitude is not a critical factor. Finally, the importance of the conscious integration of regenerative phases between the training sessions must not be forgotten.

Possible Structure of Training for the Ascent of an 8000 m Mountain
(e.g. Gasherbrum II):

- The structure can be divided up into a micro-cycle (weekly plan*), a macro-cycle (monthly plan) and a meso-cycle (six-monthly or annual plan). Different intensive training sessions are undertaken in the different phases. Intensive endurance training phases can, however, be combined with less intensive strength-building phases. The aim is to achieve an overall performance capability by way of a build up to the expedition.

- The scope of training (ordinate) is tantamount to the number of hours of training per day or per week. The optimum individual range is, on the one hand, dependent on the preconditions relating to training status before the actual start of training; on the other, a reasonable possibility must exist for integrating any sporting ambitions in social life (family, career etc.). The intensity of training in the

* Sometimes a single day is also specified as a micro-cycle in the weekly planning.

endurance range is dependent on speed or the steepness, for example, of the surface over which the running, in-line or cycling activity is taking place; in the area of strength-building, the training stimulus is dependent on the number of repetitions or sets and the weight moved (or own weight).

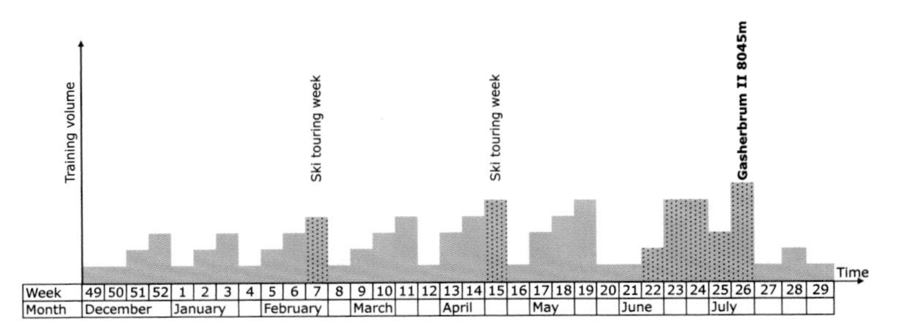

Figure 1.4: *Possible training structure for the ascent of an 8000 m mountain (e.g. Gasherbrum II)*

The micro-cycle (weekly plan) can be broken down further (example)	
Monday:	Day off
Tuesday:	Endurance training
Wednesday:	Strength-building training
Thursday:	Endurance training
Friday:	Strength-building training or day off
Saturday:	Tour Application
Sunday:	Tour Application

Bibliography:

1) Training fundiert erklärt, Handbuch der Trainingslehre, Jost Hegener, Ingold Verlag.
2) Theorie und Praxis der Trainingsherapie, Hans Spring et al., Thieme Verlag.
3) Katula JA, Rejeski WJ, Marsh AP, Enhancing quality of life in older adults: a comparison of muscular strength and power training, Health Qual Life Outcomes. 2008 Jun 13;6:45.
4) U. Granacher, Neuromuskuläre Leistungsfähigkeit im Alter (>60 J): Auswirkung von kraft- und sensomotorischem Training, Dissertation 2004, Albert-Ludwigs-Universität Freiburg i. Br.
5) Clyde Soles, Climbing: Training for Peak Performance, The Mountaineers books.
6) http://www.swimmersden.com/TubblyLynn/vo2_max.htm.
7) Schoene, Hornbein in RJ Shepard, Ausdauer im Sport, Dt. Ärzteverlag, Kap Bergsteigen).
8) Werner Kandolf, Walter Schenk, Alpine Trainingslehre, Verband alpiner Vereine Österreichs.
9) Hazell T, Kenno K, Jakobi J, Functional benefit of power training for older adults, J Aging Phys Act. 2007 Jul;15(3):349-59.
10) Burtscher M, Brandstätter E, Gatterer H., Preacclimatization in simulated altitudes; 1: Sleep Breath. 2008 May;12(2):109-14.

2. The Great Gait – with or without Poles

U. Wiget

The human body is preprogrammed to move about and function on uneven ground; the ability to do these things on a flat, paved road represents a relatively recent achievement.

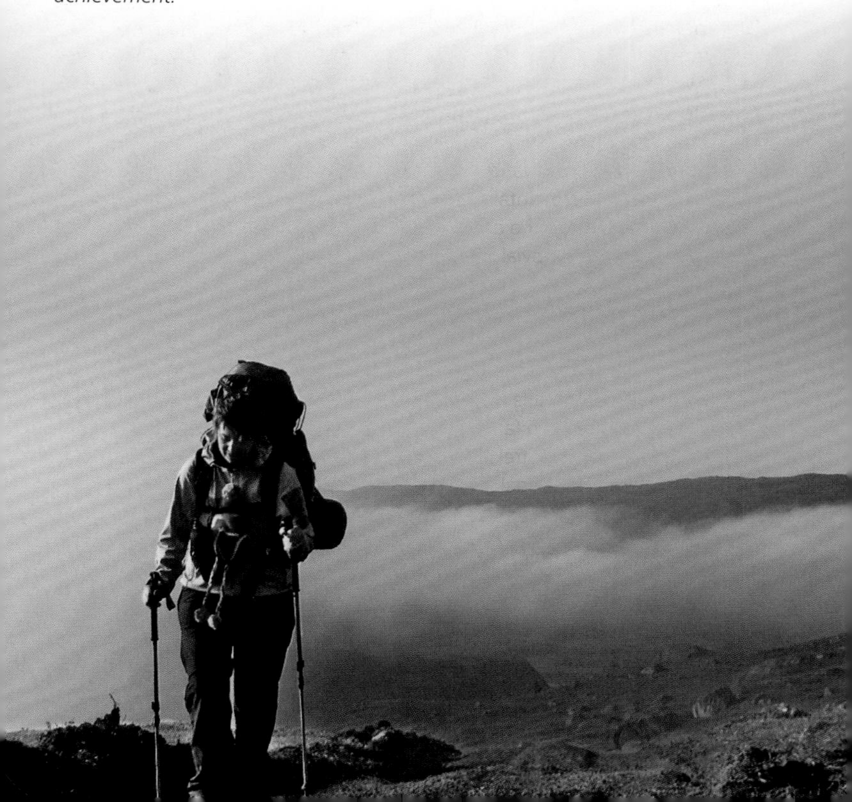

Walking and running consists of a complex interplay of a number of elements (bones, muscles, cartilage, nerves), all controlled by a highly developed regulatory system *(proprioception, sensorimotor functions)*. All these mechanical functions and their associated regulatory systems are built up and strengthened mostly during the early years of life. They are the fundament for elements like sure-footedness and the ability to descend from a mountain without becoming fatigued.

⇨ The entire neuromuscular system requires constant training based on the principle of development physiology: "use it or lose it."

Nevertheless, many prospective trekking enthusiasts have a set of deceleration muscles (located to the front of the thigh) that are seriously undertrained for the simple reason that they never need to use them. For untrained persons this subsequently results in "knee-shaking" when walking downhill for a lengthy period of time.
The stress peaks that occur when walking downhill are absorbed by the muscular system. This work needs to be carried out perfectly for several hours at a time so that no damage to the joints occurs and the body does not become overly fatigued. However, these load peaks are also essential not only for the preservation of strong bones but also for maintaining joint cartilage which relies on the application of pressure to the synovial fluid for its nourishment.

The secret to walking downhill has been known to mankind for many thousands of years; even today, we see this in the technique adopted by mountain farmers and porters in the various trekking regions of the world. In Nepal you often come across men weighing 40 kg themselves who have been used to carrying 80 kg weights up and down mountains for many years. What immediately

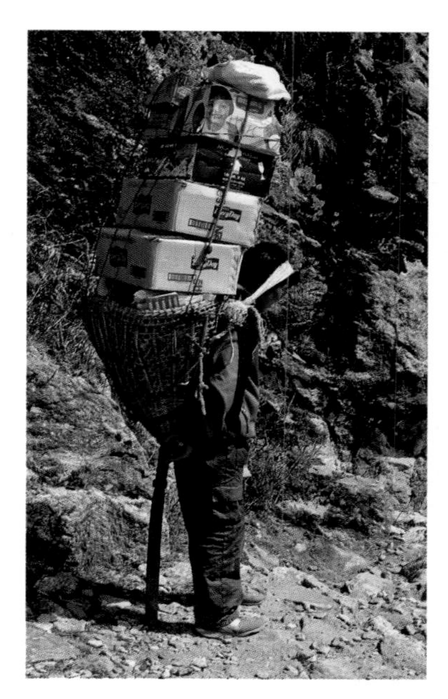

Figure 2.1: *Nepalese porters frequently use just a short, strong stick on which they can set down their loads every now and then at regular intervals (U. Wiget).*

strikes us when we observe them is the fact that, when they are coming down, they always avoid keeping their knees in the stretched position. Instead, they cushion each step by ensuring that the knee is slightly bended.

⇨ When walking uphill, it is a good idea to keep the height of the step as small as possible to avoid any risk of exaggerated knee flexing which could lead, as a result of the leverage, to a significant additional load on the joint.

An almost fatigue-free ascent is also possible by not bending the knees at all but merely by abducting the legs and shifting one's body weight. Fatigue while walking leads to uncontrolled sequences of movements and hence to strain on the joints. So remember to include sufficient breaks for eating and drinking in your schedule. Professional porters don't use poles either; instead they opt for just a short, strong stick on which they make a point of setting down their loads every now and then at regular intervals (see Figure 2.1, Page 37).

In our opinion, poles are not necessary for a healthy individual. They instil a false sense of security, undermine the element of training that is so important for the neuromotor regulatory system and to an extent intercept the load peaks that are important for healthy bones. This is especially true in instances where poles tend to be used automatically on any walk or mountain tour.

On the other hand, there are no objections to an aid of this nature being used when descending in snow and ice on expeditions that involve carrying a heavy backpack.

People who suffer from **orthopaedic problems** associated with the legs or feet or who are seriously overweight should discuss the problems associated with poles with their doctor and make adjustments at an individual level when using trekking poles. The same applies to older mountaineers (see also Chapter 6, Page 69) who feel safer with poles.

⇨ Practice is important when it comes to using poles. The poles need to be individually adapted to terrain and body size. For instance, not the same length of poles would be used for the descent as for the ascent.

It also needs to be possible to shorten the poles quickly and easily and to stow them away on the rucksack so that the hands are left free to cope with the demands of the terrain.

3. Diet and Nutrition

U. Hirsiger

It is a feeling with which the majority of mountaineers are only too familiar. During and toward the end of a long mountain tour of several hours duration, hunger and thirst begin to gnaw at our energy reserves because we ourselves have had nothing to "gnaw at" for far too long. Our legs and arms feel like lead! An early opportunity to listen to one's body and to enjoy a snack may well help to anchor the rosy glow of confidence that comes from having conquered the peaks all the more firmly in the memory.

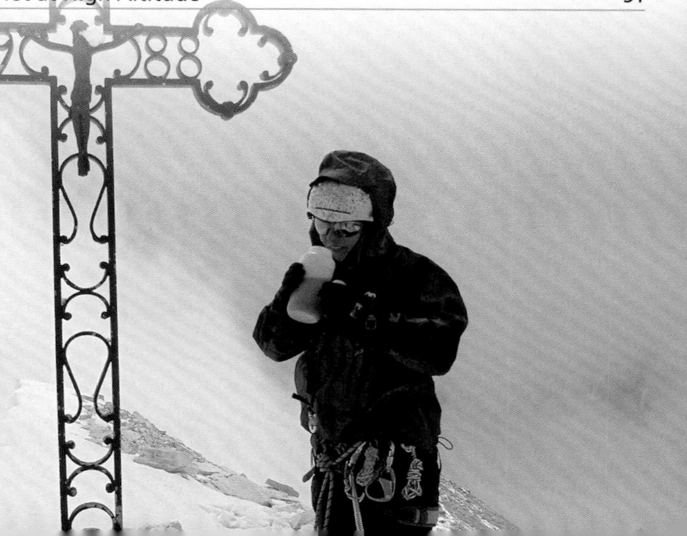

3.1 Principles

Diet in relation to mountaineering is, like the sport itself, highly complex and broad-based. Is the tour a one-day event or will it extend over several days, is it to be conducted at less than 2500 m or more than 4000 m? What sort of conditions are to be anticipated? Hot, cold or a combination of wind and rain? Questions that do not only affect the equipment and clothing we take with us but which will also have an effect on supplies of energy and fluid, because failure to feed ourselves properly will lead to premature tiredness. This section on diet deals with healthy nourishment based on the foodstuffs pyramid **(www.sge-ssn.ch)** and this means the focus will be on sections specifically relating to a nutritious diet in the mountains.
People often talk about an "optimum" diet. This theoretical option does, however, tend to have more to do with reassuring the person performing the feat or an effort to instill confidence in the competence of those who propound this theory. In addition, catering from hut to hut is basically as different as the location and seldom permits any comparable conclusions in relation to catering status to be drawn for the coming tour. What a human being needs in what situation and what s/he does not need cannot be clearly defined. Personalized results are arrived at by adding reference values to one's own experience.

Training status, metabolism and, by derivation, the diet of a **mountain guide** (someone who spends 200 to 300 days a year out and about in the mountains) is no good at all as a point of reference for a weekend mountaineer. Any potential shortfalls incurred by a mountain sports enthusiast at a weekend can be rapidly made up by means of an uncompromising and healthy everyday diet.

Thus there is not only a difference in terms of performance between a Sunday walk and a high altitude tour, but also in terms of consumption and therefore diet. The choice of quantities, menu or components, not to mention quality, needs to be adapted to individual possibilities and requirements without anything been banned.

3.2 Calorific and Fluid Requirements

Calorie consumption (also known as energy consumption) is, compared with other types of sport, high. Under "Recommendations" I have given the proportionate range for sports persons. The diet is divided up into three nutritional groups in accordance with the foodstuffs pyramid and duly specified as follows: **carbohydrates (CH), fats (F) and proteins (P).**

Carbohydrates (CH)

• **Examples:**	Vegetables, fruit, starch, confectionery, sports drinks and nutrition bars etc.
• **Energy:**	4 kcal (Kilocalories) or 17 kJ (Kilojoules)
• **Recommendation:**	45–60 percent energy from food ingested

Purely for reasons of tolerance during exercise or due to weight, vegetables and fruit far too seldom play a part in a mountaineering diet. Dried fruit and, more recently, also some vegetables, occasionally account for a small proportion of the contents of the rucksack.

This leaves the group comprising starches or complex carbohydrates (CH) and polysaccharides as the main supplier of carbohydrates. Speaking in terms of energy, this is the most important group in a sports diet but tends to be replaced by fat to a large extent, depending on the specific mountain sport.

It is divided into the natural "wholemeal/whole-grain products" and the refined "standard products."

• **"Wholemeal products"**	Wholemeal bread, wholegrain pasta, brown rice, bulgur wheat, potatoes
• **"Standard products"**	Wholemeal or white bread, white pasta and rice

Wholemeal products, vegetables and fruit supply, together with the dietary fibers (for a feeling of repleteness and to promote a healthy intestine), the well-known vitamins, minerals and trace elements, but also the less well-known secondary plant substances. In addition to these indispensable features, they are chiefly responsible for promoting a slower rise in blood sugar than standard products and confectionery. The longer a tour, a trip or expedition lasts, the more regularly these natural groups should appear on the menu in order to ensure sustained personal health and performance capability.

⇨ The more the digestive tract becomes used to these products the more they will be tolerated during exercise.

Confectionery or specific sports nutrient options incorporating mono-, di- and polysaccharides should be encountered only rarely in daily life, but there is justification for them and they have their own fixed place when it comes to a sports diet. Ease of administration, high energy density and the fact that they are readily tolerated make

them ideal companions in the mountains. During exertion or in the regeneration phase they are capable of supplying available energy quickly without placing additional load on the distribution of insulin. In addition, substances containing CH can reduce degeneration of muscular mass and shorten regeneration time.
One or two thin slices of bread (with black coffee, 1 serving of UHT coffee creamer and 25 g of cheese spread) in the hut in the morning are hardly a balanced breakfast which will set you up for the day's sport ahead. In addition, this somewhat homespun diet tends to be high in fat, something which in turn "suppresses" the CH.

Reference values for carbohydrate in the diet

Duration		Exertion	Recommendation	
1–4	days	Before	7–12 g	CH per kg BM* per day
Breakfast	1–4 h	Before	1–4 g	CH per kg BM*
On the	day	During	30–80 g	CH per hr
On the	day	During	400–700 g	CH to be spread
Directly	15–30 min	After	1.0–1.2 g	CH per kg BM*
Over the	day	After	5–>10 g	CH per kg BM*

Table 3.1: *Adapted in accordance with Hot Topic 06, 12, 13, 14, www.sfsn.ethz.ch; 2008*
**BM = Body Mass*

200 g risotto cooked	55 g	3 teaspoonfuls Muesli	20 g
200 g pasta cooked	70 g	6 dried apricots	20 g
200 g white bread	100 g	4 dried dates	25 g
200 g 5-grain bread	85 g	1 litre apple juice	100 g
200 g potatoes	35 g	1 litre soft drink	100 g

Table 3.2: *Examples of carbohydrates*

Dried fruits (all variations), fruit slices, Muesli or energy bar, bread etc. Top up regularly with proteins and fats.

Fat (F)

Examples:	Hidden fats = nuts, seeds, kernels, proteins, sweets, snacks, visible fats = butter, margarine, oils
Energy:	9 kcal (kilocalories) or 38 kJ (kilojoules)
Recommendation:	30–45 percent energy from food ingested

Some fats make ideal supplements to ensure meeting the high requirement for energy in the mountains and, in addition, supply the fat-soluble vitamins and fatty acids that are essential to life. These essential fatty acids, as they are called (linoleic and linolenic) cannot be synthesised by the body itself and so have to be provided through diet (e.g. linseed, rape oil, nuts, wheat-germ and fish). Depending on the performance requirement, 1 – 1.5 g fat needs to be ingested every day for each kilogram of body weight.
After a week's tour people often realize that their muscles have become more visually apparent. The subcutaneous fat available for energy recuperation has been used up and this is something that lady mountaineers often find particularly gratifying. The reduction of fat is, however, also an indication that there has been inadequate provision of calories, both in terms of quality and quantity. Because the good mountain guide who has completed a course in endurance training will also exhibit a higher level of fat oxidation (burning of fat in the muscle cell), including at high intensities, there will automatically be less of a reduction in his body's own stores of sugar (*glycogen*).[1] This means his *glycogen* will be stored in the liver and in the muscles and this may well be one of the reasons why he will feel much fresher than his customers after a tour. The traditional diet of cheese, bacon and sausage may therefore, as experience with long stomach rest periods and the intensive process of digestion shows, form an addition to the menu over several days. With more intensive exercise these supplements are automatically reduced. Nevertheless, in all lengthy undertakings, fat is the most important supplier of energy. On tours of several hours' duration, 50 – 80 % of energy is obtained through lipometabolism and, in the case of a mountain guide, it may be up to 90 %. This means that the amateur mountaineer will derive a somewhat greater benefit from the optimized approach to nutrition that characterizes the sports diet than the mountain guide with his trained metabolism.

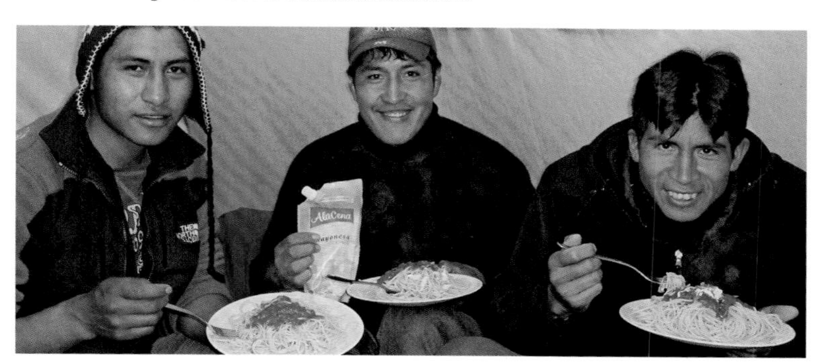

Figure 3.1: *Spaghetti dinner on a round trek in the Cordillera Huayhuash, Peruvian Andes (A. Brunello).*

Proteins (P)

Examples:	Milk and milk products, meat, fish, eggs, tofu, nuts, seeds, kernels, cereals and pulses
Energy:	4 kcal (kilocalories) or 17 kJ (kilojoules)
Recommendation:	10–15 percent energy from food ingested

The main function of protein is in relation to constructive metabolism (e.g. the muscular system, hormones, enzymes, transport proteins, immune defense system). The protein reservoirs (muscle system) will only be reduced in the event of an inadequate supply of energy derived from carbohydrate (CH) or fat (F) (mainly) or should a lack of protein occur. Thus protein, in the sense of balanced energy metabolism, has no relevant effect, although it may, for example, ensure better maintenance of concentration capability (important on long and difficult routes). On the other hand, a weakened or degraded muscle system is not efficient and is more susceptible to injuries as a result, for example, of instability. In most cases the protein group is adequately or even overrepresented in a standard homespun diet and thus the recommended 1–2 g of protein per kilogram of body weight per day is often achieved in mountain sports, regardless of whether more endurance or strength are required for mountain climbing. The dynamic effect of protein breakdown and conversion, more heat production by comparison to carbohydrate (CH) and fat (F), makes itself comfortingly noticeable in cold conditions.

⇨ Small snacks between meals should in each case be a combination of (e.g.) bread (CH) and meat (P), fruit and cheese or Tuttifrutti (fruit and nuts) etc.

A main meal without any meat is, on the other hand, only to be regarded as balanced if the missing proportion is replaced by a sufficient quantity of egg, tofu or fish, for example.

Fluid

In addition to regulating the body temperature, fluid acts as a transporter and is a fixed component of the various categories. But how much should I drink each day? Ultimately, it is an inescapable fact that we do have to carry every drop up the mountain and during the tour concentration will be focused on the next foothold. You should carry enough in your rucksack to enable you to produce a minimum of 1 to 1.5 liters of urine, spread over a period of 24 hours. Dark urine that stains the snow is cause for concern. In addition to this quantity of urine, additional fluid is lost through respiration, sweat and the stools. A trained person sweats more, electrolyte excretion tends to be less but nevertheless varies from person to person.

Depending on performance and conditions, it is possible that far more than a litre of sweat will be lost over a period of an hour.

If your throat is dry and sore, this is a clear indication of an inadequate supply of fluid. So as to save weight, fewer fresh products are consumed on the mountain and this is something that suppresses the water balance even more.

Sign of a lack of fluid: in a warm environment and with only a 1–2 % loss of bodily fluids (at a weight of 70 kg this is already ~1.5 litres) a reduction in performance, dizziness, headaches may develop; where greater levels of loss are involved, such manifestations may be accompanied by fatigue, exhaustion, irritability and nausea, loss of vitality and appetite. Muscle cramps may frequently develop due to a lack of water, salt and CH.

Drink before you start to feel thirsty because this will improve your performance!

Unfortunately, however, only around eight to ten deciliters per hour can be absorbed by the intestine in an optimum manner. In ordinary everyday practice, 1 – 2 liters of fluid is recommended a healthy diet. Should your mountain tour be equivalent in terms of performance to the performance level to be expected in standard everyday practice, then you can take these recommendations as your basis. With the help of the sports diet pyramid **(www.sfsn.ethz.ch),** you can factor in an additional four to eight deciliters of sports drinks for every hour of sport. Based on this calculation, any number of empirical values obtained from individual ambitious Alpinists and anything else you like to add to the mix, the result will be a minimum of two to three liters spread over a high Alpine day tour during the course of the tour and two or more liters of fluid before and after the tour (including soup and milk).
The beverage of choice for mountain sport may be water, tea with or without sugar, a classic sports drink or a drink you have made up yourself. Water and tea without sugar should only be taken in conjunction with meals. This can help to get the morsels ingested down, taking into account the lack of saliva. Whether a modified juice spritzer is suitable as a drink on a tour depends on the degree of tolerance (e.g. upset stomach).

Because large quantities stay longer in the stomach, smaller portions should be consumed on a regular basis.

Ingredients	Drink 1	Drink 2	Drink 3	Drink 4	Drink 5	Drink 6
Water			1 litre	1 litre	1 litre	
Peppermint tea*	1 litre	1 litre				
Fruit juice						7 dl
Raspberry syrup		30 g	30 g			
Sugar	30 g			15 g		
Fructose		30 g		15 g		
Maltodextrin	50 g	50 g	50 g	90 g	50 g	20
Kitchen salt	1.5 g	1.5 g	1.5 g	1.5 g	1.5 g	1.5
Total CH g/l	**78**	**78**	**73**	**111**	**78**	**6**

Table 3.3: *Homemade sports drinks[2)] modified in accordance with Mettler S. ETHZ, HotTopic 17, 2006; *or otherwise tea*

However, if there is a lack of time or appetite it is all the more important to pay attention to a sensible balance in relation to drink. So that the drink can be retained in the body, it should have just the right amount of salt added to it that you can still enjoy drinking it. Glucose also improves absorption of the salt in the intestine.
Where short- or long-term exertion is concerned it is worth ingesting energy in liquid carbohydrate (CH) form (without fat F or protein P) because this will help to maintain the stocks of CH (glycogen) through regularly topping up and will compensate for loss of fluids. To improve tolerance and utilization, a range of different carbohydrates should be introduced [glucose, fructose (fruit sugar), sucrose (cane or beet sugar in the form of household sugar), maltose (malt sugar)]. Ratio glucose to fructose to sucrose: 2 to 1 to 1.
If the drink is intended to supply energy for a long period or to be more nutritious in its effect, then it can be enriched with maltodextrin (polysaccharide), protein or milk powder.
Contrary to common belief, **coffee** only acts as a diuretic in drinkers who are not used to it. Those who use it regularly do not necessarily have to reckon with excessive urine excretion. On the contrary, caffeine is likely to have an even more supportive effect on performance and concentration where the "uninitiated" are concerned.

Homemade sports drinks made from watered-down fruit juice should have salt added in quantities of 1.5 g of salt per liter of fluid (check what you can tolerate). For any exertion over a number of days, sports drinks powders or tabs to supplement the tea in the hut and for good measure top up from the salt cellar. The sports-specific additives not only incorporate important sugars of different types but also minerals and vitamins.

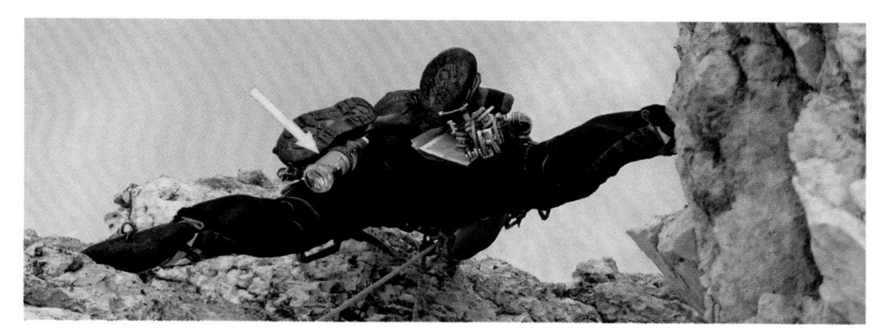

Figure 3.2: *Drink before you start to feel thirsty: Urs Hirsiger in the Gelbe Kante, Kleine Zinne, Dolomiten; Italy (I. Weber).*

Keep some salt to hand for times when you run low on fluid while hiking. Fill your bottle with snow and add some salt, pop it under your jacket while you are walking along and ten minutes later enjoy the first swig. If available, supplement with sports drink powder, dried fruits or sweets.

The Camelbag is a very practical drinking bottle, however, it tends to lead to uncontrolled drinking in the initial phase of a tour, something which may lead to shortages as you near the end of the tour. Non-carbonated drinks (sports drinks, tea, water) are better tolerated.

Avoid alcohol on the tour because it impedes concentration and condition and changes one's perception of cold. An alcohol-free beer may go down well after the tour as its mineral composition is relatively beneficial, although nowhere near sufficient to provide a full replacement.

3.3 Secondary Plant Substances, Minerals, Trace Elements and Vitamins *(Micronutrients)*

This group constitutes an essential component in the intake of foodstuffs which need to be introduced regularly via the diet because the body is unable to store them itself. The exception is vitamin K in modest amounts and, in instances where there is adequate exposure of the skin to merit it, vitamin D. This group is also known as adjuvants or protective substances. What is it that they are protecting us from? Long-term physical exertion, spending lengthy periods at high altitudes, intensive exposure to

the sun or to the ocean will prompt the growth of ***"free radicals."*** These radical oxygen compounds are capable of destroying (for example) cells, fats etc. by way of he domino effect and thus weakening our system. Acting as antioxidants, the micronutrients engage in this domino effect by interrupting the chain reaction and protecting our entire system from its consequences. This means that these micronutrients play a part in energy metabolism and bone metabolism, within the nervous and the immune system, in all the organs as well as in relation to healing processes.
In the forefront of these foodstuffs are vegetables, fruits, grain and nuts, seeds and kernels. Although sports nutrient bars frequently have a similar and fat content to biscuits or chocolate, in the main they contain more micronutrients, something which is of primary benefit on tours stretching over several days with no fresh supplies.

⇨ The micro-nutrient additives must not be allowed to come into contact with hot tea etc. because this will have the effect of destroying up to more than 70 % of the heat-sensitive nutrients.

A generalized depletion seldom occurs on mountain tours of four to eight hours' (h) duration. However, should, during a long and hard tour, there be a marked output in terms of sweat or even losses due to vomiting and diarrhea, this will mean a tangible reduction in an individual's availability and make him or her immensely weak. Here natrium, together with potassium and magnesium, is particularly worth bearing in mind. Dried fruit or glucose after a soup or salted juice is a quick way to restore the balance. Simply recommending the minimum quantity of vegetables and fruits (five a day), it is possible to ensure that the "secondary plant substances" are covered.
In sport, although **magnesium** is an important factor in muscle metabolism, there are still interactive complexes which may have an effect on one another and of which we should be aware. Going in for sport after a meal with magnesium in the digestive track can trigger stomach cramps and diarrhea. Many mountaineers on tours of several days' duration have noticed that the tea often seems to have lost its flavor. If this happens, adding a powder with a mineral content before the tea bag to (what is often) tea made with meltwater will give a stronger taste in a trice. The most important electrolytes/ions are natrium, potassium, chlorine, bicarbonate, sulfate, magnesium and calcium.[3)]

In cases of dehydration, the **World Health Organisation (WHO/FAO)** recommends a solution of the following by way of a substitute:

- 1 litre of water
- 3.5 g cooking salt (natrium chloride)
- 2.5 g baking powder (natrium carbonate can be dispensed with at altitude because it forms in increased quantities in such locations)
- 1.5 g sylvite (potassium chloride)
- 20 g glucose (or 40 g household sugar)

Obtainable at the pharmacy, on its own or already mixed.
Should the supply of natural foodstuffs not be sufficient to prevent a shortage over a number of days, then a natural complex **supplement** (capsules, effervescent tablets, powder etc.) will compensate or may even influence performance directly or indirectly.

For a precise resumé of all important details relating to vitamins and minerals see **"Energy & Nutrients"** at **www.sfsn.ethz.ch**.

3.4 Diet before, during and after the Tour

If your aim is regeneration with maximum expedition, this will begin in advance of and carry on during the tour. Which means that that you should regularly consume items from all the groups of foodstuffs wherever possible in all phases, taking into consideration the individual priorities.

Don't try out anything new before or during a serious mountain tour.

Before the Tour

On the day before your big tour starts your priority should be to ensure that you schedule a massive increase in your carbohydrate (CH) intake (400 – 700 g per day). In Table 3.2, Page 42 we have given a few examples together with their duly rounded-off carbohydrate (CH) content (these can be found under CH). Make sure, if possible, that you are relaxed when you arrive at your accommodation on the day before the "ascent" because this will mean that the CH stores (*glycogen*) will not be depleted and any shortages can be made up as quickly as possible directly on arrival at the hut. The first meal before the tour should be an easily digestible meal which means that you should only eat and drink things with which you are familiar. Here's an example of a breakfast before the big tour:

- Light muesli (cereal flakes, fruit, nuts) with yoghurt and/or milk, bread with "lots" of butter and lots more jam or honey instead of cheese, always ensuring that it does not lie heavily on the stomach. Round it off with a juice.
- Drinking "lots" will mean a short "pit stop" ~ 1 to 1.5 hours later

During the Tour

By consuming several small meals at intervals during the day it is possible to prevent any problems with tolerance or lack of appetite and relieve the pressure on blood sugar levels.

Because carbohydrates deliver the energy required, depending on source, up to four times as fast as fats, it will be obvious why this group is repeatedly recommended during exercise and will counteract a fall in sugar levels. For drinks see fluid.

Every two hours: Biscuits (Swiss "Willisauer Ringli", "Basler Leckerli"), Gummi bears, rice cakes or waffles, "Tuttifrutti", nut mixtures, cereal bars, sports bars, "Appenzeller Biberli" (a type of spiced biscuit from Switzerland), "Birnenweggen" (a pastry concoction), dried fruits (fresh fruit for people who don't mind carrying it), chocolate, bread, crispbreads or chocolate, wholegrain crackers with cheese or cold meats, sandwiches or "salty" protein savouries from the sports nutrients sector.

Lots of things can be carried in the pocket of a jacket and consumed slowly either while walking along or at a stand along the way.

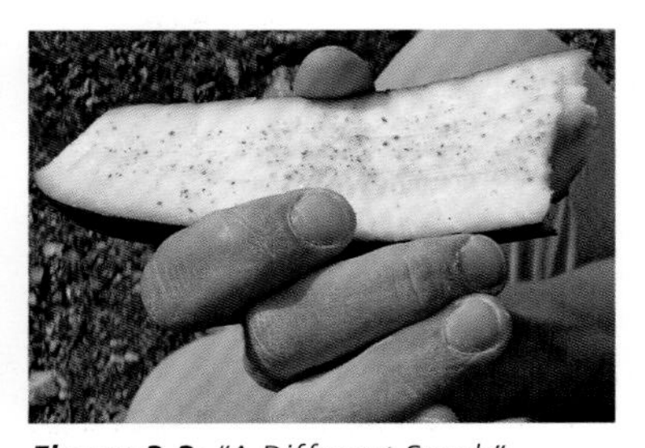

Figure 3.3: *"A Different Snack" (U. Hirsiger).*

Powder for shakes can be mixed up quickly and easily in the bottle using water from a mountain stream to reinstate enhanced performance capability following temporary exhaustion.

Post-tour

The first meal (carbohydrate CH and protein P) should be eaten in the first 15–30 minutes after the tour.

If a strenuous tour is to be continued on the following day or if you are keen to shake off the feeling of tiredness as quickly as possible, regeneration drinks/shakes should be used in your tent **directly** following exertion. Because the muscle cell absorbs sugar better in the first 1–2 hours, you can be sure of acquiring a feeling of well-being faster. A good fruit flan or some hot soup with a juice spritzer in the hut can have a similar effect. Fruit juice with cheese and bread. Fruit juice with protein powder and a spot of salt.
Mountaineers who have encountered their limits will, depending on the goals they have set themselves and the type of exertion, will need several weeks to regenerate. Time required for a recovery to take place at cell level.

Please visit **http://www.dopinginfo.ch/faktenblatter-nach-klassen.html** to read about the effectiveness of macro- and micronutrients as well as other possible aids to performance.

3.5 Diet at High Altitudes

The most important point of all in this chapter is the reference to fluid. Maintaining the flow of liquid as described above in order to counteract the risk of dehydration due to sweating and accelerated exhalation. Cold, dry air is heated by the lung and becomes entirely saturated with water vapor inside the bronchial tubes. In addition, despite the presence of dry skin, the loss of fluid through sweating must not be underestimated because more rapid evaporation takes place at cold altitudes.

At high altitudes it is also possible not to recognise the feeling of thirst even once the loss of fluid has become advanced.

It will frequently be necessary to catch up on one's fluid intake in the evening and many people are still unable to understand why they should have experienced such performance lows during the day.
A requirement of around 3500 kcal is calculated as the amount a person weighing 70 kg is likely to need on a day's hike. On a tour lasting several days this increases to approx. 4000 kcal and, for climbers in high alpine latitudes, to more than 4500 kcal. The allowance is approx. 100–150 kcal for every 100 meters altitude.
Extreme environmental conditions such as heights above 4000 meters and the physical

stress associated with such conditions will change the metabolism in a different way to what was anticipated, much to the surprise of the explorer of the heights. Although a higher level of oxygen consumption is required for reducing fat than for reducing carbohydrate, the body tends to fall back on its reserves of fat. The reasons and explanations for this still lie in the deep dark depths of conjecture.[4)]

The Calorific Equivalent (CA) or energy equivalent of oxygen means the energy yield per liter of oxygen [5)] resulting from the breakdown of foodstuffs.

- Carbohydrate breakdown: supplies per litre of oxygen (O2) CA: 5.01 kcal/lO2
- Fat breakdown: supplies per litre oxygen (O2) CA: 4.69 kcal/lO2
- Protein breakdown: supplies per litre oxygen (O2) CA: 4.48 kcal/lO2

Thus it is not possible to pinpoint the amount of oxygen extracted from the breakdown of carbohydrate (CH) at high altitude in the hitherto accepted sense. This will please everyone who has in the past sworn by their cheese, sausage or nuts and chocolate. The extent to which the carbohydrates have a part to play in major achievements alongside the new, high altitude diets rich in fats is something that promises to be a subject for future research.[6)]

Because, as of around 2000–2500 m, a sizable number of people already experience a lack of appetite and, as a result, fewer quality foodstuffs (not to mention hardly any fresh products) are being consumed, it may be advantageous from the point of view of the energy balance, the immune system etc. if, to accompany lengthy periods of exercise, corresponding micro- and macronutrients are taken into account. This often enhances the feeling of well-being and improves performance capability. Based on the altitude training of endurance athletes, it has been shown that an increasing number of free radicals are created and that a vitamin E substitute has been recommended to neutralize them.[7a)] More recent findings, however, indicate a broader based supplement (not only Vit. E) as protection against the free radicals.

At least at the beginning, a diet rich in iron should be adopted in order to cover the increased iron required for the formation of more red blood cells.[7b)] Lean meat may represent a readily available source of iron *(hemoglobin iron)* which will enable adaptation to the altitude to take place at a faster rate. The important thing to note when taking it is that it is not to be taken together with milk products, black tea or coffee. The thermogenic (heat inducing) effect of protein is capable of tempting people to consume too much of this group, something which would be counterproductive at altitude. An "excessive" reduction of protein in the liver will lead, for example, to an increase in the quantity of urine being flushed out via the kidneys, which would in turn call for more water for the flushing operation. The water is, nevertheless, required by the body more urgently for other processes in order to enable it to cope better with the altitude.

In the high mountains, on extreme trekking trips or on expeditions, it is possible, in the upper performance segment, to rapidly consume 5000 to 10000 kcal per day. Undoubtedly, the extreme climbers, even those on a high fat diet, incur a deficit that will be balanced out over the subsequent days and weeks.

If it is not possible to acclimatize slowly, then the immune system will be weakened and as a result it makes sense to take increased daily quantities of micronutrients in order to increase one's resistance to infections. However, this practice is attracting an increasing number of critics because this involves auxiliaries (such as oxygen) which are not ingested by means of a natural product (vegetables etc.). Anyone who reacts with problems of tolerance, stomach pains, diarrhea etc. which is not necessarily associated with a lack of hygiene or infection should note the following:

Cook or peel before you eat it or forget it!

Sometimes BioflorinaTM capsules can help. These back up your own intestinal flora.

Food intolerances and allergies: In the meantime there are, on the home pages of the major distributors and the health food chains, reliable lists itemising dietary products for use by coeliacs (gluten intolerance), those with lactose intolerance or allergies etc. Despite the majority of dietary modifications there is nothing to stop Mahomet going to the mountain. For example, many gluten-free foodstuffs are refined products, something which tends to be an advantage in performance sport due to the improved level of tolerance. If you feel uncertain about this topic, then you are most welcome to visit the homepage of our qualified dietary advisers (university diploma in health sciences) **(www.svde-asdd.ch)** where you will be able to make contact with a competent adviser in your vicinity.

Summary: When it comes to making a success of your tour, don't make yourself dependent on your diet, adapt to the given situations and make the best of them!

Bibliography:

1) Knechtle B; Aktuelle Sportphysiologie, Leistung und Ernährung im Sport; Karger-Verlag, 2002, 60.
2) Spahr C, Mannhart Ch; Müesli und Muskeln, Essen und Trinken im Sport; Ingold-Verlag, 2008, 10.
3) Williams Melvin H; Ernährung, Fitness und Sport; Dt. Ausg. hrsg. von Rost Richard, Berlin; Wiesbaden: Ullstein Mosby, 1997, 302.
4) Huber A, Pichler J, Hefti U, DIE ALPEN März 2011, S. 30–33.
5) Suter Paolo M; Checkliste Ernährung–Stuttgart; New York: Thieme-Verlag, 2002, 9.
6) Knechtle B; Akt. Sportphysiologie, Leistung und Ernährung im Sport; Basel: Karger-Verlag, 2002, 57.
7) (ab) Williams Melvin H.; Ernährung, Fitness und Sport; Dt. Ausg. hrsg. von Rost Richard, Berlin; Wiesbaden: Ullstein Mosby, 1997, 109, 245, 279.

4. Mountaineering for Kids

S. Kriemler

Mountaineering and trekking with children has the potential to be a once-in-a-lifetime experience for the whole family. So as to avoid any disasters, the following should be borne in mind…

4.1 General Aspects

Children differ from grown-ups in terms of a number of physiological and psychological features. Thus, for example, there is a factor of 20 between a baby weighing 3.5 kg and a youth weighing 70 kg. This means that doses of medication and fluid balance need to be adjusted. If you, as a parent, do not know the weight of your child, you risk running into serious difficulties.
Heat regulation in children is less efficient than in adults, something which exposes them to greater risk in a cold or a hot environment. Because children have more body surface per mass or body weight, they compensate more quickly for differences in temperature between their body and the environment. As a result they cool down faster and their bodies overheat more quickly.

⇨ Children's bodies are subject to more rapid cooling and overheating.

In cold conditions factors such as a lack of subcutaneous adipose tissue or absence of movement, in particular as regards infants who are carried immobile on their backs by parents who are mountaineering enthusiasts, constitute further risk factors.

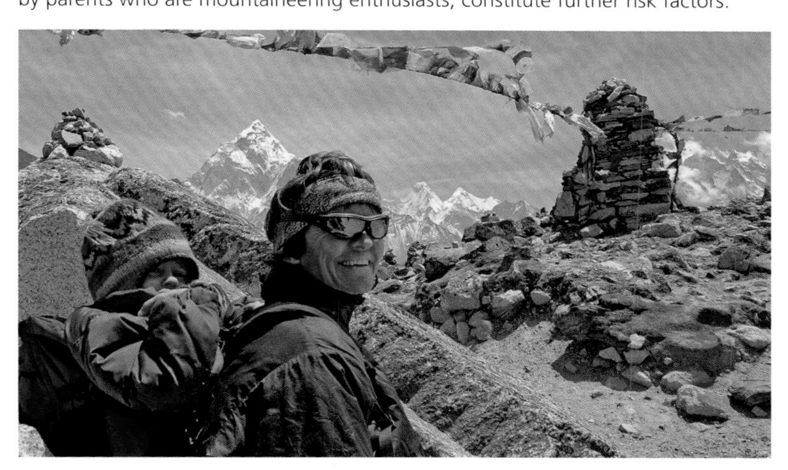

Figure 4.1: *Trekking on the Ama Dablam, Nepal (U. Wiget).*

In hot conditions, the fact that sweat production is not yet sufficiently developed before puberty leads to the body heating up further. In our latitudes it is predominantly the cold that is a problem. In this context the principle of "*windchill*" should be taken into account.

Wind Chill: This means nothing more than that the effect of cold on the skin or the general loss of heat from the body is influenced to a major extent by the wind speed. For example, wind travelling at 40 km/h at a temperature of 0 °C will lead to a loss of heat similar to that if the temperature were -16 °C in calm conditions.

In addition, the loss of heat through the skin may increase many times over if the skin is damp because the conductivity of water is 20–25 times higher than that of air. How often does this happen in the mountains when the child is romping about and perspiring or when it is raining? A spare set of dry clothes, especially not forgetting parts of the body that are not primarily exposed (damp socks, undergarments) is every bit as essential here as emergency supplies on an expedition.

⇨ People are exposed to 80 % of all the sunshine they will experience in their lives before their 20th birthdays and the risk of developing a malignant melanoma is at least twice as high if a child or young person has suffered one or more bouts of sunburn (see Chapter 19.2, Page 249).

Children experience more **infections** than adults and these often run a more problematic course on initial exposure and also because of anatomical differences. Children have a narrower system of airway-tubes which, due to the fact that they are narrower, become congested more quickly with mucus and swelling. Any type of fever is capable of leading to febrile convulsions, loss of appetite, nausea, sickness, diarrhea with **dehydration** and weakness.

⇨ These are all symptoms that can mimic altitude sickness of one type or another.

Diarrhea and sickness are hard nuts to crack on any trip, especially when they persist over several days. Children dehydrate very much more quickly than adults; an absence of urine over a period of six hours is an unmistakable sign of dehydration. It is important that the child should if necessary be coerced into imbibing liquid in small sips, but continuously over a number of hours even if he or she objects or is sick. Wise parents have an adequate therapy to hand for every possible ailment so that they can be sure of being able to avert a catastrophe should a situation of this kind arise. If the symptoms do not disappear within a few hours, it will be necessary to call for help and in case of exposure to altitude, immediate descent is essential.

One of the most important things to remember is that one must be careful not to spoil children's enjoyment of nature and the opportunity to move about. To this end, an age-adapted travel schedule is to be recommended that is geared to the physical and mental circumstances of the children. Everything needs to be hands-on.

Smaller children are experts when it comes to discovering their surroundings. It is helpful to search the neighborhood for toxic plants that can disappear into children's mouths all too quickly, or to attach a bell to a shoe so that the little explorers can be located once again. Older children are enthusiastic students when it comes to practicing emergency situations in an emergency bivouac, heat insulation or pathfinding. Any child will be proud to carry his or her own rucksack.

A child's rucksack should not exceed 20 % of his or her body weight.

Children should not be overstrained, in particular when climbing. Each episode of anxiety has the potential to subsequently lead to the child withdrawing from activities of this nature. Children under 12 years of age should not be made responsible for securing a partner on a rope without supervision because they are simply not old enough to take personal responsibility.

In any event, an emergency plan must be drawn up. This should include the local rescue facilities, an emergency pharmacist and the quickest way back. It is only when you take precautions that nothing happens.

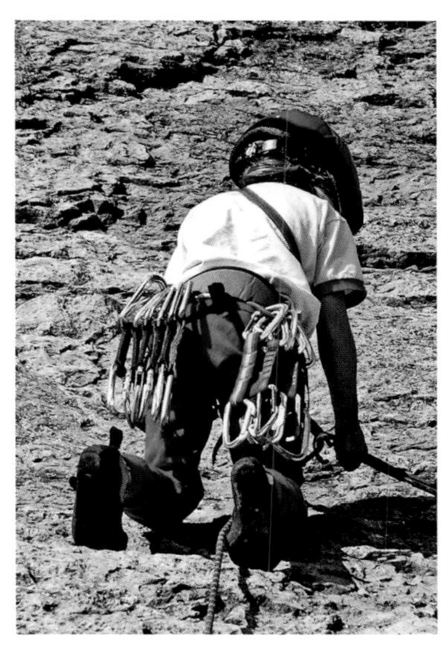

Figure 4.2: *Young climber scaling a rock (U. Wiget).*

4.2 At High Altitude

Whether it is right to take children along when hiking at high altitudes will always be contraversial and provoke lively discussions and recommendations range from strict tut-tutting and finger waving to ecstatic endorsement of such undertakings, depending on whether you have just been reading about the frostbitten extremities of an infant or have just come from standing with your 12-year old son on the summit of Switzerland's Mönch. A major international group of experts published a consensus[1] recommendation in 2001 that was directed at doctors. Many of the details are, nonetheless, of interest for all parents and persons who head for the mountains accompanied by children.

General

Even today there are only a small number of scientific studies that are concerned with temporary and relatively short stays at high altitude involving children. Many recommendations are based on research carried out on adults at high altitudes and are not surveys conducted directly in relation to children at all.
Altitude is capable of triggering three different acute disorders or medical conditions in the human body, the clinical presentations of which are described in detail in the chapter entitled "Altitude:"

"Acute Mountain Sickness AMS"[2]
"High Altitude Pulmonary Edema (HAPE)"
"High Altitude Cerebral Edema (HACE)"

4.3 AMS (Acute Mountain Sickness)

Based on studies carried out to date with children, the frequency of Acute Mountain Sickness in children and adolescents is no different from that which affects adults. In two studies carried out in the Rocky Mountains, infants aged between three months and three years were studied at a height of 2800 m. In order to record AMS, a specially developed questionnaire was developed for preverbal children (see Appendix 22.2, Page 300). The frequency with which children and their parents tended to succumb was the same, 1 in 5 fell ill. Two independent studies at a height of 3450 m investigated the frequency of AMS in schoolchildren and adolescents, including compared to adults. In both studies and using the Lake Louise Score, AMS was recorded in healthy, non-acclimatised children and adolescents aged from 8–16 years within 18–20 and 42 hours of arriving at an altitude of 3450 m. One third of the children and adolescents and even a third of the adults fell sick with a form of AMS at some stage during the time spent at high altitude. The number was at its highest on the first day, 6–8 hours after arrival, and declined steadily on day 2 (21 %) and day 3 (8 %). There was no difference noted between prepubescent children and adolescents.

If we consider the distribution of the altitude symptoms, there were more manifestations of stomach/intestinal complaints in pre-pubescent children by comparison to adolescents and adults, but at the same time fewer headaches and less disturbance to sleep.

Generally speaking, serious medical conditions occur only rarely at a height of 3450 m (Jungfraujoch), but can nevertheless occur, in particular on even higher climbs. Two children (aged 9 and 11) nevertheless had to be treated with Dexamethason on the Jungfraujoch following a serious attack of AMS.
Specific questionnaires are used for recording altitude sickness, which register the individual symptoms and indications of altitude sickness. **The Lake Louise Score** is the questionnaire most frequently deployed and this can also be used without problems where older children are concerned. For infants the use of the CLLS (Children's Lake Louise Score) is recommended (see Appendix 22.2, Page 300), for small children of school age an adapted version of the LLS (Lake Louise Score) for adults can be used. The latter makes use of child-oriented language and integrated Smileys to describe the severity of the symptoms in a way that is easier for the children (see Appendix 22.2, Page 301).

4.4 HAPE and HACE (High Altitude Pulmonary Edema and High Altitude Cerebral Edema)

There are no studies relating to the frequency of HAPE or HACE in children. Experienced specialists in high altitude medicine from Colorado, however, report definite instances where HAPE was encountered in healthy children who had undergone acute exposure to altitude. In the studies described above on the Jungfraujoch (3450 m) not a single case of HAPE occurred, something which is also unlikely due to the fact that there was only slight exposure to altitude. Nevertheless it is important to note that such an instance is quite capable of arising and that both forms of altitude sickness may well be life threatening.

Risk Factors

As far as the risk factors for the various forms of altitude sickness are concerned, the same risk factors apply as with adults. The crucial factors are the speed of ascent, the altitude reached and the personal susceptibility. Respecting the guidelines for prevention of altitude sickness,[1] a minimum risk may be assumed. However, three situations exist which constitute more or less child-specific risks:

- Acute or only recently experienced **conditions affecting the airways** (cold, bronchitis, pneumonia) seem to increase the dangers of falling ill with a high altitude pulmonary edema. This is of course a frequent situation which is important to take notice of – especially where children of preschool age are concerned. It may be assumed that, as a result of the inflammation in the lungs, the porosity of the blood vessels increases, especially at high altitudes where there is a deficiency of oxygen, as has been shown in studies using animals as models.

- Children who, during the birth process or shortly afterward, have experienced a regulatory disturbance of the pulmonary blood flow in the form of **an inadequate supply of oxygen,** have a higher risk of developing a pulmonary edema at high altitude as a result of increased pressure in the pulmonary circulation system. This situation is rare. In cases of doubt, parents should contact their paediatrician who cared for their child during and shortly after birth. Special attention should be paid to those children in particular who needed to be placed on a ventilator during their first few days of life.

- Children who suffer from *Trisomy 21 (Down's Syndrome, Mongolism)*, from a **heart defect** or from a **serious chronic lung disease** *(cystic fibrosis)* appear to be more prone to suffering high altitude pulmonary edema than healthy children. This is associated with the inadequate ability of the heart and lungs to adapt to the reduced pressure of oxygen at high altitude.

4.5 Indications or Symptoms

Older children display the same indications of altitude sickness as adults. As is the case with adults, the symptoms do not commence until 4 – 48 hours after ascending to a high altitude.

⇨ Where smaller children are concerned, the development of altitude sickness can be difficult to identify because children under the age of around 8 years are not able to give specific details of their symptoms, their statements do not always tally with what the body is actually feeling at a given time.

For this reason a specially adapted system of points (**"Lake Luise Score for preverbal children"** – see Appendix 22.2, Page 300) has been developed for small children at the preverbal stage (up to 3 years) which is based on indications such as general restlessness, lack of interest in eating, reduced play behavior and sleep disturbances. In general each symptom and every change in behavior, in particular affecting small children at altitudes higher than approx. 2500 m, should be assessed as altitude sickness and a descent will be called for.
Nevertheless, there are a number of other causes that may be responsible for the "altitude symptoms," as they are called: travel sickness, lack of motivation, overexertion, infections of any kind, poisoning by berries, plants or fungi or inhaling a small foreign body which may subsequently be misdiagnosed as a high altitude pulmonary edema.

4.6 Prevention

When it comes to preventing high altitude problems in relation to children there are three crucial elements to be borne in mind. These are to ascend slowly, to avoid physical overexertion and to organize an undertaking suitable for children.

- As with adults, the recommendation is, from 2500 to 3000 m, to increase the sleeping altitude each day by no more than 300 to a maximum of 500 meters of altitude. For every 1000 meters, one extra night should be spent at the same altitude for purposes of acclimatization. The effect of administering a prophylactic dose of **Acetazolamide** (Diamox®) has never been tested on children and should therefore be considered only in special individual cases and following discussion with the family doctor. What appears to be more important is that parents should know their children inside out, are well-informed when it comes to the presentation of the various forms of high altitude sickness and also know how children generally react to journeys so that they are able to distinguish travel symptoms from high altitude symptoms.

- Any overexertion increases the risk of altitude sickness. This is something to watch out for, especially in small and "hyperactive" children. The first commandment as far as the venture into high altitude territory is concerned should be that the child should be having fun, is feeling good and is not completely at the mercy of record-busting parents. Longer, "boring" daily stages must be broken up by an overnight stay and children's natural instinct to play must be satisfied anew at every opportunity along the way.

- As an aid to prevention, a precise medical history will be required for each child as well as an **"emergency plan"** in the event of an accident or illness. This should include precise information on rescue potential and the name of a pharmacy with child-specific medications, complete with a dosages list based on body weight or age. If children are present, in my opinion both as a mother and from an ethical point of view, the possibility of descending immediately with the child should be a requirement on any such trip.

4.7 Treatment

The treatment of altitude sickness in children is the same as it is in the case of adults. The most important element is the **descent**, assuming that the patient is still able to walk. Seriously ill children will need to be carried in order to keep the degree of physical exertion to the minimum possible. To make the descent easier for the children, pain relief (Dafalgan®, Brufen®) or medications designed to counteract nausea and queasiness (Itinerol®) may be helpful and can be used without hesitation. However, they are not an alternative to actually making the descent! In cases of severe mountain sickness oxygen, Diamox®, (Dexamethason®) or a therapy involving the use of a hyperbaric chamber may be deployed in the event of an acute attack of AMS and oxygen, Nifedipin® (or Tadalafil) in the event of HAPEs. However, this is only by way of a stopgap–the most important thing is to get down as quickly as possible! The doctor will be able to use the consensus paper to obtain more precise information about the dosages which–it goes without saying–will need to be adapted to the child's body weight. The following check list includes the most important medications that can be put together with a family doctor. In general, care should be taken to ensure that as many multifunctional medicaments are taken along as possible. Every pharmacy holds detailed instructions for use by laypeople and a list with the age and weight of any children who may be involved (see recommended child pharmacy in Appendix 22.1.4, Page 293).

Bibliography:

1) Pollard AJ, Niermeyer S, Barry P, Bartsch P, Berghold F, Bishop RA, et al. Children at high altitude: an international consensus statement by an ad hoc committee of the International Society for Mountain Medicine, March 12, 2001. High Alt Med Biol 2001; 2: 389–403.
2) AMS, HAPE and HACE are the international designations/abbreviations used in each case.

5. Mountaineering for Women

S. Kriemler

A group of international experts has been attempting to provide scientifically based answers to questions posed by women planning to spend some time at high altitude or a lengthy journey off the tourist beat. The information is based not only on scientific knowledge but also on practical empirical values supplied by female scientists and/or experienced female mountaineers.

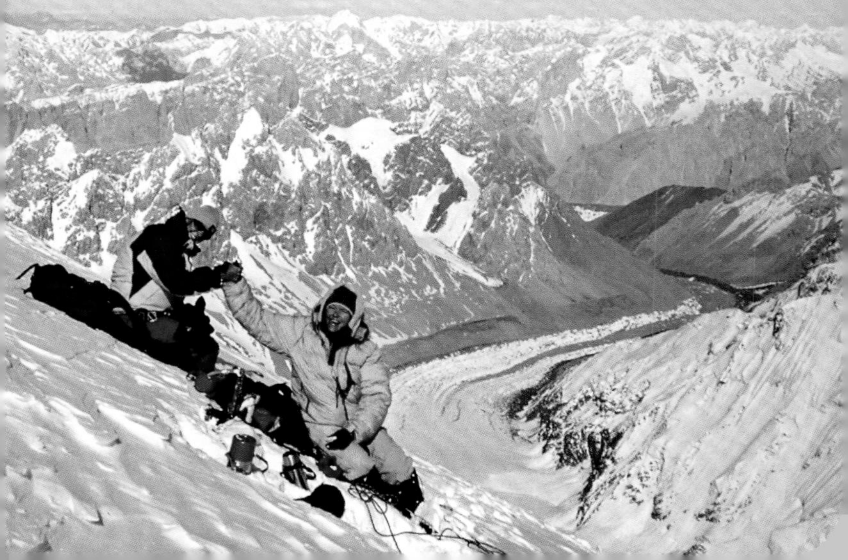

5.1 Differences between Women and Men in Extreme Environments

Adaptation to Altitude and Forms of Altitude Sickness

The time taken to get used to (= period of acclimatization) high altitudes may be described as equal as far as men and women are concerned.

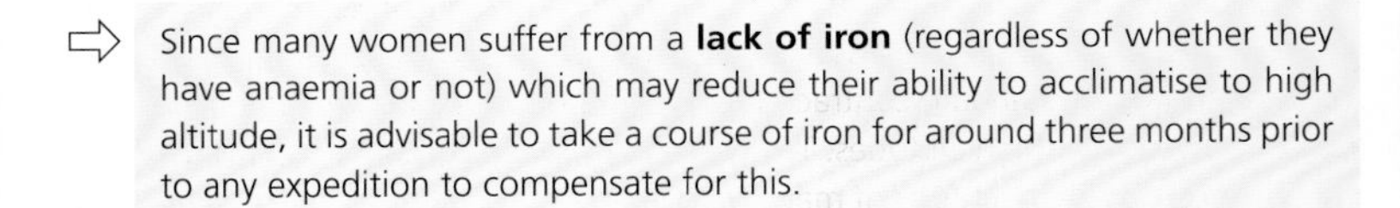

Since many women suffer from a **lack of iron** (regardless of whether they have anaemia or not) which may reduce their ability to acclimatise to high altitude, it is advisable to take a course of iron for around three months prior to any expedition to compensate for this.

Acute altitude sickness occurs with equal frequency in both women and men. However, women are more inclined to exhibit **swellings** in hands, feet and face, something which is probably connected with a different structure of the subcutaneous tissue. The menstrual cycle in women does not seem to affect the frequency of altitude sickness. High altitude pulmonary edema seems to occur less frequently in women. It is not clear whether this has something to do with the lower exposure of women generally or whether there are physiological differences which protect women against high altitude pulmonary edema. To date there is no scientific information available on the question of whether women and men are equally susceptible to high altitude cerebral edema.

Menstrual Cycle

⇨ A woman's menstrual cycle frequently alters on expeditions.

It may be assumed that the trip *per se* with all its accompanying manifestations such as changes in hygiene, cold, eating habits, loss of weight etc. by way of a prime example of a physical stress situation play a crucial part in this, presumably more than the altitude itself. In most cases there is total or partial amenorrhea, or the cycle becomes irregular.

⇨ The effectiveness of pharmacological and mechanical methods of contraception is not affected by the altitude.

For those who do not benefit from this advantageous side-effect of altitude, menstruation can become a real headache taking into account the lack of water, the cold, the accommodation in tents and the restrictions in terms of spare clothes. One must never forget either that an absence of periods does not give protection against pregnancy! Every woman should sit down and ask herself before setting out whether she is prepared to put up with the less pleasant aspects of menstruation or whether she would prefer to opt for a standard contraceptive (the pill, oral contraceptive, estrogen ring, estrogen patches, diaphragms, the coil). In the former case an adequate supply of hygiene items (cleaning-up cloths, tampons, sanitary towels) can save the situation. In such instances it is also worth considering whether to shave the genital hair in order to make it easier to keep the area down below clean. As far as we know today, the standard contraceptives do not undergo any change in terms of their effectiveness at high altitudes. The use of oral contraceptives does not alter the ability to acclimatize to altitude, it may however, theoretically speaking, promote the formation of blood clots (thromboses) and embolisms in conjunction with a loss of water (dehydration), cold and lengthy stays at high altitude. Nevertheless, neither scientifically based reports nor clearly documented cases exist in relation to this.

The oral contraceptives have various advantages in addition to preventing menstruation: they offer full protection against the risk of pregnancy and reduce the **discomfort associated with menstruation.** In addition, the pill can be taken continuously over several months which reduces the number of days' bleeding to a minimum or none at all.

In order to keep the **risk of thrombosis** low, second generation oral contraceptives with 30 µg of estrogen and not those of the first (with 50 µg of estrogen) or the third generation (with 20 µg of estrogen) should be used. The irregular eating and sleeping times on expeditions will, under certain circumstances, make it more difficult to take the pill regularly, something that reduces the reliability of contraception. In addition, antibiotics (especially broad spectrum penicillins and tetracyclines) which may be taken, for example, to combat an attack of bronchitis or diarrhea, may weaken the effect of the pill during the period when it is being taken and for up to seven days afterward. The medication Diamox® can also have an adverse effect on the reliability of the hormonal contraceptive.

5.2 Trips/Exposure to High Altitudes in Pregnancy

Travel – general

Anybody who embarks on a trip while pregnant must remember that it is often difficult to obtain specific professional advice in relation to pregnancy.

Certain infectious diseases such as malaria, hepatitis E or diarrhoea can progress to a more severe form during pregnancy and may also endanger the unborn child.

Many medications that are taken to prevent tropical diseases and ailments during the trip (anti-malaria medicines, antibiotics such as Quinolone or Sulfonamide) must not be used during pregnancy as they could endanger the child in the womb. Both pregnancy and high altitude stimulate breathing which has the effect of removing more water from the body. This is enormously important, particularly at high altitude, because air humidity is very low and the feeling of thirst is often suppressed. For this reason special attention must be paid to ensuring an adequate intake of fluid.

Forms of Altitude Sickness

Pregnancy has no effect on the frequency of occurrence of altitude sickness. However, if they occur, they may endanger the child. Medications aimed at the prevention of and/or the treatment of altitude sickness like Acetazolamide (Diamox) and other Sulfonamides are prohibited during the first three months of pregnancy due to proven damage to the unborn child and during the last three months of pregnancy because of an increased risk of neonatal jaundice.

Complications for the Mother and/or the Unborn Child

The majority of scientific studies into this particular problem area have been carried out on mothers who actually live at high altitudes. Significantly less is known about the reaction of the unborn child and the mother who normally resides in a lowland area and goes off to higher altitudes for short periods of time lasting for days or weeks. For this reason the recommendations are based on incomplete data. It may be assumed that there is an increased risk of a miscarriage during the first three months of the pregnancy. Women who have already lost one child during the early stages of pregnancy should not go on climbs involving ascents to high altitudes during this time. Short periods of time spent at levels of up to 2500 m or major physical exertion over a number of hours/days at heights of up to 2500 m for mothers who have up to now experienced no complications in their pregnancies and without any known risk factors in the second half of pregnancy do not present any problems. To date there is no information available on periods of time spent by such subjects at heights in excess of 2500 m.

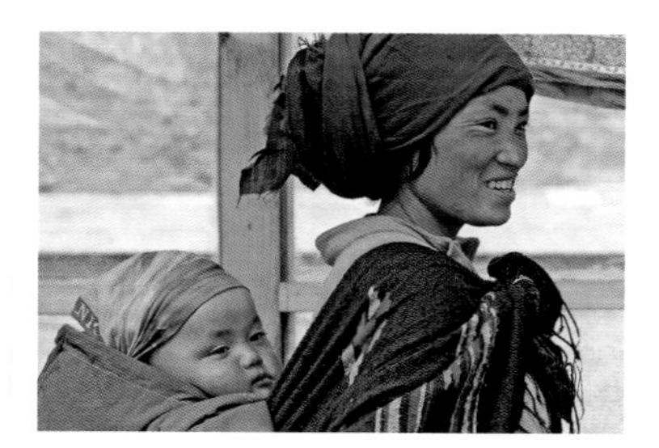

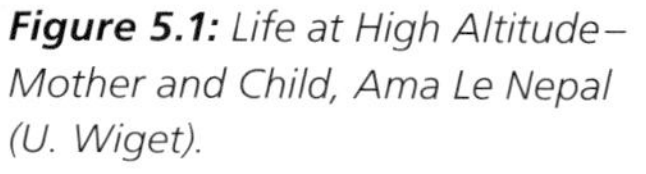

Figure 5.1: *Life at High Altitude–Mother and Child, Ama Le Nepal (U. Wiget).*

Expectant mothers at risk of **miscarriage** or disturbances affecting the development of the child, or who suffer from high blood pressure, anaemia, heart or lung disease as well as heavy smokers should, on the other hand, avoid spending even short periods at altitudes above 2500 m.

We also know that, in the case of mothers who reside for lengthy periods (weeks and months) at heights of more than 2500 m, susceptibility to the complications of pregnancy increases. For this reason the recommendations are that expectant mothers, if it is impossible to avoid spending a lengthy period of time at high altitude, should present themselves frequently and in sufficiently good time for specific medical tests in order to identify any prospective complications and to be able to react appropriately. Because physical exertion at high altitude could, theoretically, lead to premature onset of labor and to a lack of oxygen for the child as a result of the mother's own needs, pregnant women are recommended not to overexert themselves at heights in excess of 2500 m for two to three days and to wait for the full acclimatization period of two weeks before indulging in more intensive **physical activities.** In general, pregnant women should be advised against very strenuous activities at extreme altitudes because it is there that the marked lack of oxygen in the maternal and the fetal bodies can lead to injury.

Climbing and Skiing

There are no specific studies in relation to these questions. In general it can be assumed that such activities will not pose problems during the first three months of the pregnancy. The climbing belt must not be allowed to exert pressure on the abdomen at any time. Later on it is important to remember that the increase in weight, the increased elasticity of the ligaments and the shift in the body's center of gravity as the circumference of the abdomen increases may lead to accidents and falls with potential risks to the unborn child.

5.3. Practical Tips for Women Mountaineers

Clothes and climbing belts should incorporate an easy-to-operate opening system to enable the wearer to relieve herself quickly even at very low temperatures and in windy conditions. Sealable plastic bags (zip bags) and bottles with a wide opening make urinating in the tent not only possible but easier. Not to be scorned either are the plastic systems you can buy in trade shops that enable you to pass water in a standing position using a hosepipe or a funnel with a bag suspended from it. Some experienced female mountaineers recommend shaving the public hair for hygienic reasons. On lengthy expeditions every woman should prepare herself for the possibility of having to treat cystitis, inflammation of the vagina and/or an attack of urinary incontinence herself. And, last but not least, there is still no getting away from the fact that the condom is the best way of guarding against venereal diseases.

6. The Mature Mountaineer

U. Wiget

We are as young as we feel
and as old as others perceive us.
(Reinhard Ernst)

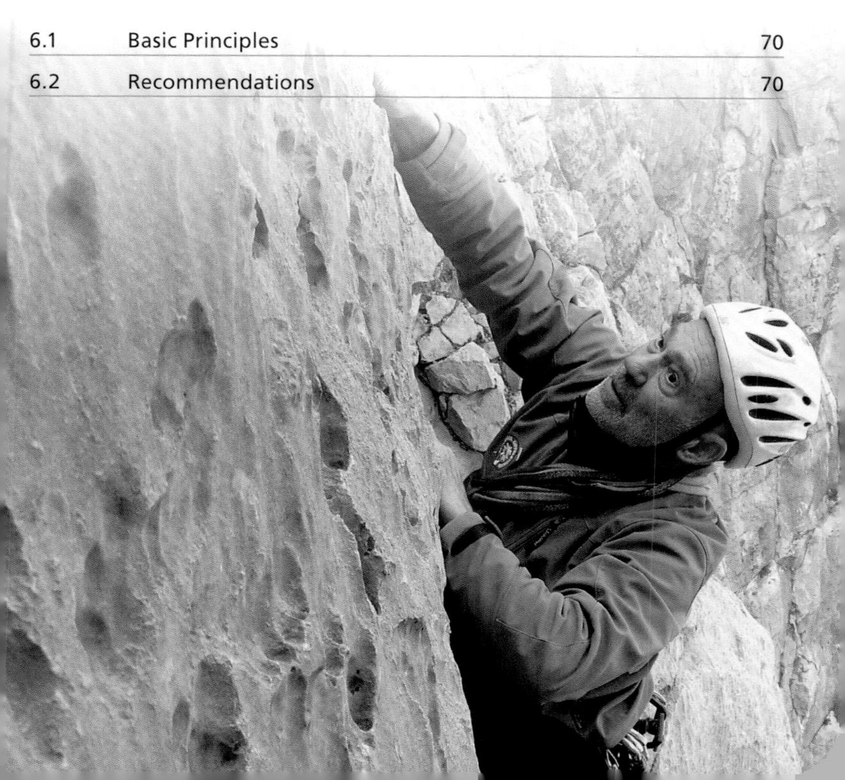

6.1 Basic Principles

We can't stop the clock, however, the aging process differs from one individual to the other.
Aging is not an illness and keeping on the move is the foundation stone for staying able-bodied right into advanced old age. Some elements of the aging process start in early adulthood (arteriosclerosis, loss of raw muscle power), others only become evident once the individual has reached the age of 40 (reduction in metopic vision and keenness of sight, reduction in the speed of reaction of the coordination system). Around the age of 60 it is likely that the majority of people, although their basic health may be good, will also become aware of constraints in relation to their locomotor system (joints, muscles). So when the mountaineer of retirement age finds himself on the move in the mountains with young friends, he will undoubtedly need a little more time to complete the ascent to the hut although he will not necessarily "lag behind" when rock climbing. So what actually happens is that our bodies, as they change, automatically become more attuned to Mother Nature, all we have to do is listen to what she is telling us…
However, age does bring many people a host of benefits that, generally-speaking, improve their lives considerably:

- An increase in the enjoyment of mountaineering and the desire to climb mountains
- Mountaineers who have retired mostly have more time and money
- Many "mature" yet active people are more experienced in the mountains, are more economical in terms of their climbing and "have a better nose" for the dangers associated with it

6.2 Recommendations

Sport Climbing

Sport climbing is one of the very best forms of movement for the more mature individual.

In most cases it does not entail any long descents with heavy rucksacks, it provides an opportunity to move the whole of the body, it maintains and enhances coordinative capabilities, it is practically injury-free–and, quite simply, it's lots of fun! And there's another factor that always pleases me: in my experience I have never known "Juniors" say anything disparaging about the "Seniors," either in the gym or when

negotiating a climbing wall or rock face, let alone laugh at them; quite the opposite, in most cases what emerges is a friendly rapport which encompasses all age groups. Sport climbing has also encouraged the older generation to think more about safety; most people who "before" might have coolly embarked on 40 m lead climb without any intermediate fixing point, are today giving some thought to how they can best guard against risks without losing a great deal of time in so doing.
No specific recommendations are needed for sport climbing because mother nature will automatically take revenge if the climber in his "youthful" overeagerness is hanging on too long to handles that are too small ...

High-Alpine Tours, Treks and Expeditions

Treks are absolutely ideal for supplementing the mountaineering experience as we grow older. You can take more time for the proper enjoyment of hiking at high altitude and in a different cultural environment.
Mature mountaineers suffering from pre-existing illnesses need to discuss their trekking plans with an experienced medical practitioner (see also Chapters 7 and 16, Pages 74 and 195). The trek leaders also need to know how older trekkers are likely to react and what to do should an emergency arise.
The most important point has already been mentioned: each individual must listen to his own body–and that is something that the more mature person is generally better able to do than the "Junior" ...
Regular, all-the-year-round **endurance training** is essential. As everyone knows, the fact that the older sports enthusiast is simply not as fast means that he has to keep moving for longer than a 20-year old. So sports that are easy on the joints like cycling, swimming, cross-country skiing are ideal by way of a change from mountaineering sports.

Ensuring that well-managed **power training sessions** are a regular part of life right into old age can significantly slow down the unavoidable changes in and degeneration of the muscles as one ages (from around 60 onwards) and is, together with coordination ("senso-motoric") training, the best way of preventing falls and injuries in old age.

By way of an additional observation to "gait-related tactics" (see also Chapter 2, Page 36) and something that is particularly relevant for the older mountaineer: it is beneficial, when setting out and after each break, to deliberately go very slowly for the first few minutes and progressively increase your pace to normal. You need to make sure that you avoid incurring an "oxygen debt" that will need to be "repaid" later when you may already be somewhat tired. It is also important to approach gradients very cautiously at the beginning.

When it comes to equipment, the more mature trekker needs to know about the sleeping arrangements: a small inflatable sleeping mat can provide excellent service, as can portable seating (e.g *Kelty Camp Chair®* or *Crazy Creek® Chair)* which make sitting on the ground so much more of a pleasant experience.

Diet and the more Mature Individual

When it comes to diet for the older person, it is especially important to remember that older people no longer need so much energy in the form of calories (up to 30 % less) and therefore energy input needs to be reduced in old age. The basic metabolic rate, that is, the metabolic process, slows down as people become older.
In order to maintain a healthy appetite, a varied diet, particularly one rich in vitamins, minerals and protein, is to be recommended. The protein requirement in old age is similar to that in younger people (see also Chapter 3, Page 39). The need for fat and carbohydrate falls as people grow older parallel to their requirement for energy. It is particularly important to keep an eye on cholesterol in older people.
Aging affects adsorption, utilization and elimination of nutrients. Recourse to vitamins and minerals is to be recommended.

Many older people frequently forget how important it is just to keep **drinking**. As people age they experience the feeling of thirst less. Allowing the body to dry out rapidly leads to a decline In one's overall condition which may proceed to mental confusion *(dehydration)* (see also Chapter 3, Page 45). It is important for older mountaineers in particular to consciously make sure that they drink enough.

The passage of clear urine several times a day is an indicator of adequate hydration.

What in particular does the "Junior" need to notice when he finds himself in the mountains with a "person of more mature years?"

- As the group makes its getaway from the hut before daybreak the "Junior" should remember that his "Senior" teammate does not have such good **mesopic vision** as he does. Without a torch, the older mountaineer will be constantly stumbling over stones and will tire more quickly merely due to the fact that, in the twilight, he does not see the obstacles so well…

- The "Junior's" **cardiovascular system** will respond much more quickly to the stress of exertion than that of the older person–the latter will require considerably more minutes for his body to warm up so that it is able to respond to exertion. If the "Juniors" make too fast a start it may happen that a very well trained older mountaineer may experience a conditional collapse and need to call off the tour.
- There are many older people who no longer enjoy coming down–for this reason it is better to let the senior member start earlier with the descent (if this is acceptable from the point of view of terrain) and for the "Junior" to happily bring up the rear.

7. Pre-existing Ailments

Ch. Marti, A. Kottmann, Th. Szeless, A.G. Brunello

There are 1000 diseases, but only one health
Arthur Schopenhauer

7.1 High Blood Pressure (hypertension)

Arterial pressure is measured in the arteries. It is made up of two values: the so-called "systolic" pressure is measured during contraction of the heart muscle (heartbeat, heart muscle output pressure) and is represented by the higher value, whereas the diastolic pressure (measured during relaxation/heart muscle incoming pressure) is represented by the lower value. The pressure of the blood in the arteries is determined by the volume of blood, the strength of the heart (volume of blood in circulation that is pumped out at each beat) and the resistance of the vascular tree. We talk about high blood pressure where the systolic values are in excess of 140 millimeters Hg (mmHg) and diastolic values above 90 mmHg.

Indications: The signs of high blood pressure are typically to a large extent silent. High blood pressure is associated with an increased cardiovascular risk, for example, of myocardial infarction, stroke and renal insufficiency. If peak values are reached the hypertension can become symptomatic in the form of headache or of serious complications such as Angina Pectoris, cardiac insufficiency (heart failure) meningeal or retinal hemorrhage.

Mountaineering and High Blood Pressure: [1] The fall in the partial oxygen pressure at altitude coupled with physical activity causes activation of the sympathetic nervous system. This leads to an increase in heart rate, in vascular resistance and arterial pressure, even in healthy people. The consequences depend not only on the altitude itself but also on the speed of ascent.

Recommendations: People who suffer from hypertension but who display normal values when receiving treatment with medication do not need to be dissuaded from mountaineering. However, caution is recommended where unstable or poorly controlled blood pressure levels are concerned. In such cases specialist medical advice is recommended before embarking on a mountain tour involving unusually high ascents (obtainable, for example, through the Swiss Mountain Medicine Association SGGM).

7.2 Coronary Heart Disease

Also known as "ischemic cardiopathy," coronary heart disease is the primary cause of death in the western world. The cause is due to a narrowing of the coronary arteries with atheromatous plaques, promoted by the consumption of nicotine, by diabetes, hypertension and too high a cholesterol level. Narrowing of the coronary arteries results in insufficient flow of blood to the heart muscle which causes the typical chest pains or **angina pectoris,** as it is known, which are contingent on exertion. Plaques can also break away and encourage the formation of a blood clot (thrombus) which may seal off the coronary artery completely. The area of heart muscle supplied by this vessel dies and a **myocardial infarction** (myocardial = heart muscle) occurs. Without immediate treatment disturbances to the heart rhythm can lead to the death of the patient.

Indications: Angina pectoris is usually a pain dependent on exertion, localized behind the breastbone. Typically the pain is described as a "feeling of tightness and pressure." It is not dependent on deep in- or exhalation and cannot be reproduced by pressure on the rib cage. It may radiate out into the lower jaw and into the left arm. The pain associated with cardiac infarction can be very strong and unleash the fear of death. Keeping the patient calm can reduce the symptoms.

Mountaineering and Coronary Heart Disease

With altitude comes a reduction in partial oxygen pressure and an increase in the activity of the heart along with raised heart rate and vascular resistance. As a result of this mountaineers may experience an imbalance between the availability and the consumption of oxygen in the heart muscle and hence the pains associated with angina pectoris.

Recommendations: Mountaineering is contraindicated where unstable angina pectoris (where pain is also experienced when at rest or increasing duration of pain or intensity of pain) or known heart failure is present.
If a patient's coronary heart disease is stable (no pains and under treatment) mountain climbing may be practiced with caution. However, a slow and optimal acclimatization to altitude is of particular importance. Before (re-)commencement of physical activity, it is recommended that specialist medical advice be sought. In certain cases, heart screening concurrent with exertion (cycloergometer) may be indicated before a planned mountaineering tour.

Angina pectoris-type pains on a mountaineering tour are a medical emergency! The alarm should be raised immediately and physical rest is also indicated.

Where delays in rescue time are likely to occur, vaso-dilating medications such as nitroglycerin may, if available, be given by way of pain relief (two shots of a spray administered sublingually NB: check the pulse!) Oxygen and inhibitors of platelet aggregation (aspirin) are also a useful alternative.

 Good tolerance of exercise does not necessarily mean a good tolerance of altitude and its consequences (altitude sickness, cerebral or pulmonary edema).

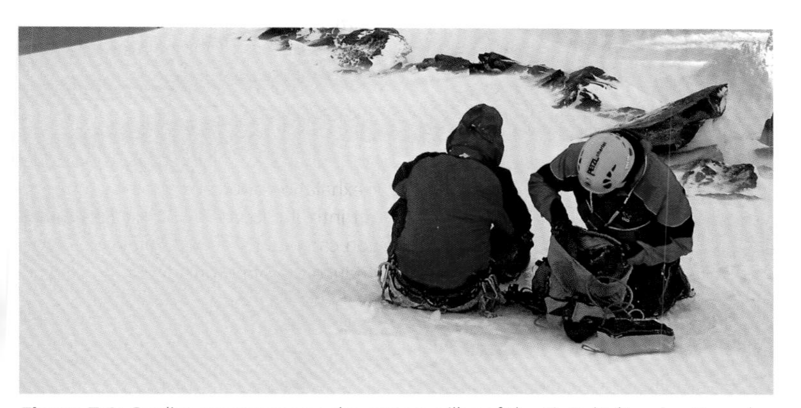

Figure 7.1: *Cardiac emergency on the eastern pillar of the Piz Palü (Bernina Group), approx. 3700 m (D. Hunziker).*

7.3 Convulsions (Epilepsy)

Definition: An epileptic attack is a sudden, periodically recurring disturbance of brain activity caused by uncontrolled and pathological electrochemical activity of the nerve cells. There are many kinds of epilepsy. A broad differentiation: some are partial attacks (only one part of the body is affected) with or without loss of consciousness and others are generalized attacks with loss of consciousness. Attacks are typically accompanied by twitching convulsions (affecting the entire body or one part only), a tendency to falls, foaming mucus, uncontrolled defalcation/urination, biting the tongue. Persons affected may feel unwell before an attack (abdominal pain), disturbances of perception and behavioral disorders (feelings of anxiety, unpleasant smell, an attack of shouting or crying out) may occur. The majority of attacks last for less than four minutes. If an attack lasts for longer than 30 minutes or if consciousness is not regained between two attacks, we talk about an epileptic state *(status epilepticus)*.

Causes: Frequently convulsions occur in association with diseases of the brain; in the majority of cases however a clear cause cannot be identified. However, there are many factors that may be favorable to an epileptic attack–stress, lack of sleep, extreme exhaustion, dehydration, fever, electrolyte disturbances, hypoglycemia, withdrawal of alcohol and drugs, the menstrual cycle are just some of them.

Treatment: Acute treatment follows the ABC rules (see Chapter 9.2, Page 97). It is important to be aware that a considerable loss of blood can result from biting the tongue and can obstruct the airways. The affected person must be protected from potential injury (falling) and be restrained in the event of danger.

⇨ An epileptic fit is invariably a life threatening emergency. Medical help must be summoned immediately.

Recommendations: [2)] Patients who are not allowed to drive (e.g. during a change of therapy) should also be very careful when taking part in any type of mountaineering.

⇨ Depending on the place where it happens, any attack has the potential to lead to an accident.

Nevertheless, if well managed, epilepsy does not have to represent a contraindication as far as mountaineering is concerned. Accidents are very rare while indulging in physical activity and sport can even reduce the risk of an attack. High altitude is, in itself, not regarded as a potential trigger for an attack *per se*. However, during physical activity at high altitude, there may be an accumulation of typical triggers (stress, exhaustion, dehydration).

⇨ Conditions and diseases associated with height (e.g. cerebral edema) may provoke an attack of epilepsy.

It can be difficult, on tours or treks lasting several days, to be meticulous about taking medication at specified times. The taking of additional medications must always be discussed with a medical practitioner since certain medications can lead to specific reactions with medications for epilepsy (weakening of the effect).

7.4 Stroke (Cerebral Infarct) and Cerebral Hemorrhage

Stroke is one of the leading causes of invalidity and death in industrialized countries. Stroke (also known as Cerebral Infarct) occurs as a result of a sudden insufficient supply of blood to one region of the brain or, more rarely, as a result of a cerebral hemorrhage, either of which may lead to the death of brain cells. Disturbances to

the flow of blood may be caused by clots or constrictions in the vascular wall.
If a state where the supply of blood is insufficient is of only temporary duration and the corresponding neurological disturbance is demonstrably evident for (typically) less than an hour, we talk about a "TIA" (transient ischemic attack or "mini-stroke,") if it persists for more than 1 day, we talk about an ischemic stroke. Recovery after a TIA is rapid and leaves no damage behind. A TIA, on the other hand, is a warning symptom and sometimes a full stroke may follow. Risk factors for the occurrence of a stroke or a cerebral hemorrhage are high blood pressure, disturbances to the heart rhythm, diabetes and smoking.

Indicators: The individual regions of the brain fulfill a very wide range of functions so that a stroke may present with sudden and diverse manifestations:

- Reduced strength and/or feeling in one half of the body, the muscles of the face, arm or leg
- Reduced vision, disturbances to the ability to turn the head or in relation to the field of vision
- Disturbances in relation to language and/or the ability to speak (slurred speech)
- Disturbances to balance and to movement sequences
- Convulsive fits
- Disturbances to memory and awareness right through to unconsciousness

Headaches may occur but are not a typical indicator for a stroke.

Treatment: TIAs and strokes are medical emergencies and call for immediate evacuation. This therapy only offers any prospect of success within a narrow time window and is carried out in specialized departments (stroke units.)

Intra-cerebral bleeding in the brain itself is described as a **cerebral hemorrhage.** This may happen suddenly, in particular in persons with high blood pressure, and manifests itself in the form of a stroke. Another form of cerebral hemorrhage occurs when small aneurysms burst and this typically manifests itself in terms of particularly strong neck pains ("stronger than ever before.")
These are life-threatening ailments that are associated with a high level of mortality.

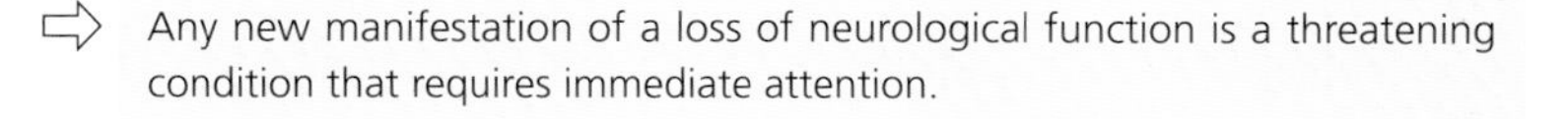
⇨ Any new manifestation of a loss of neurological function is a threatening condition that requires immediate attention.

7.5 Chronic Bronchitis (Chronic Obstructive Pulmonary Disease/COPD)

Chronic Obstructive Pulmonary Disease (COPD) is a chronic inflammation of the airways. It is characterized by a persistent cough, in addition to which a paroxysmal shortage of breath is evident at the beginning, followed in the later stages by shortage of breath when at rest. The disease is almost always caused by smoking.

Indications: Since healthy lungs have plenty of reserves, the symptoms only become evident at an advanced stage or at an increased age with a decrease in the physiological reserves. Symptoms include intolerance of physical exertion, chronic and productive cough and frequent infections of the airways.

Treatment: The only way to improve life expectancy is to stop smoking. In the event of an attack of dyspnea see treatment for asthma.

COPD and mountain climbing: If COPD patients (as well as other persons suffering from pulmonary diseases) suffer from dyspnea even when they are in flat country or at medium altitude (2000 m) due to the reduction in partial oxygen pressure and dry, cold air, serious respiratory problems can occur more quickly, especially under exertion. For this reason such patients should avoid exposure to altitude or, if unavoidable, ensure that they have oxygen with them. In particular they will, due to chronic pulmonary hypertension, be at increased risk of developing HAPE (see Chapter 17.3, Page 213). If patients experience no problems when in flat country, a consultation with a medical specialist is recommended, as is also the case for plane journeys. Heights of 2000–2500 m should not pose problems for patients with moderate levels of COPD. The reduction in atmospheric density may even be of benefit. Particularly slow acclimatization makes sense in all cases!

7.6 Bronchial Asthma

This is characterized by a temporary obstruction of the airways in an oversensitive respiratory system which makes it difficult to exhale. Trigger factors may be allergens (see Chapter 21.4, Page 286) or nonspecific stimuli such as cold and exertion.
Indicators: Difficulty in breathing with extended exhalation, whistling respiratory noises, coughing, feeling of claustrophobia in the chest, bluish coloring to lips, restlessness and anxiety. A serious lack of oxygen may lead to failure of the circulatory system.

The possibility of pulmonary edema should always be considered in any occurrence of respiratory problems at high altitude.

Treatment: Fresh air, loosen clothing, make the patient sit down with the upper part of the body bent forwards (preferred position). Patients who suffer from asthma should always have medication with them. Such items consist of so-called broncho-dilators (e.g. Ventolin®) which reopen the narrowed airways. In serious cases steroids are indicated.

Asthma and Mountaineering: Sport is an important component of rehabilitation in the case of asthmatics. As regards alpine sports (hiking, mountain climbing, ski sports) which can be interrupted at any time in the event of asthma attacks for administration of appropriate medical therapies, there are no restrictions.
At high altitude the air contains fewer hazardous substances and fewer allergens, as a result the majority of patients benefit from spending time at levels of around 1500–2500 m. On the other hand, an increase in the rate of respiration contingent on exertion can trigger an attack in cold air. This Is also demonstrated by the high proportion of asthmatics among competitive skiers. If the disease is properly controlled by means of therapy there is no additional danger from exercising at high altitude. Additional emergency medication must be taken along. If the asthma is at an advanced stage, destinations that are particularly off the beaten track or situated at especially high altitudes should be avoided or, if this is impossible, only attempted after completion of an intensive course of preventive treatment (steroids). Specialist medical advice is recommended.

Take sufficient medications along and take them, even if the symptoms improve; slow acclimatisation.

7.7 Diabetes (Diabetes Mellitus)

It has been described as the "honey-sweet flow" and is a disorder of the metabolism which is characterized by too high a sugar content in the blood (hyperglycemia). The cause may be either an insulin deficiency (type I), a nonsusceptibility to insulin or both (Type II). Diabetes Type I occurs mostly in young people whereas Type II affects older, often overweight patients. Diabetes, along with high blood pressure, excess weight and the consumption of nicotine, is one of the risk factors for cardiovascular diseases. A normal and constant blood sugar level is made possible by a delicate interplay between a fall in sugar (after meals) and an increase in sugar (when fasting).

Insulin is responsible for the storage of glucose (breakdown module for carbohydrates) in the liver, the muscles and the fatty tissues and thus for reducing the sugar level. People who have diabetes need to take insulin as required in order to keep their sugar levels constant or medications that improve the utilization of their own insulin. Over the years diabetics can expect to develop incurable diseases of the vascular and nervous systems which, in addition to a heightened susceptibility to frostbite, also lead to disorders of the visual and sensory systems and to impaired healing of wounds.

Hypo-/Hyperglycemia: Too little sugar (hypoglycemia) occurs as a rule in insulin-dependent patients who ingest too little sugar or use up too much sugar (physical stress).

⇨ If there is a diabetic patient in a group of mountaineers (ask!) the signs of sugar deficiency must be known – restlessness, decline in performance, pallor, palpitations, rapid pulse, nausea.

The brain in particular is highly sensitive to sugar deficiency; personality changes, conspicuous behavior, double vision, disturbances to memory, convulsions and unconsciousness may potentially develop. The lack of sugar should be identified and treatment given before the occurrence of any neurological symptoms.

⇨ If, having absorbed sugar and following a sufficiently long break, the patient feels better, the activity being pursued can be continued. If convulsions and/or unconsciousness have occurred, the affected person must be evacuated and given medical treatment.

Lack of insulin and persistently high levels of blood sugar may lead to hyperacidity **(diabetic ketoacidosis)** in type I diabetics: extreme thirst and frequent urination, stomach spasms right through to fits and unconsciousness are some of the indicators for this disease. Excessive sugar (hyperglycemia) in patients with diabetes type II is more difficult to identify than hypoglycemia and may be the first sign of a form of diabetes. A definite feeling of thirst, frequent need to pass water, stomach pains and visual disturbances are indicative symptoms. Hyperglycemia must and can only be treated in hospital.

Diabetes and Mountaineering: In maturity-onset diabetes some kind of regular physical activity (e.g. hiking) is an excellent way of moving about so as to stay in shape and lose weight. A young type I diabetic of normal weight is just as well suited as a healthy person to strenuous types of alpine sport and even expeditions. Indeed, as regards physical exercise, all that is different is the consumption of energy and the need for sugar and insulin. A more precise adjustment in the supply and reduction of glucose is required. The following factors should be borne in mind when dealing with sports enthusiasts who also happen to be diabetics:

- It is important to appreciate that sugar levels must also be monitored at night and to even closer tolerances. Instances where levels of sugar fall at night following a long and gruelling tour are not rare occurrences.
- Readily absorbable carbohydrates and drinks must always be within reach (see Chapter 3, Page 39).
- During lengthy tours over cold and windy stretches, the calorie intake must be increased: shivering with cold uses up a lot of calories!
- Insulin is not effective in cold conditions and must be carried on the person.
- The measuring devices are as a rule only validated up to heights of approx. 4000 m. Altitude, cold, UV radiation may cause error values to be generated.
- Make sure you organise sufficient stops; ensure that everyone is in training and don't forget the importance of packing a good measure of self-esteem!

Before spending time at high altitudes, an examination by the optician is obligatory for diabetics because of changes in the **ocular fundus:** advanced damage is inclined to result in bleeding at high altitude (see Chapter 17, Page 224).

7.8 Ear, Nose and Throat Ailments

Colds and Influenza: everyone is familiar with the signs that are typical of a cold or flu. Anything that obstructs breathing through the nose can be very tiresome when it comes to sporting activities: decongestant sprays and gel offer only temporary respite. If you catch cold on a trek or on an expedition, it is difficult to ensure that you get physical rest. It is a good idea to give some thought to treating the symptoms and taking antibiotics (e.g. in cases of fever) somewhat earlier than would be the case at home. Unless you feel 100 % fit, you should not go any higher. In addition, flu-like infections also rank as risk factors in relation to pulmonary edema (see Chapter 17, Page 220).

⇨ If you do not feel well at high altitude, then you will, in the absence of any evidence to the contrary, be assumed to have altitude sickness.

Inflammation of the paranasal sinus (Sinusitis): The paranasal sinuses are sacculations of the mucosa filled with air which are located between the two cover plates of some of the cranial bones. They are linked with the nasal cavity and form part of the respiratory system. Inflammations are mostly caused by viruses. Treatment consists of decongestant sprays or gel and rinsing with sea salt. Alarm indicators for bacterial inflammation include instances where the illness has persisted for more than a week despite treatment with decongestants or where blood-tinged mucus is a feature, in which case antibiotic treatment will be indicated (e.g. Augmentin®).

Nose bleeds (Epistaxis): The most frequent causes are violent nose-blowing, picking the nose or following a fall or impact. The very dry air on altitude can dry out the nose mucosa and encourage nose bleeds. Nose bleeds can be stemmed by adopting a bent forward position, cold compresses on the nose and/or neck and by compressing the nostrils for at least five minutes or, if this is not sufficient, by plugging both nostrils with cotton wool to stop the flow of blood. After this do not touch the nose again for two hours.

⇨ It is only on rare occasions that the above treatment fails to contain a nose bleed. If the treatment is unsuccessful a doctor must be consulted.

Preventive therapy: Nose ointment (e.g. Bepanthen®)

7.9 Gastrointestinal tract

Travel diarrhea and how to treat it is described in the chapter entitled Trekking – (see Chapter 16, Page 195).
Patients with stomach or duodenal ulcers may be developing complications (bleeding) on longer journeys or expeditions. Where problems of this nature exist in a patient's history a gastroscopy, followed by appropriate treatment before departure may be recommendable. Very little is still known about the direct effects of altitude-related shortages of oxygen on such ailments or on the overall gastrointestinal tract. A reduction in appetite has been observed even in healthy persons spending time at heights of above 5000 m. This symptom is part of the so-called **"maladaption syndrome,"** which is a decline in a person's overall state of health and failure to achieve any further acclimatization after lengthy periods of time spent at extreme altitudes. In addition, a progressive loss of weight ensues as well as difficulty in sleeping and increasing apathy (lethargy). The lack of oxygen at high altitudes can provoke the onset of maladaption syndrome. The underlying mechanisms are not known.

Bibliography and sources:

1) People with pre-existing conditions going to the mountains Medical Commission of UIAA Official Guidelines Vol. 13 2008 Cardiovascular adjustments for life at high altitude Respiratory Physiology and Neurobiology 158 (2007) 204-11.
2) P.W. Berry, A J Pollard: Altitude Illness. BMJ 2003, 326:915-9.
3) Moderne Berg- und Höhenmedizin Th. Küpper, K Ebel, U Gieseler, 1st edition Gentner Verlag, 2010 Bergmedizin Höhenbedingte Erkrankungen und Gesundheitsgefahren bei Bergsteigern A.J. Pollard, D.R. Murdoch 1st edition 2007 Huber Verlag.

8. Mountaineering after Operative Procedures

U. Hefti

Even after operations and especially for people with an artificial limb a moderate amount of mountaineering is still a possibility. The wearer of a prosthesis, however, needs to accept that he is to a major extent responsible for himself and has to be aware of the risks. Quality of life and good health can, nevertheless, be enhanced with a moderate amount of sporting activity.

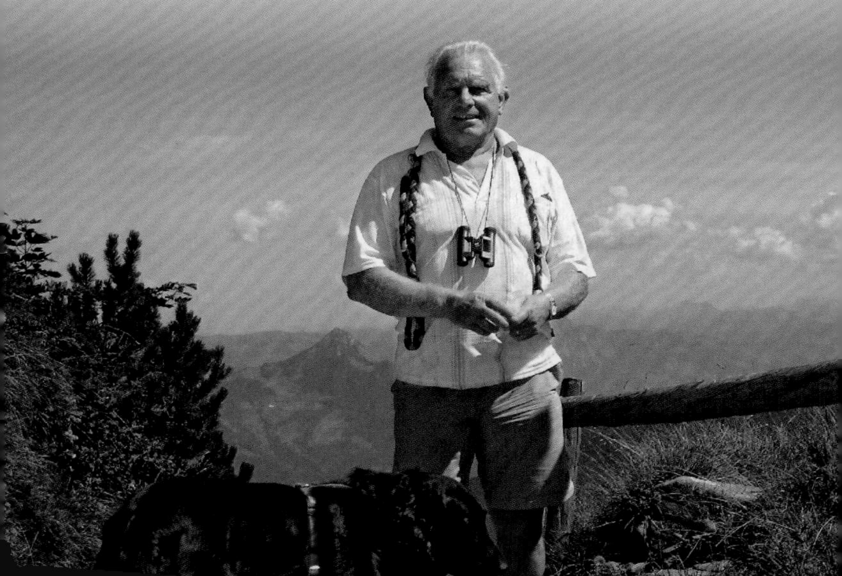

8.1 Mountain Climbing with an Artificial Joint (Hip, Knee, Shoulder)

There are thousands of people with "artificial joints" (so-called endoprostheses or joint replacements) of the shoulder, the hip, the knee or the ankle joint living in Switzerland. The replacement of joints by prostheses is one of the most impressive achievements of modern day medicine. The primary aim of the operation was and still is to free the patients from years of pain which can sometimes turn them into invalids. Up to a few years ago, the patients were in the main very old and only rarely still active on the sporting front. However, it is becoming evident that younger patients, between 40 and 60 years, are receiving a replacement joint more and more frequently. This group of patients, who are still often active sporting enthusiasts, expect not only freedom from pain but also a functional capability that is as normal as possible in the affected limb, in other words, the ability to continue with sporting activities. Since the "service life" of a hip prosthesis, for example, is 15—20 years, one must assume that, in the case of a young patient, it is likely that it will be necessary to change the prosthesis at least once more and probably on two or three further occasions. As a continuance of further exertion means that the material will be exposed to a greater level of wear, prosthesis wearers were until recently being dissuaded from indulging in any sporting activity as a matter of principle.
Today we evaluate the situation as to whether someone with an artificial limb should actually go in for sport or not somewhat differently, in particular because the advantages tend to outweigh the disadvantages, although there are still some possible serious disadvantages.

Advantages to sporting activity with prosthetic limbs

- The improvement in wellbeing achieved through sport enhances quality of life
- Improvements to quality of life promote an increase in good health
- Sporting activity strengthens and conditions the muscular system. It also enables the joints to better fulfil their function as shock absorbers.
- Sporting activities have positive effects on the cardiovascular system, metabolic activity, bone density (reduces the likelihood of osteoporosis due to inactivity), health in general

Disadvantages

- Exertion of increasing loads on the prosthetic material
- Material fatigue and fracturing of the prosthesis (extremely rare with new implants)
- Increased risk of dislocation of the artificial joint

Sporting activity is an important part of the perception of life of many people who wear prostheses. Based on this knowledge, it does not make sense to ban such active people from participating in sport.

However, we do need to recommend to prosthesis wearers that they make some adjustments to their lifestyle:

Recommendations

- A slow period of **rehabilitation** after the operation under the supervision of physiotherapists and doctors who are themselves sports enthusiasts
- Regular on-going exercise and good muscular stability
- Avoidance of extreme exertion (jumping from great heights, training if in pain, ultra-endurance exercises, extreme turning/shear stresses etc.)
- Go for those types of sport which are most suitable for prosthesis wearers (cycling, hiking, mountain climbing)
- Go for the types of sport that you were used to prior to the operation
- Avoid new types of sports that are complex in terms of coordination (such as, for example, various ball sports, snowboarding, skiing)
- **Keep a** consistent **eye on your weight**

⇨ Basically, the decision as regards who should be indulging in sporting activities with which prosthesis and to what extent is a personal decision on the part of the wearer of the prosthesis.

Sports medicine practitioners and orthopedists are in a prime position to outline and point the way to achieving the right balance as regards everyday sporting activities for prosthesis wearers and may on occasions find that they need to apply the brakes slightly where motivated sports enthusiasts are concerned. Enthusiasm is great but remember, you do have to be reasonable!

8.2 Sport after Operations

The question of resuming sporting activities after an operation is, unfortunately, hardly ever broached before the operation or, if it is, it is often not specifically answered. It has to be not only in the interests of the patient but also in the interests of the doctor who is responsible for the treatment that this question is discussed before or after an operation.

In principle, with the majority of operations, you can expect to resume the sporting activities to which you are accustomed **after a period of six weeks.**

Simpler exercises, activities involving less exertion such as, for example, power training or endurance training (e.g. on a cycle home trainer) are, however, in the majority of cases possible very soon after the wound has healed, even as early as **two weeks** after the operation.

The precise details of the rehabilitation plan and the resumption of sporting activity are, nevertheless, individual and depend on the operation that has been carried out. The doctors responsible for treatment, the physiotherapists and the patient her- or himself need to have an interest in sport and be highly interested in obtaining the appropriate information as well as in setting up a training schedule. If the doctor is not interested in sportsmen and -women he will probably not have any meaningful recommendations to make.

So, before the operation or during the period of rehabilitation, make contact with sports medicine practitioners, sports physiotherapists and give some thought yourself to how you can actively become involved in designing your own rehabilitation programme.

9. Accidents in the Mountains

Various authors

The following chapters illustrate the most important aspects of First Aid when walking off the beaten track, from raising the alarm right through to identifying and treating injuries, illnesses and transport for evacuating the casualty to safety.

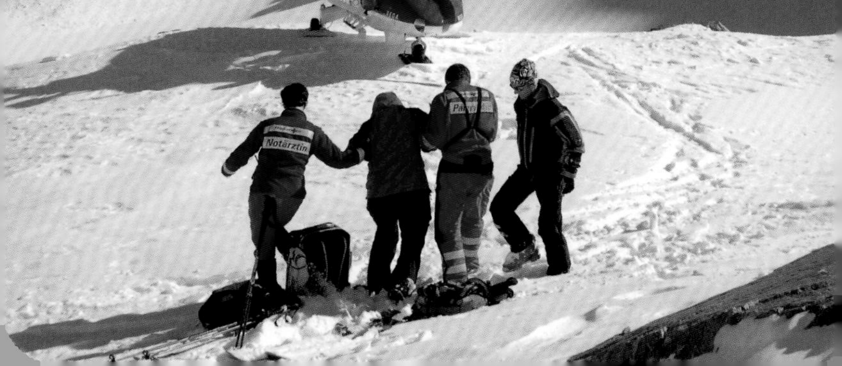

9.1 Basic Principles in the Event of an Accident

When accidents occur, a state of shock, panic and confusion often takes over. Together with the paralyzing feeling of loss of control, a distinct stress situation may develop: hectic, uncoordinated and sometimes even pointless or counterproductive activity can be observed. In addition, factors such as individual exhaustion, group dynamics or environmental factors tend to compound the issue.

Immediate Action

To stimulate an appropriate response to the situation, algorithms and mnemonics are often helpful–aids of this kind are also used by professional rescuers–for example, the ABC in cases of cardiopulmonary arrest or in the emergency room.
Hence the **first principle** in any accident situation is:

SAFETY–LOOK–THINK–ACT

Safety: What is my own position and/or that of my companions? Is there any direct risk of further danger? Implement your own safety procedures (secure footing, ensure that your companions are safe, belaying material, warn any other persons).

Look: i.e. try and acquire an overview of exactly what has happened, whether any objective hazards are present (fall hazard, rock fall, ice falls, avalanches) as far as both the injured and the uninjured are concerned, how many injured people are there altogether, how serious are their injuries, who can do what and what resources are available?

Think: It is worth investing time in acquiring an overview and developing a subsequent plan of action (stand still and get your thoughts together). How you plan your course of action will depend on the objective hazards, the extent of the damage/injuries that have occurred and the resources that are available in terms of personnel and materials. In the event that a number of persons who are capable of doing something are present on the scene of the accident, the rapid selection of the most competent leader will make the greatest contribution toward ensuring a successful outcome and enabling a targeted and coordinated solution to the problem. Delegating tasks within a group is the way to ensure that abilities and training are fully utilized, to improve efficiency and ensure that a targeted course of action is adopted and to take the pressure off the team leader. Responsibilities can be shared from an early stage and immediate action can be taken while the "team leader" is still thinking about raising the alarm or keeping notes. Of course, group dynamics can also have negative effects on the operational capability of any group.

 In any exceptional situation one person must assume the function of leader.

Action: Only once an overview of the situation has been achieved should the problem be tackled by adopting a specifically targeted approach. It is very important to ensure that there is no risk of endangering either oneself or uninjured members of the group.

The **second principle** in any accident situation may therefore be summed up as follows:

RAISING THE ALARM–SAFETY–RESCUE–FIRST AID

Raising the Alarm: In the Alps, where professional help can in most cases be called in from outside within a relatively short period of time, raising the alarm is one of the most important factors in an emergency. If there is only one rescuer available it makes sense to send an alarm call very early on, maybe even with only a minimum of detail, as resources will certainly be limited and there is the risk of losing valuable time as a result of delaying or even forgetting to raise the alarm. Of course, not every minor injury will require help from outside–however, it is important to ask this question every time an accident happens. In the case of simple injuries such as a sprained ankle it is, of course, acceptable to wait before raising the alarm until it is absolutely clear that the casualty can no longer walk.
In a group, this task can be delegated and the individual concerned can first of all acquire the necessary information (in most cases this takes just a few minutes) before putting through a correct and complete alarm communication.
In remote areas abroad, raising the alarm can have completely different implications. It is possible that an individual will be totally reliant on himself or herself and with a bit of luck it may be possible to organize external help to assist in any evacuation. In all cases, information regarding the options for raising the alarm and the rescue organizations in the region (in overseas locations rescue is frequently the sole preserve of the army) should have been acquired before an accident occurs!

Safety: As far as possible every effort must be made to avoid endangering the rescuers. Heroic acts placing a rescuer, (who could be on his own) at risk, are pointless and will expose any persons already injured as well as the rescuer himself to danger. For this reason, it is essential to ensure that the rescuers are protected from any risk of falling as well as from rockfalls, ice falls and avalanches. It is only once this has been attended to that there will be any assurance of reliable protection for the injured.

Rescue: In order to protect the injured from objective hazards a rescue will often be necessary. The aim is to remove the injured parties from the direct proximity of a hazard zone. Naturally, care must be taken to ensure that, in so doing, no additional injuries are caused (for example, in the event of injuries to the spinal column). Where immediate threats are present, it will, however, depending on the situation, be necessary to make compromises.

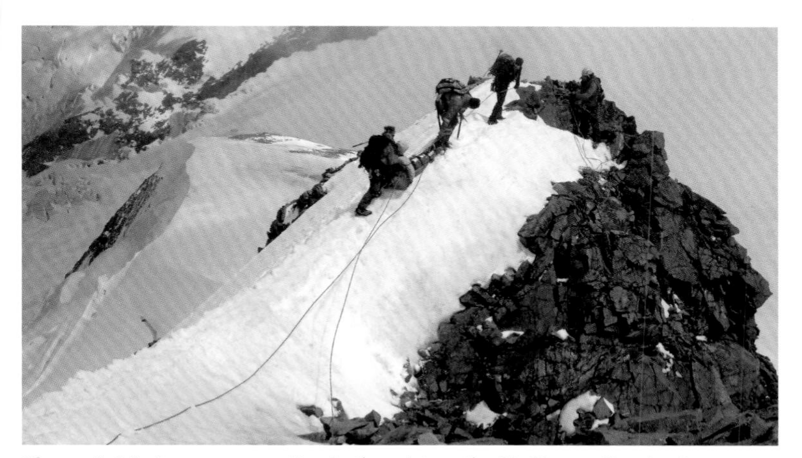

***Figure 9.1.1:** A rescue operation in the mist on the Piz Bianco, Bernina Range. Challenging rescue in high Alpine terrain (D. Hunziker).*

First Aid: It is only once the safety of the rescuer and the injured party have been objectively guaranteed that administering First Aid can commence.

The First Aid sequence will depend on the injuries suffered and the condition of the casualty. In the event of a simple sprain this will not be difficult and there are many options when it comes to responding. There are few instances that may give rise to problems. Where injuries are more complex or with multiple injuries *(polytraumas)* the following procedure is recommended:

- ABC and immediate life-saving action
- Body Check
- More comprehensive First Aid measures
- Preparations for transporting and positioning the casualty
- Monitoring

Emergency Message, Raising the Alarm, Emergency Signals

For the sake of completeness, the most important features that need to be borne in mind when raising the alarm will be explained here and listed in the form of a summary. Please ensure that this section is dealt with in detail in all alpine textbooks* as well as in the SAC tour guides.

The Emergency Message

Regardless of whether the message relates to an accident, illness or a different type of emergency it must be systematic and structured in terms of its layout. Alarm message protocols exist** which can be of valuable help in an emergency and these should always form part of any emergency kit. Most of the questions asked begin with a "W" word:

Who has raised the alarm?
What has happened?
When?
Where? Location/geographical coordinates
How many injured casualties/persons?
Any other info? e.g. visibility, wind, helicopter landing area

If the alarm is raised via a professional emergency response center in Switzerland (tel. nos. 144, 1414, 1415, or 112, 117, 118) this information will be specifically requested and checked for completeness. At the same time steps will also be taken to coordinate various services in case, for example, a helicopter rescue is out of the question because of weather conditions or if specialists or other emergency services are required.

* "Bergsport Sommer und Winter" (Mountaineering Summer and Winter), Winkler et al. published by SAC Verlag

** e.g. Federal Office for Sport (BASPO) 2532 Magglingen

Overseas, emergency numbers tend to differ widely and it always makes sense to acquaint oneself with them prior to setting out. Assistance may be summoned at any time via the Switzerland-based Rega Abroad alarm no. **Tel. +41 333 333 333.**

Resources for raising the alarm

Mobile telephones: These days the mobile telephone is the method of choice for raising the alarm in alpine regions. Although there are – even in Switzerland – still some areas where there is no network coverage (so-called "black holes") these can nevertheless frequently be circumvented by changing position. Normally an emergency call can be made to the established emergency numbers, even on PIN-protected mobiles or if the SIM card has been removed. Since 2002 there has been a Europe-wide emergency call number (Tel. 112) that can also be used in Switzerland (here the call will be diverted to the regional police emergency call centers (Tel. 117).

For accidents in the mountains, raising the alarm via direct contact with an air rescue organisation is recommended: Tel. 1414 and 144 (in Canton Valais). These organisations will waste no time in coordinating the necessary resources and are able to retrieve the information specifically required for the Alpine rescue services. Direct contact with the person raising the alarm can be made from the rescue helicopters (e.g. Rega). This shortens the time required for pinpointing the location in the mountains where the accident has occurred, something which can, depending on the situation, be very useful.

Radio equipment: The use of radio equipment in Switzerland is invariably subject to licensing. There are items of radio equipment available through commercial outlets with which, thanks to an emergency channel, it is possible, via a defined selective call facility, to establish a link to the Rega emergency call center. These are free of charge. However, this is only possible where no other radio channels are programmed and the equipment meets the specifications of the Federal Office for Communications (BAKOM). Such devices can be of benefit in areas with patchy cellphone network coverage but, even here, the so-called "black holes" can be found. One definite advantage is the possibility of a direct radio telephone link with the helicopter via the **emergency-channel** or, if available, via the **K-channel** or the **heli-channel.**

Before visiting mountain ranges abroad, it is essential to familiarize oneself with the established alarm notification frequencies and telephone numbers in advance and to purchase the necessary technical equipment (frequencies are in most cases treated as confidential data).

Alternative ways of raising the alarm: the use of distress rockets and light signals are highly dependent on the weather and geographical factors, while acoustic signals (whistles etc.) depend on distance. For these reasons, the use of these resources tends to be restricted and may, under certain circumstances, be limited to a major extent.

International emergency calls

Internationally recognized distress calls, which are subject to compulsory acknowledgment have been adopted from maritime practice and may be used even today in exceptional cases despite the most modern technologies. However, because of the high density of mobiles and radio equipment, they have lost some of their importance in mountaineering even though they may offer the only possibility of broadcasting an emergency situation from a distance and calling for help.

The internationally recognised and compulsory distress signals may be delivered either acoustically or visually and are derived from the Morse code used by the ships' wireless operators in the past.

Wireless operators on ships were not allowed to accept radio calls or even distress calls from ships with other systems. In order to bring this state of affairs to an end, **SOS** (three short, three long, three short: · · · – – – · · ·, expressed as dididididahdahdahdididit) was specified as the international emergency call sign at the International Wireless Telegraph Convention in Berlin on 3rd October 1906 and, following confirmation by all seafaring nations, introduced officially as of 1st July 1908. SOS was easy to remember as well as being readily distinguishable from other signals, even for inexperienced wireless operators. The emergency call sign is not made up of three individual letters, as is widely assumed; rather, the SOS code is transmitted in one block, i.e. with no character silent time between the letters, viz.:
···–––··· (SOS). Purported meanings of SOS as an abbreviation for Save Our Souls or Save Our Ship were only ascribed to the signal at a later date.

Alarm raised: • • • – – – • • • (SOS)
Confirmation: • • •

Derived exclusively from maritime radio applications, acoustic and visual procedures based on the use of light or sound or even the human voice have been developed. Today the result is an emergency signal which is independent of any language constraints and can be identified both nationally and internationally.

9.2 First Aid

Medical emergencies in the mountains and rough terrain represent a particular challenge. In most cases there may only be a few lay persons present who, as a rule, will not have any medical training. The "rucksack pharmacy," if indeed there is one available, will probably only be sufficient to cope with minor injuries. In addition, those concerned often experience a great deal of emotional tension and stress due to the fact that the individuals affected are, in most cases, close to them and this applies particularly where injuries to children are involved. Frequently, people find themselves in an area where the only way of achieving a speedy rescue is by helicopter or, if the weather is poor, by recourse to the ground-based rescue services, something which often takes even more time and means a great deal of stress for everyone concerned.
The following section illustrates some immediate lifesaving measures that can be implemented and the situations that may lead to them.

The reasons for serious health problems in an "outdoor environment" are many and diverse. These reasons can be divided up into external influences and internal disorders (see Table 9.2.1). In addition to accidents, the external causes include adverse weather conditions (cold, heat, lack of oxygen), bites from animals and infections. Internal disorders may well be pre-existing and can worsen gradually or suddenly. The most significant here are disorders of the cardiovascular system.
Despite all the difficulties mentioned it is possible to help very ill people and, in certain circumstances, even ensuring their survival. This section is intended to act as a guide for those who would describe themselves as medical lay people. The internationally applicable procedures relating to "basic life support" (BLS) have been set out here clearly and concisely for this purpose.

External Influences			
Causes		**Effects**	**Clinical Signs**
trauma	fall / crash avalanche rockfall	broken bones / fractures vertebral fractures brain injury injuries to spinal cord injuries to airways and thorax injuries to internal organs hypothermia	pain malalignement of extremities paralysis, palsy disorientation unconsciousness
thermal influence and radiation	cold	hypothermia	shivering, disorientation unconsciousness
		frostbite	white, blue acra, loss of sensation eventually blistering
	heat	dehydration, overheating	circulatory collapse unconsciousness
	radiation	sunburn	reddening, eventually blistering
		sunstroke	headache, disorientation, unconsciousness
animals	bites, stings	infection	reddening, swelling overheating, pain loss of function
		poisoning (snakes, scorpions, jellyfish, fish)	circulatory collapse paralysis, palsy, unconsciousness tissue decomposition, blood decomposition
general infections			fever, circulatory collapse organ failure
lack of oxygen	high altitude	see chapter 17, altitude and mountain sickness	
	cooking in tents	carbon monoxyde poisoning	unconsciousness
Important internal medicine diseases			
circulation		angina pectoris cardiac infarction heart rhythm disorder hypertensive crisis	thorax / breast pain, difficulty in breathing anxiety, perspiration
vascular disease		cerebral haemorhage stroke	headache, palsy unconsciousness
		leg vein thrombosis	leg pain leg swelling
		pulmonary embolism	thorax / breast pain, difficulty in breathing anxiety, perspiration
		circulatory disorder in the leg	leg pain, white and cold extremity, paralysis
various disorders	convulsions migraine diabetes metabolism	low blood sugar values electrolyte disorders	unconsciousness, mental changes headache heart rhythm disorder

Table 9.2.1

Critical vital functions and how to monitor them

Consciousness: In the narrower medical sense, a definite state of awareness is indicative of the waking state of a living organism which is to be distinguished, among other things, from the sleeping state or from a state of unconsciousness. Unconsciousness has already been mentioned here on one or two previous occasions. However, there are various different levels of awareness between a person who is alert and free of any adverse effects and a deeply comatose casualty and these can be checked by means of a range of tests. The AVPU scale provides an approximate starting point:

A	Alert:	Casualty who is awake and responsive
V	Voice:	Responds when addressed
P	Pain:	Reacts only to pain*
U	Unresponsive:	Does not react

⇨ Impaired awareness is an indicator of serious damage to health.

The reason for this may lie with the brain such as in an accident involving the skull or in the event of a cerebral hemorrhage/blow to the head. However, the cause often lies elsewhere, for example, with inadequate supplies of glucose, serious derangement of blood electrolytes, vascular collapse, hypothermia or poisoning. Clouding of consciousness will then be the secondary result of any such disorder.

* Inflict pain stimuli: pinch inside of upper arm or the shoulder/neck muscles.
Don't box the casualty's ears!

Respiration: A healthy adult breathes 10 to 20 times a minute. As s/he does so, movements of the rib cage and abdomen are clearly visible. An impaired respiratory system may be indicated by the rate of breathing, the pattern of breathing or the depth of breathing (see Table 9.2.2); in addition, the airways may generate noises that point to an obstruction.

Breathing frequency	too fast	stress, anxiety difficulty in breathing bloodloss lack of oxygen fever pulmonary disease exertion, physical stress
	too slow	poisoning impairment of respiratory brain areas
Breathing pattern	irregular	elevated brain pressure cerebral insult poisoning
Breathing strength	strongly elevated	metabolic disorders exertion, physical stress
	diminished	entrapment of a person poisoning
Sounds	gargling	fluids/foreign body in upper and lower airways
	inspiratory whistling/wheezing	narrowing/constriction of larynx or trachea
	expiratory whistling/wheezing	asthma
	hoarseness	swelling of the larynx
Thorax	intercostal/thorax wall retraction	fractured ribs/serial fracture of ribs
	unilateral respiration	air in the thorax/pneumothorax

Table 9.2.2

Any impediment to breathing will trigger massive stress and anxiety in casualties who are awake and this will increase the body's oxygen requirement. If the gaseous exchange in the lung is disturbed, the skin of the casualty will take on a bluish discoloration ***(cyanosis)***. Every breath taken involves major physical effort and all the muscles of respiration are needed to assist (abdominal muscles, throat muscles plus all the thoracic muscles).

Cardiovascular System: A healthy adult at rest has a regular pulse of 60 to 100 beats per minute. The best place to take the pulse is on the inside of the wrist. If the cardiovascular system is impaired, this will have an adverse effect on all parts of the body through which blood flows and thus on the whole of the organism. At the same time, the pulse rate may change in terms of its frequency, strength and rhythm and may no longer be detectable at the periphery (e.g. at the wrist artery on the same side as the thumb). If this happens, the carotid artery will need to be checked (central pulse, see Figure 9.2.1).

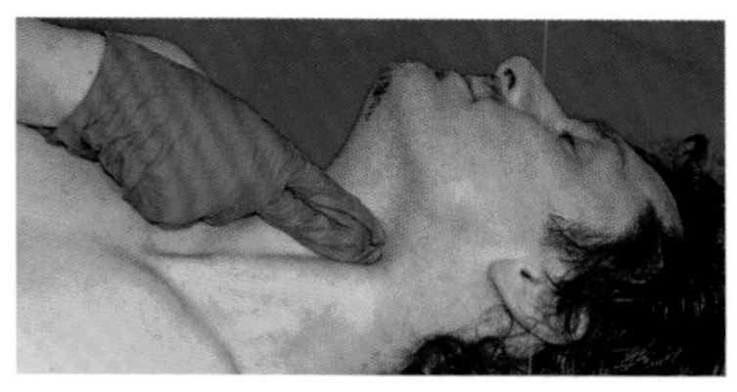

Figure 9.2.1: *The carotid artery is located in the middle of the throat between the larynx and the sternomastoid muscle. This blood vessel lies only about 2–3 cm below the surface of the skin and normally demonstrates a powerful pulse beat. It is important that the pulse is taken with the tips of fingers two to four and not with the thumb, because it is possible for the person taking the pulse to detect his or her own pulse.*

With babies and infants the pulse is normally taken on the inside of the upper arm. If a casualty presents with a total absence of respiration and no further signs of life, action to resuscitate must be commenced immediately. Waste no time and start looking for a pulse immediately! The situation is different for casualties who are alive where there will be sufficient time available for assessment.

An irregular pulse may indicate a diseased heart, metabolic derangement or poisoning, whereas a shallow, fast pulse may occur in response to significant losses of blood or fluids. If the cardiovascular system is disturbed to a major extent, the skin of the casualty will assume a pale to white color. The casualty may be restless and/or confused at the very least, if not completely unconscious.

Causes of cardio-vascular impairment

Major loss of blood: not only visible external bleeding but also internal bleeding fall into this category, such as, for example, a bleeding stomach ulcer or a ruptured aorta.

Disturbances to heart rhythm or cardiac insufficiency: The heart is either beating too quickly, too slowly or irregularly and is as a result no longer in a position to maintain an adequate flow of blood.

Dehydration: Excessive loss of fluid due to vomiting, diarrhoea or a long period of sweating. In addition, this may also give rise to shifts in the balance of ions in the body which, in turn, may lead to disturbances in heart rhythm.

Low blood pressure for any other reason: The following fall into this category–instances of poisoning and serious conditions relating to an infection (blood poisoning) or rapid onset paraplegic symptoms. However, in these casualties, the skin tends to be warm.

Causative Factors for Disturbances of Consciousness and Failure of the Cardiovascular System

A wide range of factors exists that present a threat to Vital Parameters.* As already stated in the Introduction, these may be divided up into internal disorders and disturbances caused by external influences (see Table 9.2.1, Page 98).

The most important factors that may lead to a rapid decline in the condition of the sick person and which therefore need to be dealt with quickly are:

- impaired breathing
- impairments to the gaseous exchange in the lungs
- cardiac insufficiency
- massive blood and fluid losses
- hypothermia

Resuscitation (cardiopulmonary resuscitation = CPR)

A sudden failure of the cardiopulmonary system is one of the main causes of death in Europe. More than 25 % of these casualties demonstrate ventricular fibrillation (VF) during the initial ECG recording by rescue personnel (= life-threatening impairment of cardiac rhythm with no pulse). VF can in most cases be converted back into an adequate cardiac rhythm using a defibrillator (device for delivering electric shocks to the heart). Today, **automated external defibrillators (AED)** are being used more and more to complement rescue techniques and also as part of efforts to promote resuscitation by lay people in public places and buildings, (see Figure 9.2.7 a and b). These devices analyze a casualty's heart rhythm and deliver verbal instructions using language that a lay person can understand. If required, the rescuer may be requested by the AED to deliver an electric shock.
Immediately after vascular collapse, significantly more casualties have VF than the

* Vital Parameters: respiration, blood pressure, circulation, level of consciousness

above initial documentation might lead us to assume. Had the ECG been recorded at this early stage, it might have been possible to record VF in up to 65 % of casualties. Pending arrival of the rescue services (average response time 10 minutes), the symptoms may worsen to the extent that the chances of successful defibrillation (and with it the chances of survival) are reduced. If a minimal flow of blood is maintained by applying **cardiac massage (CM)** while waiting for an AED to arrive, the heart may continue to respond well to defibrillation. The casualty's best chance of survival therefore relies on immediate resuscitation by lay helpers.
Should the cause of a cardiopulmonary arrest not be the heart itself, consideration must be given to a possible disturbance of the respiratory function or even suffocation (rib cage trauma, drowning, avalanches). In such cases opening up the airways and/or giving artificial respiration to the casualties is just as important as cardiac massage.

Lay Resuscitation Concept

- A **cardiopulmonary arrest must be identified as soon as possible** (see below). Because cardiac incidents (caused by the heart) are often preceded by feelings of tightness in the chest, it is best to call the emergency services before the victim collapses. Approximately a third of those affected suffer a cardiopulmonary arrest an hour after starting with pains caused by a heart attack!
- It is therefore essential that the **rescue sequence** is set in motion as quickly as possible.
- If a cardiopulmonary arrest is presumed, **resuscitation measures** (Basic Life Support–BLS) must be initiated immediately. This can triple the likelihood of survival. It is important to remember that even a cardiac massage without additional artificial respiration (see below) is better than not performing any resuscitation at all.
- Cardiac massage is always particularly important if there is no possibility of defibrillating in the first few minutes following collapse.

Defibrillation with an AED should take place as quickly as possible. In VF, immediate mechanical resuscitation plus defibrillation within the first 5 minutes will increase the likelihood of survival to 75 %, whereas every minute without resuscitation reduces the likelihood of survival by 10 %. If you are on your own, the call to emergency services must therefore be made before commencement of cardiac massage.

- The time you can expect to wait for the emergency services to arrive is 11 minutes in urban districts. In rural areas or in rough terrain this period will be considerably longer.

During this time the survival of a casualty suffering a cardiopulmonary arrest depends on the response of lay people (bystanders or other non-medical personnel who may be present).

Standard Procedure for Lay Persons in the Resuscitation of Adults and Children over one month of age

- Pay attention to your own safety and to the safety of others. This applies in particular when you are in terrain subject to rockfalls or avalanches or where there is a danger of falling, as well as accidents involving drowning, if the victim is still in the water.
- Simply talk to them and/or apply pain stimuli to see if the person reacts. The pain stimuli are best delivered by intensive pinches to the upper arms. Under no circumstances should the defenseless person be slapped in the face!
- If the person fails to react, help must be summoned.
- The person must now be turned over on to their back with the neck extended (Figure 9.2.3) and the airways cleared if necessary (snow, vomit).
- Check breathing: any respiratory noises and movements of the rib cage. If **breathing** appears to be **normal** the person should be placed on their side in a stable position (see Figure 9.4.1, Page 127) and help organized (Tel. 144 or local emergency numbers see Page 94).
- Even if there is only a small degree of doubt as regards normality of breathing, proceed as though the person has suffered a failure of the cardiovascular system:
- Alert the rescue services (Tel. 144 or local emergency number) and arrange for an AED to be picked up.
- Perform **Cardiac Massage (CM)**: min. 100 compressions/minute, not more than 120/minute (Figure 9.2.6): to center of breastbone, apply compressions to a minimum depth of 5 cm or 2 inches (in the case of children, $^{1}/_{3}$rd of the diameter of the rib cage).
  - **Cardiac Massage (CM) with Artificial Respiration:** after 30 compressions using cardiac massage, follow up with two short ventilations as described in Figure 9.2.5, don't spend more than 5 seconds on this and immediately continue with performing cardiac massage.
  - **Cardiac Massage (CM) without Artificial Respiration:** If there is no possibility of artificial respiration (capability, hygiene) deliver continuous cardiac massage (CPR) at 100/minute, but not more than 120/minute. This variant is equally effective following a cardiopulmonary arrest that has not been caused by choking.
- As soon as the **AED** has arrived, apply adhesive electrodes to the naked rib cage of the lifeless person and follow the instructions issued by the device.
  - **AED: "shock recommended:"** deliver a **defibrillation** and afterwards continue **immediately with further CM** with or without artificial respiration (see above).
  - **No shock recommended:** immediately perform more CM with or without artificial respiration (see above).
- **Wherever possible avoid any interruption to the efforts at resuscitation.** (For reasons justifying termination of CPR, see Page 113)

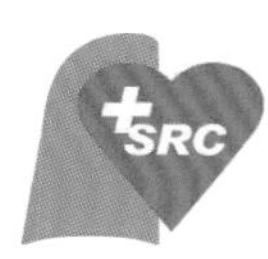

Algorhythm BLS (Basic Life Support) + AED for adults, children and infants older than 1 month

Resuscitation Guidelines 2010 Swiss Resuscitation Council (SRC)
according to ILCOR recommendations

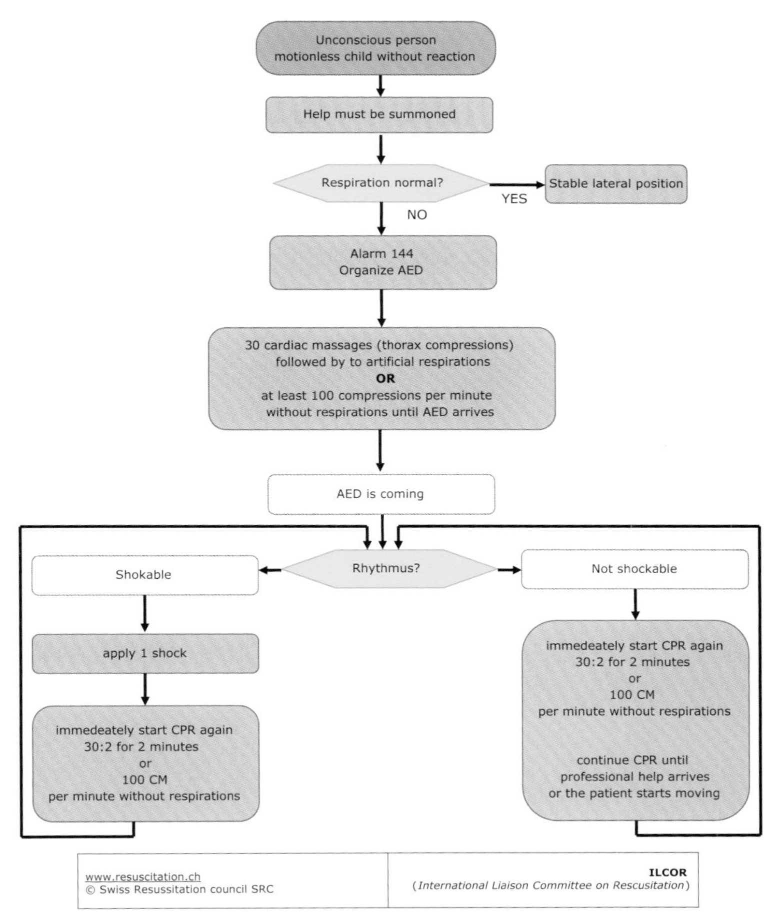

www.resuscitation.ch
© Swiss Resussitation council SRC

ILCOR
(International Liaison Committee on Rescusitation)

Schematic 9.2.1: *Process Algorithm Resuscitation Guidelines 2010 (Swiss Resuscitation Council).*

Resuscitation Measures without Artificial Respiration

Many first aides are reluctant, either due to revulsion or fear of transmittable diseases, to carry out mouth to mouth or mouth to nose artificial respiration, in particular if they do not know the person affected. As reassurance it may be said that there have been only a few instances described where it has been possible to associate any transmission of disease with the performance of artificial respiration. In particular, there has never been any evidence of the transmission of hepatitis B, hepatitis C, HIV or cytomegalovirus infection as a result of the above-mentioned artificial respiration techniques. Studies on animals have shown that, in the case of a cardiopulmonary arrest that has not been caused by choking, cardiac massage (CM) without respiration in the first few minutes is just as effective as cardiac massage combined with artificial ventilations. Where adults are concerned, the likelihood of survival as a result of receiving cardiac massage alone is significantly higher than without any type of resuscitation treatment. However, cardiac massage without any artificial respiration is probably only adequate in the first few minutes and then only in instances where cardiopulmonary arrest has been caused by something other than choking. It has been shown by research in the central European regions that, as a rule, CPR without artificial respiration is sufficient to bridge the period while awaiting arrival of the rescue personnel.

⇨ If the airway is completely blocked by a **foreign body** (e.g. snow in the case of avalanche victims), then the ensuing cardiopulmonary arrest is mostly caused by the lack of oxygen in the blood. Helping these persons will require artificial respiration as a complement to cardiac massage.

Here the following algorithm applies:

Procedure for laypersons to treat airway obstruction due to foreign bodies (adults and children)

⇨ NB: Avoid fishing about with the fingers in the mouth of the person. Only visible foreign bodies should be removed.

- If the person is still responsive when spoken to, thumps on the back may be employed or compressions applied to the upper abdomen and rib cage **(Heimlich Manœuvre)** in order to dislodge the foreign body.
- Should the choking **person become unconscious,** commence **cardiac massage** as described above, partly in order to dislodge the foreign body by means of the ensuing high pressure on the rib cage.

- In the event of **cardiopulmonary arrest as a result of choking** (e.g. victims of avalanches who have had to be dug out) a **combination of cardiac massage and artificial respiration** is also important (see diagram 30:2).

⇨ In the case of **children**, an alternative is to start with 5 breaths followed by cardiac massage (CPR).

- Before administering each individual breath, remove any foreign bodies that have become visible from the mouth cavity.

Lay persons often have difficulty in ascertaining whether a person's lifeless state has been caused by a sudden cardiopulmonary arrest, choking or another cause. Where there is the slightest doubt, the standard resuscitation sequence should be applied for both adults and children.

Free airways:

⇨ Complete blockage of an airway will result in unconsciousness within the space of 1–2 minutes.

The airways include the nose, the mouth cavity, the pharynx, the larynx and the windpipe.

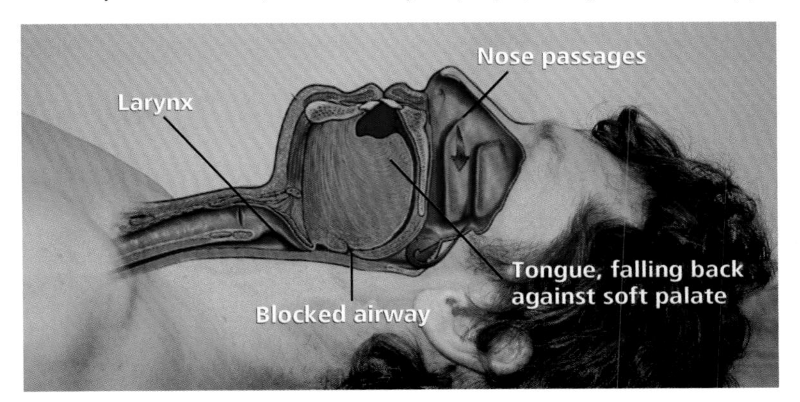

Figure 9.2.2: *Illustration of the upper airways, here blocked by the tongue falling backwards.*

A sick person who is fully capable of speech will, as a rule, have no problems with the airway because the voice travels to the outside via the airway.
In the case of casualties who experience difficulties speaking and breathing or where, for example, gurgling sounds are to be heard each time they take a breath, the mouth will need to be opened. If this reveals the presence of blood, vomit or a foreign body/ bodies in the mouth cavity, these must be wiped away and removed from the mouth using a cloth or tissue. Dentures that are firmly anchored can be left in place.

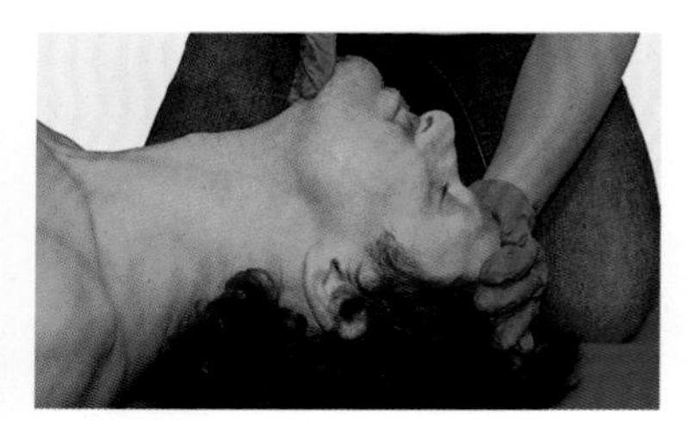

Figure 9.2.3:
Opening up the airway using the "Head-Tilt-Chin-Lift" technique. Keep one hand on the forehead and use the fingers of the other hand to lift the chin. This will ensure that the tongue is lifted away from the posterior pharyngeal wall and the airway opened.

⇨ Don't waste time trying to remove items that are difficult to reach.

If the airways cannot be opened up in this way the head will need to be bent backwards and the chin lifted.

⇨ In the majority of cases the airways of unconscious persons tend to be blocked by the tongue falling backwards.

Airways and cervical spine: with all unconscious casualties who have experienced trauma (impact, a fall, collision, avalanche) an injury to the cervical spine (CS) must be presumed. In 10 % of cases, accident casualties who are unconscious will have an accompanying CS injury. Moving an injured CS increases the danger of damage to the spinal cord by a factor of 7 to 10. It is important as far as rescue personnel are concerned that the CS of accident victims is stabilised by means of a hard neck collar. When it comes to lay rescue operations, it is important to ensure, taking advantage of all existing experience/training, resources (rescuers) and materials (e.g. SAM® splints) that the CS is stabilised as early as possible by resorting to makeshift means if there is any suspicion of an injury to the CS (see Section 9.4, Page 140).

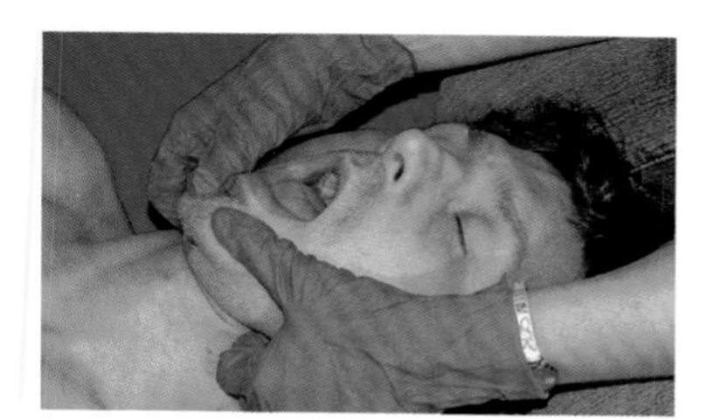

Figure 9.2.4: Opening up the airways using the "Esmarch Jaw Thrust Manœuvre."

If a CS injury is suspected, then the Esmarch jaw thrust manœuvre is to be recommended. This involves pushing the lower jaw forward without turning the head on the CS.

Artificial Respiration:
When the casualty is undressed to the waist, breathing activity is readily identifiable from the upward and downward movements of the rib cage. Because unconscious or sick casualties or those who are victims of accidents are seldom undressed when roaming in a wilderness environment, the jacket at least should be opened to check the breathing and give a better view of the rib cage. The check on breathing is then carried out with the rescuer's ear against the casualty's face and observing the casualty's chest and abdomen while they take two breaths on their own: Listen, Look, Feel.

Breathing in gasps, other sporadic noises similar to breathing or an inconsistent see-sawing movement of the rib cage must not be confused with normal breathing. In cases of doubt or uncertainty, proceed as if no breathing were present.

If a disturbance to breathing cannot be resolved by the above measures (tilting the head all the way back, Esmarch jaw thrust manœuvre) and a lay rescuer decides to follow the BLS Algorithm and opts for discretionary artificial respiration, there are various possibilities when it comes to getting one's own breath into a casualty without any external assistance.
The best known option is mouth-to-mouth artificial respiration (see Figure 9.2.5).

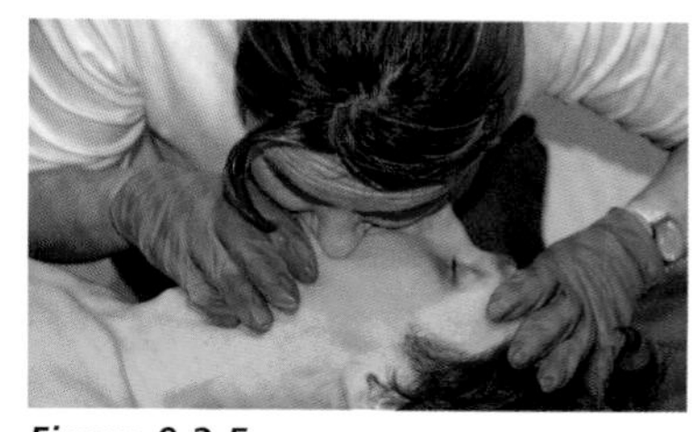

Figure 9.2.5: Mouth-to-mouth artificial respiration.

To perform this, the rescuer kneels beside the casualty's head and opens his mouth by pushing the chin downwards with one hand. Placing the other hand on the casualty's forehead he tilts the head backwards. The casualty's nose is blocked by the rescuer's cheek when the air is forced in so that the air exhaled cannot escape via the nose. A further possibility is mouth-to-nose respiration, which is used primarily on children. In addition, ventilation can be made easier and more hygienic by the use of auxiliary means (e.g. a pocket mask).

⇨ Only perform artificial respiration if you are in possession of all the facts! Do not perform artificial respiration if there is blood or vomit in the mouth. Pay attention to your own safety. Rescuers who are either not able or not inclined to carry out mouth-to-mouth resuscitation should conduct any attempt at revival using rib cage compressions only.

Circulation of the Blood:
If the affected person has suffered a complete cardiopulmonary arrest s/he will quickly become blue to purple in the face and will no longer be responsive.
In the absence of any definite signs of life, raise the alarm by contacting the emergency call center and start cardiac massage immediately after this (see Schematic 9.2.1, Page 105).

Nevertheless, in certain conditions, artificial respiration is of the utmost importance (infants, children, drugs overdoses). In addition, artificial respiration is in any event relevant after a few minutes of cardiopulmonary arrest, irrespective of the cause. With regards to any attempts at reviving adult casualties and children aged over one month, the following **rules for cardiac massage** apply:

- Casualty lies on his/her back on a hard surface
- Apply pressure to the centre of the sternum, the palms placed one above the other, arms outstretched, the shoulders of the person administering the cardiac massage vertical above his/her hands (see Figure 9.2.6).
- 5 cm rib cage compression for adults, ⅓rd of rib cage for children, then relax fully
- 100 rib cage compressions per minute, maximum 120/minute
- Min. 100 rib cage compressions/minute without artificial respiration or
- Ratio: 30 compressions: 2 ventilations until a definite airway exists (e.g. resuscitation tube applied by an emergency doctor)
- Counting out loud: 1-and-2-and-3-and-4-and… 30

 Any interruption of cardiac massage must be avoided (no massage = no circulation): rapid resumption of cardiac massage after 2 ventilations.

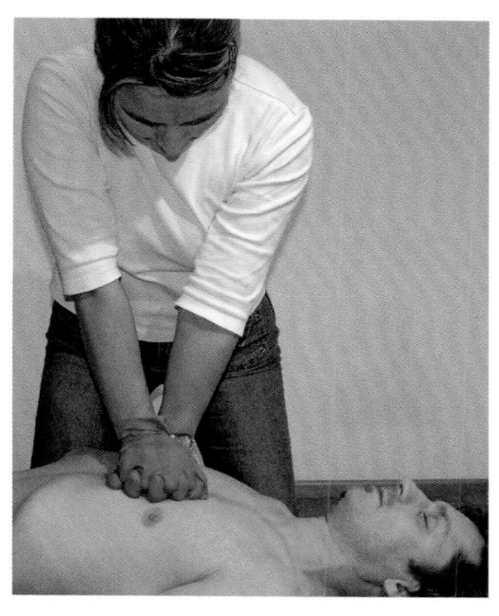

Figure 9.2.6: *Cardiac massage.*

Where a number of rescuers are present, it is important to take turns at cardiac massage every two minutes even if the rescuer does not yet feel tired.

Major bleeding may be the cause of the circulatory problem ("C Problem") and must be stemmed as quickly as possible, since a marked fall in blood pressure may ensue due to loss of blood. (See also Section 9.4, Page 130). Stemming the bleeding takes place in parallel to cardiac massage and must not be allowed to delay or to hamper this.

AED – Automated External Defibrillator

It is extremely unlikely that people venture into a wilderness environment or into the mountains with a defibrillator to hand. These devices are pretty heavy because of their batteries. However, it is feasible that AEDs may well be available, for example, in a public mountain hut or in major skiing areas. This is why we refer to them at this point.

Automated external defibrillators (AEDs) are devices that can be connected via adhesive electrodes to a casualty's (unclothed) rib cage.
The heart rhythm is then determined automatically and, depending on the result, a recommendation made for defibrillation (discharge of energy/shock). The defibrillation corresponds to a sudden discharge from a capacitor, when the electricity flows across the casualty's heart muscle. At the same time, a predefined level of energy is applied (expressed in Joules [J]) which ensures that the electrical status of all the heart cells is identical, and this facilitates resumption of a normal heart rhythm. Defibrillation has an anti-arrhythmic effect on *ventricular fibrillation*, a life-threatening disturbance of cardiac rhythm. Delivery of a shock will only be authorized by the device if the AED acknowledges the heart rhythm as suitable for defibrillation.

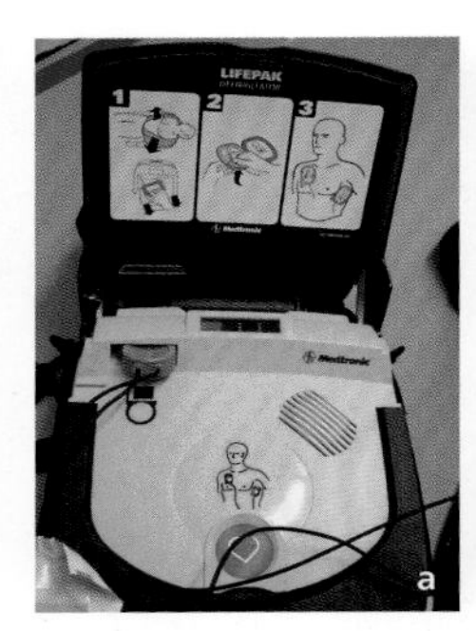

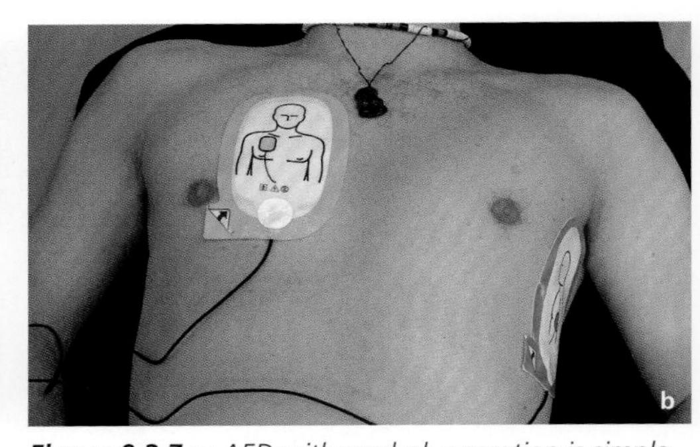

Figure 9.2.7 a: *AED with symbol: operation is simple, the instructions are clear.*
Figure 9.2.7 b: *The electrodes are connected to the casualty as shown in the drawing.*

⇨ If there is an AED available this must be used as specified in the algorithm.

A case of ventricular fibrillation has the best chance of being converted into a normal cardiac rhythm if defibrillation is carried out within the first 5 minutes following occurrence of the emergency. Approx. 85 % of casualties can be saved if the first shock is delivered during this period. However, since even the best rescue services cannot guarantee arrival within the optimum time window, AEDs are becoming increasingly available within the public sector (stadiums, railway stations etc.). In addition, the fact that they are easy to handle makes them particularly suitable for lay rescuers. The locations where these items of equipment are kept are marked with an international symbol (see Figure 9.2.7 a).

Once a shock has been delivered, CPR must be resumed for 2 minutes, regardless of the heart rhythm displayed on the AED's monitor. This is because following ventricular fibrillation and delivery of the shock, there may be impaired cardiac function which leads impaired blood flow to all organs without CPR (see also Schematic 9.2.1, Pages 104 and 105). It is important to realize, the primary ABC rules remain valid during CPR.

⇨ The AED is a supplement for cardiopulmonary resuscitation, not a replacement for it!

Frequent errors in relation to resuscitation measures:
- The biggest mistake is not to do anything at all!
- Too much time lost before starting cardiac massage; pauses that are too long between artificial respiration and cardiac massage.
- Alarm raised late or not at all

Reasons for termination or non-initiation of CPR
- Personal safety is not/no longer guaranteed
- Personal exhaustion
- Handover of casualty to professional rescue team
- Casualty comes round –> monitor!
- Injuries sustained are not compatible with life
- Definite signs of death (rigor mortis, livor mortis, decomposition)

 It is a doctor's job to establish/confirm that death has occurred.

9.3 Body Check and Primary Survey

Basic Information about the Body Check

Once the vital functions (using ABC) have been assessed, treated by immediate action and stabilized during the primary survey (as described in Section 9.2), casualty treatment and care moves on to the Body Check. This is a full body examination that needs to be carried out systematically from head to toe.

 The aim of the Body Check is to ensure that no injuries requiring therapy are overlooked.

If the alarm has been raised early and the flight time has been short, the Body Check is, in most cases, not something that we need to be unduly worried about because the professionals often take over before the ABC on the casualty has been completed. However, with lengthy waiting times or if, perhaps, an overland rescue has to be mounted or if the individuals concerned are reliant on their own resources in remote areas abroad, things may be very different. Also, lay persons with limited equipment will be subject to numerous constraints when it comes to possible therapies–however, there are some types of injuries that are life-threatening but which we can still tackle using simple, improvised methods. For this reason, in casualties with a number of injuries and/or injuries that are serious as well as those who are unconscious, the Body Check is an absolute necessity. A head-to-toe check on those who are assumed to have sustained only minor injuries is also to be recommended.

Where painful single injuries are a feature, it is possible that these may mask an associated injury (e.g. to the spinal column or the internal organs) which may consequently be missed.

Systematic Body Check from Head to Toe

To guarantee a complete examination, a systematic approach is recommended. Of course, an examination of this kind should be carried out on the casualty when naked in order to deliver the most reliable and indicative information. However, when in an emergency situation, we need to take account of the situation and wherever possible we need to avoid any chilling of the casualty. We frequently find that we have to resort to palpation through the clothes or, at the very least, only expose those body parts where examination with clothes is impossible. If the casualty is responsive, it may be possible to ask at each relevant point before examination if the casualty is experiencing any pain or particular sensations.

Normally, an inspection takes place first (visual examination) during which external bleeding, swellings or abnormal movements can be established. Then comes what is initially a superficial palpation (examination using the sense of touch) of the relevant area during which any bleeding (to the rear of the body), swellings, indurations, abnormal positions (joints) and painful areas can be identified. Deep palpation can be painful to alert casualties and should therefore be carried out with appropriate care. This step will provide information on any deeper injuries such as broken bones, pelvic injuries or internal injuries. The application of a full range of motion to the joints at the end of the examination of the extremities can provide us with information regarding joint fractures or any other injuries to joints that may not yet have been identified.

Last but not least, the casualty–subject to sufficient people being available to help–can be turned on to his or her side exercising appropriate care and using the correct technique (see Figures 9.3.1, Page 115), so that the whole of the casualty's back can be examined. This measure is justified if we need to exclude open wounds or sources of bleeding due to the mechanics of the accident. Failure to identify bleeding can lead to heavy blood loss and a subsequent state of shock.

The Body Check and the most significant injuries are described in the following. Both medical and functional aspects will be explained, along with the diagnostics and treatment options pointed out.

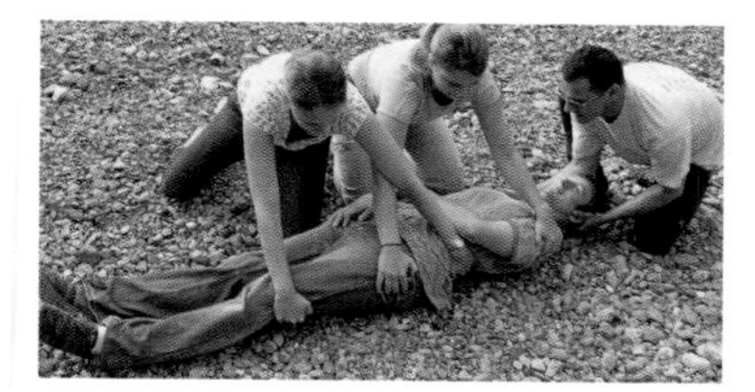

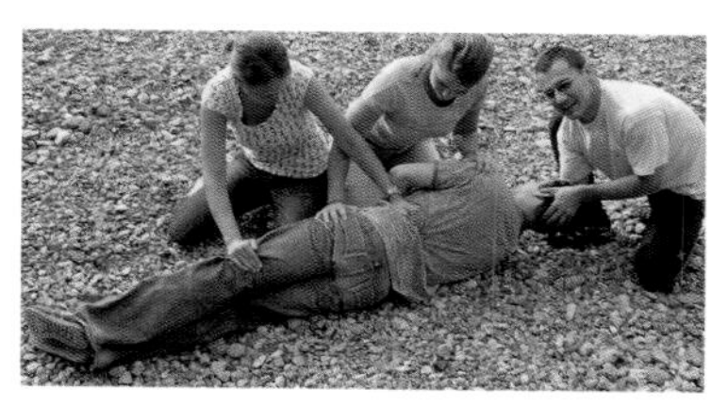

Figures 9.3.1: *An illustration of how the casualty can be turned over with minimum pressure on the spinal column so that the back can be examined: turning "en bloc" or by deploying a "log roll." Note cross-body grip. The rescuer at the head is the one who issues the instructions.*

Head and Neck Injuries

Commence examination of the part of the head covered with hair. Injuries to the skin of the head may be followed by heavy **bleeding** and this may lead to considerable blood loss. If such bleeding is localized at the rear, occasionally this may not be noticed until later.

Treatment: a compression dressing can be difficult to fit; sometimes the simplest solution is to apply a ligature to the main vessels of the scalp, although this is not recommended for fractures of the skull.

Eyes: Injuries to the eyes as a result of direct trauma (impact, splinters) are rare. The eye is protected by reflexes and, anatomically speaking, very well protected too. More frequent are small foreign bodies due to the accidents such as splinters of stone or glass (spectacles).

Treatment: Serious injuries to the eyes cannot be treated in an emergency environment in the field. A clean, protective bandage will prevent contamination and minimise any movement of the eye. Foreign bodies can be removed carefully using the corner of a handkerchief or a cotton wool bud. The lower conjunctival sac will unfold almost completely if you hold the lower lid down and ask the casualty to look upwards. Things are more difficult when it comes to the upper conjunctival sac; foreign bodies that are located some distance above can frequently not be removed until the upper lid (eyelid) has been pulled down – this can be achieved by placing a cotton applicator stick or similar over the eyelid to hold it firmly in place.

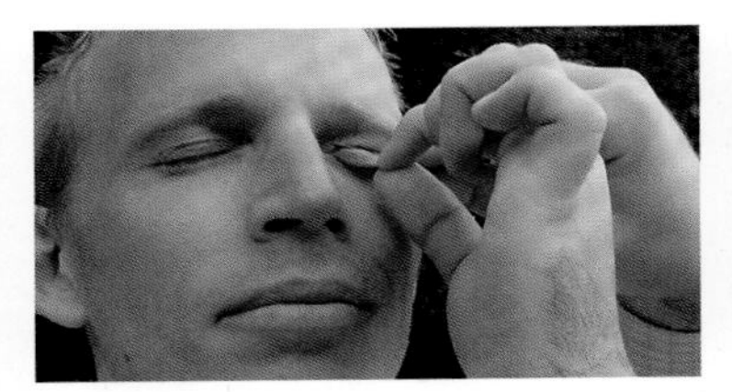
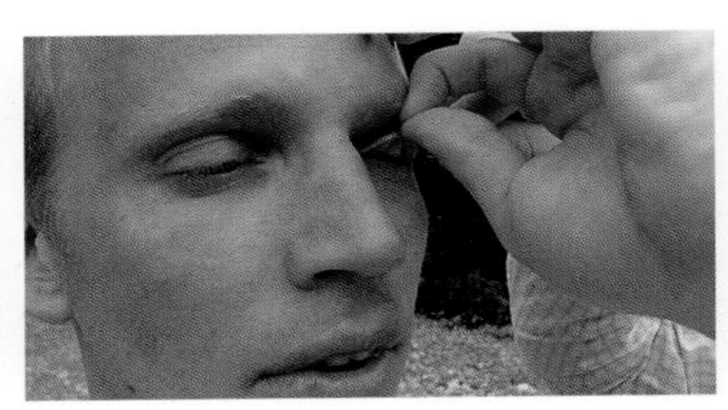

Figure 9.3.2: *Eversion of the Upper Lid.*

Cranio-cerebral Trauma: Injuries to the brain may or may not involve fracture of the skull bone. The mildest form of cranio-cerebral trauma is **concussion of the brain.** The defining factors for this are unconsciousness and partial amnesia. Additional symptoms may include nausea and vomiting. Where unconsciousness lasts for less than 5 minutes, we talk about a slight concussion of the brain. However, it is not possible to draw any definite conclusions regarding the extent of damage to the brain purely from an external examination. Depending on the effect of the energy transfer, crushing of the brain may occur ***(contusio cerebra),*** under certain circumstances with more or less pronounced bleeding into the brain **(intra-cerebral bleeding).** Injuries of this nature are mostly associated with lengthy periods of unconsciousness and, from their appearance, are indistinguishable from serious concussion of the brain.

Subsequently, intracranial bleeding may develop. The most frequent form is an **epidural hematoma** (bleeding from an artery of the cerebral membrane, commonly associated with a fractured skull). With this kind of bleeding, a "lucid interval" often occurs where the casualty is alert and responsive before a period of unconsciousness. However, over the course of time, the casualty's condition may deteriorate quickly so that he or she lapses back into unconsciousness and anisocoria (unequal pupils) may become evident. This indicates that the pressure is increasing on the injured side of the brain so that the nerve responsible for mycosis (cranial nerve 3, N. Oculomotor) becomes trapped and the pupil dilates. Another form of intracranial bleeding is **subdural hematoma,** which, particularly in the elderly, does not necessarily go hand in hand with a fracture of the skull. This type is characterized by a rapidly increasing deterioration in brain function (clouding) (see AVPU Scale, Page 99).

With any injury to the brain or skull, therefore, an examination of pupillary reaction can provide valuable information about the condition of the brain. Particularly in the unconscious casualty, no other assessment is available to us in an emergency situation; the pupil reaction test is carried out immediately after examination of the top of the skull.

If unconsciousness with anisocoria is present immediately after the accident, a serious brain injury should be assumed, predominantly on the side with a pupil that is dilated, sluggish or which is no longer reacting. Bilateral dilation of the pupils may indicate serious general brain damage with cerebral edema–however, this tends in most cases to occur only after several minutes (serious form) or even hours (less serious forms) have elapsed.

Bilateral dilation of the pupils may, however, also be a sign of lack of oxygen or underlying cranio-cerebral trauma. This may also happen, for example, in cases of respiratory insufficiency (see A and B problems, Section 9.2, Page 100) or a serious ***state of shock*** (C problem, Section 9.2, Page 101).

Another frequent manifestation of cranio-cerebral trauma are **fractures of the base of the skull.** These fractures penetrate the base of the skull where the neurocranium is connected to the face skull. Frequently there is a discharge of blood and cerebrospinal fluid from the ear or nose but a state of unconsciousness will not necessarily be present.

Treatment: Treatment is not really feasible in the field. The best results will be achieved if we are able to maintain the supply of oxygen (thus solving A and B problems) and the supply of blood to the brain (C problem). Under certain circumstances it may be possible to slightly reduce the pressure inside the skull by elevating the upper part of the body (see Section 9.4, Figure 9.4.4, Page 128).

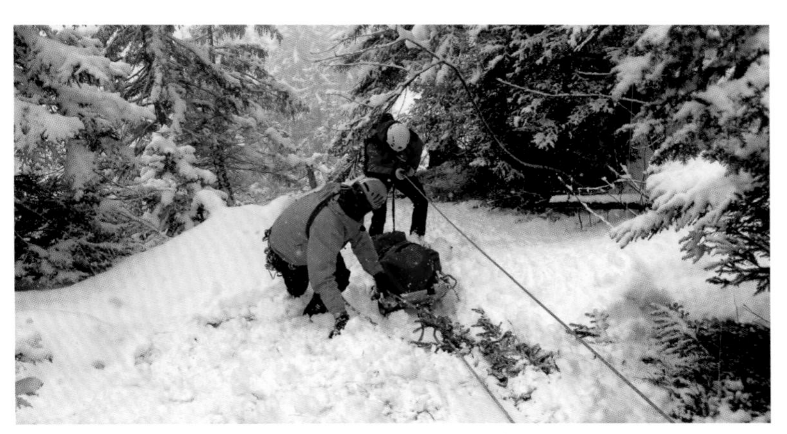

Figure 9.3.3: *Terrestrial rescue in winter conditions (M. Walliser).*

Injuries to the face skull: These are frequently associated with intense bleeding which may be difficult to stem from the outside. In such situations, particularly in the unconscious casualty, protecting the airways is vital; this can in most cases be achieved only by laying the person in the correct position on his or her side. Swelling, absence of normal facial contours, the identification of asymmetries during palpation, malocclusion and crepitation as well as double vision may constitute further clinical signs of **middle face *fractures.***

Treatment: Lay casualty down, if possible with upper part of body raised, clean bandages, staunch bleeding (may be difficult).

Continue the examination to take in the soft tissues of the neck. Swellings in the vicinity of the neck or injury to the larynx are alarm signals indicating the possibility of a threat to the casualty's airways.

Injuries to the spinal column and the vertebrae

If there is any suspicion of injury to the cervical spine (CS), attention must be paid to proper protection of the CS so as to avoid consequential damage or additional injury during transportation. Suspicious factors are primarily a compatible trauma (cranio-cerebral trauma, injury to thoracic spine or lumbar column) or pain in the area of the CS. If the casualty is unconscious, it is particularly important to protect the CS (for measures see Section 9.4, Page 140), because if muscle tension is lost, the vertebrae will be more susceptible to injury if there is an unstable fracture.

If the casualty is responsive, pains and swelling of the CS together with abnormal sensation (formication, tingling), loss of sensation or even paralysis in the arms and legs should be regarded as alarm signals as they may indicate the existence of an injury to the spinal cord ***(quadriplegia).***

This is also true of injuries to the thoracic spine and lumbar column ***(paraplegia),*** although these structures tend not to be recognized until right at the end during the examination in the lateral position (log roll). However, in an emergency environment, this examination is carried out primarily to exclude any bleeding.
The extent and the localization of neurological disturbances can provide information on the location of the injury to the vertebrae (see Figure 9.3.4, Page 119).

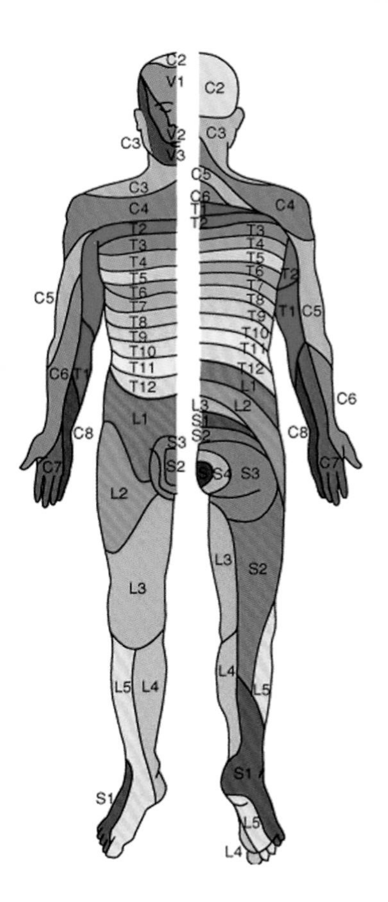

Figure 9.3.4: *Division of the human body into Dermatomes: the term Dermatome (Greek "Derma" = skin and "Tomus" = section) means the segmental area of skin innervated by a spinocerebral (spinal) nerve. Loss of sensation and paresthesia starting in a particular area of the skin indicate a certain level of injury to the vertebrae (cervical [C], thoracic [T], lumbar [L], sacral [S] spine).*

Spinal cord transection may also be associated with loss of vascular tone in the blood vessels below the level of injury. This can lead to a fall in blood pressure, even if there is no loss of blood. By contrast to the most frequent form of shock resulting from loss of blood, the skin here in the affected area is not cool and clammy but warm and dry. The pulse will also tend to be slow. This condition is also described as *neurogenic shock* and constitutes an exceptionally rare cause of shock.

Treatment: Injuries to the spinal column that occur in an emergency environment in the field necessitate the identification of the most comfortable and safe position for the casualty. Under certain conditions the casualty may even be left in the position in which they were found, if this is safe and not too unpleasant for the casualty and evacuation can take place within a short period of time.

However, if the location is vulnerable or if we need to solve a possible ABC problem, repositioning – wherever possible taking care to avoid additional injuries – is often necessary. Continuous monitoring of the casualty pending evacuation is essential.

Injuries to the chest (thorax)

In badly injured casualties, examination of the chest is normally undertaken at the ABC stage. If there was initially no evidence of a B problem but in due course the casualty displays dyspnea or pains related to breathing, the chest must be re-examined.

 Restricted breathing may develop due to pain following a broken rib.

Several broken ribs or flail segment (several ribs broken in a number of locations) can lead to a massive restriction in respiratory function. If damage to the lungs occurs (mainly due to fractured ribs) a **pneumothorax** may arise due to air leaking from the lungs. This means that there is air in the normally air-free space between the lung and the wall of the chest and this causes collapse of the respective lung. If this air is under tension due to an internal valve mechanism a **tension pneumothorax** develops. This tension then displaces the other lung, the heart is placed under pressure and the blood can no longer flow into the circulation causing distention of the neck vein. The signs of this are extreme shortness of breath, a racing pulse and congestion of the veins in the neck. It is only by initiating emergency measures to siphon off the air that this situation can be alleviated.
However, lay persons without the appropriate equipment will find that they have come to a point where they have exhausted all feasible possibilities available to them.

Another form of injury is an **open pneumothorax.** This can be caused by a stabbing injury, for example, by an ice pick or crampoon. There may be evidence of a wound to the chest through which air and blood may be escaping. In this situation the formation of a tension pneumothorax where a dressing is subsequently applied is rather unlikely:

Treatment: An airtight seal, as clean as possible (plastic sack) is fixed over the wound on three sides. In this way any penetration of air into the thorax is prevented, **whilst any excess pressure can still be spontaneously discharged.**

Injuries to the abdominal cavity (internal organs)

Additional injuries to the abdominal cavity are common, particularly where casualties with multiple injuries are concerned. These are often not discovered early, therefore it is very important to check the abdomen carefully during the Body Check.
Abdominal pain may not only be a sign of external injuries but also of internal injuries. Any swelling of the abdomen linked with a "C problem" indicates injury to an

organ causing bleeding. The most frequent injuries are injuries to the spleen and the liver; however, injuries to blood vessels in the abdominal cavity may also be encountered (see Section 12, Page 182 **"Ruptured Spleen"**). The distance from hospital facilities means that it is rarely possible to treat such injuries. If a hollow organ in the abdominal cavity (gastrointestinal tract) sustains injury, peritonitis may develop after a period of time (minutes or hours, depending on the segment injured), characterized by stiffening of the abdominal wall, guarding of muscles, fever and intense pain.

Treatment: Where internal injuries have been sustained the only feasible course of action in a wilderness environment is optimum positioning (lay the casualty in the shock position, relieve pressure on the abdominal wall) and **in all cases to administer pain therapy.**

Pelvic injuries

Exposure to high energy accidents (falling from a great height when climbing, falling at high speed while skiing) means that pelvic fractures are anything but a rarity. **Unstable pelvic fractures** (unilateral instability affecting at least the pelvic girdle) may lead to significant blood loss and shock. Intense pain and mobile iliac crests with signs of shock (depending on the time sequence) should raise alarm bells.
In most cases palpation needs to be carried out through the clothing. In order to obtain some idea of the existing pelvic injury you will need to be able to feel the symphysis (on the front of the pelvic girdle, directly in front of the bladder) and the iliac crests (at the sides of the pelvis) (see Figure 9.3.5). If it is not possible to feel the symphysis, a fracture of the pelvic girdle is likely. If the pelvic girdle is actually ruptured at the front, it may be assumed that there will also be an injury at the rear of the pelvic girdle.
If the iliac crests can be pressed together and some movement is established in this location, we can safely say that a fracture of the pelvic ring exists and we will need to assume a significant amount of blood loss internally.

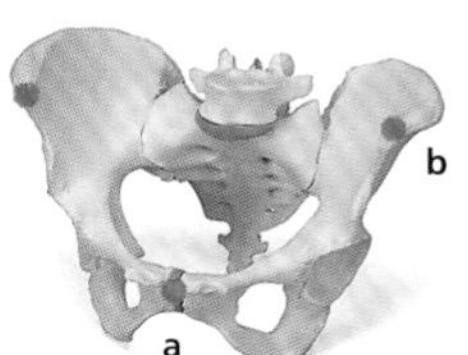

Figure 9.3.5: *Pelvic girdle, palpation points (a = Symphysis, b = Ala of the ilium).*

Treatment: The fracture (and also the pain) is usually to be found on the side with the shorter leg! By pulling on the shorter leg and rotating the feet inwards a partial reduction can be achieved. Tying the legs together whilst practising inner rotation and with the knee and hip joints bent approx. 10–20° will reduce the volume of the pelvis and the possible space for bleeding. It is possible in this situation for further pressure to be applied to the pelvic girdle from the outside by means of a pelvic compression bandage so that, under certain circumstances, the bleeding can be controlled. This measure can be implemented using belts, braces or climbing harnesses and can sometimes prove to be a life saver (see Figures 9.3.6 a–b).

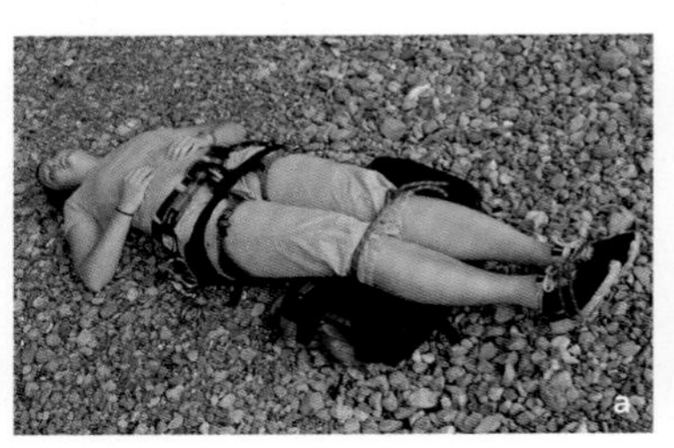

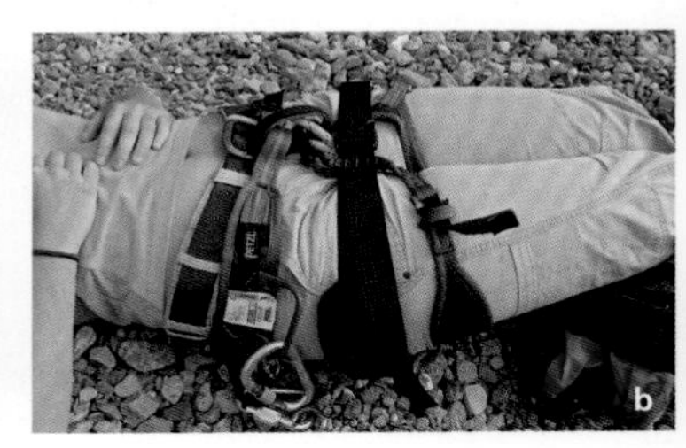

Figures 9.3.6 a–b: *Immobilization of a pelvic fracture using a belt. The legs are tied together at the knees and feet and the hips and knee are bent by approx. 20°.*

Injuries to the Arms and Legs (Extremities)

These are the most frequent injuries in the mountains and often lead to helicopter rescues as particularly with leg injuries, the ability to walk is limited or even lost completely.

In Section 9.4 there is a detailed description of a range of measures for reducing and stabilizing injured extremities.

In the following section, individual groups of injuries are first of all described in general. Then comes a detailed description of the most frequent injuries starting at the top and working down.

Broken Bones (Fractures)

Fractures to arms and legs are among the most frequent injuries that can befall mountaineers and outdoor sports enthusiasts. Pain, swelling, unnatural alignment, reduced mobility and bones rubbing together (crepitation) are the most important signs. Shaft fractures tend to be associated with a better prognosis than joint fractures. A "compound fracture" refers to a fracture associated with injury to the overlying soft tissue. Depending on the degree of contamination and the damage to the soft tissues the prognosis here may be less encouraging (risk of infection, impaired wound healing). The most important indicator as regards to the diagnosis is the information given by the casualty about the pain. The examination is carried out using the eye and the sense of touch. A comparison between the two sides will often provide information as to how far an abnormal position may extend. In the case of obvious fractures causing abnormal positioning, the diagnosis is easy. However, fractures may not be so easy to identify, for example, with cracked bones where there is no abnormal positioning.

Treatment: Up to the point of definitive treatment for a broken bone (e.g. surgical intervention) treatment in an emergency situation consists of straightening and reduction of dislocation of a markedly displaced bone or joint, immobilisation and the treatment of pain subject to the availability of appropriate resources (see Section 9.4, Page 125).
Further measures in the acute phase include placing the injured extremity in the raised position and cooling it–this helps to minimise the swelling and also the pain.

Broken collar bone: Falling on to the shoulder or direct trauma may result in a fracture of the collar bone. This is a frequently occurring injury that is quite painful; in most cases active use of the arm is no longer possible. Under normal circumstances it is an innocuous injury that can usually be treated without an operation. In the acute phase, immobilizing the arm will be sufficient (see Section 9.4, Page 138).

Fracture of the Upper/Lower Arm: The chief cause of these fractures is falls. Pain and abnormal limb positioning speak for themselves. Compound fractures tend to be rare and reduction and immobilization usually pose no problems.

Fracture of the Wrist (Radius and/or Cubitus): This is one of the most common fractures of all! Compound fractures also occur occasionally. Reduction under traction is often possible without any problems. However, in unstable fractures, reduction can be lost again. In the majority of cases, fixation in the best attainable position is usually not problematic. Maintaining an elevated position and cooling are the important factors!

Fracture of the Hand/Fingers: Entrapment, rock fall or even falling from a height often leads to compound fractures since the hands are highly exposed. Reducing, connecting and securing in a finger/forearm splint generally pose no major problems but an assessment by a specialist doctor is recommended, even if the injuries are presumed to be very minor. Taking an early opportunity to raise and cool the limb may delay the swelling that invariably occurs.

Fracture of the Thighbone (Femur): This is a type of fracture that tends to to be rare. In most cases it is closed but it can still be dangerous due to risk of major loss of blood (over two liters), especially if there are already other sources of bleeding present. Rapid reduction and fixing of this fracture can minimize the blood loss. Fixation from outside is difficult; tying both legs together seems to be the simplest measure in this situation. Some basic additional measures include monitoring the circulation and, if need be, shock positioning.

Fracture of the Lower Leg: This is a frequent type of fracture (from walking in coarse scree etc.). Due to the lack of soft tissue coverage, compound fractures are common. Reduction is in most cases readily possible and there are various options for fixation, even with simple resources. Early raising and cooling of the limb are very important with these fractures.

Fracture of the Ankle (Malleolar Fracture): The most frequently occurring fracture after fracture of the wrist. It occurs predominantly when wearing low-cut footwear in rough terrain, but may also happen with high footwear designed to protect the ankle. Compound fractures are not rare and fracture-dislocation of the ankle may occur. In this situation rapid reduction is especially important and will help to protect the delicate soft tissue (see Section 9.4, Page 146).

Dislocations

In a dislocation the joint springs out of its natural cavity and remains fixed in this position. Such injuries are relatively frequent and there are joints that are more prone to dislocation than others. However, any joint is capable of dislocating in response to enough force. Accompanying injuries often occur. In a simple case there may only be distention/strain on the joint capsule. However, more frequently there are tears in the joint capsule and in the stabilizing ligaments and sometimes even damage to nerves or blood vessels. This makes any dislocation an injury to be taken seriously which, even once successful reduction has taken place, needs to be assessed by a specialist with appropriate follow-up treatment (see Section 9.4, Page 143).

Sprains

Sprains are injuries to joints which involve distention of the joint capsules and ligaments with corresponding swelling and pains. However, there are a number of structures in and around the joint that may be damaged. In most cases in a wilderness environment we are limited with regards to further assessment of damage to cartilage, cracks to bones or soft tissue injuries. The joint may be simply sprained, swollen, painful and frequently not capable of supporting a load.

Treatment: Immobilisation can certainly never be wrong where the findings are definitive, in particular if there is the slightest suspicion of a fracture. Otherwise there is not much that can be done, apart from elevating the joint, cooling, pain killers and rest. An assessment by a specialist doctor is recommended in order to rule out any accompanying injuries.

Injuries to Soft Tissues (Skin, Muscles, Tendons)

Localized pain and loss of function following trauma may indicate deep-seated **injuries to muscles** or **tendons**. Occasionally they may lead to an inability to walk; in most cases these injuries occur in the lower limb. The precise structures that have been damaged is not something that we tend not to find out in the field and evacuation is usually necessary due to an inability to walk. Keeping the limb elevated, cooling and pain killers are all we can offer in the field; immobilization can be helpful if, for example, the extensor mechanism to one of the legs is no longer functioning and the leg can no longer be controlled.

9.4 More Comprehensive First Aid Measures

Introduction

Imagine you are with a few friends on the classic trek to the Everest Base Camp in the Khumbu Valley in Nepal. There is nobody in the group who has any medical training. During the climb there are no problems worthy of mention and the members of the group are starting to think that the extensive First Aid kit they have brought with them was probably a bit over the top after all …

Coming down the group start to run out of time so they up the tempo. Then one of the party suddenly slips, falls over the edge of the path ten meters down into the steep scree below. After the fall he does not move, does not answer, is bleeding from several wounds and his right foot is grotesquely bent at a right angle.

A similar situation may also develop in the Swiss mountains under adverse weather conditions. What can we do in a situation like this when we are reliant on our own resources? In the following, one or two points are addressed:

- Positioning of persons who are sick or injured
- Wound, cover and support bandages
- Immobilisation of injured body parts (immobilisation, fixation)
- Straightening of grotesquely displaced body parts, reduction of dislocated limbs
- Preparations for transport and improvised modes of transport

- Removal of rings from fingers in a wilderness environment
- Comments on emergency bivouac

Positioning

Special forms of positioning are used to fully optimize the casualty's medical situation while awaiting rescue, ensure avoidance of any additional dangers and make things as comfortable as possible for the casualty.

Basic notes:

- Before a casualty is placed in a stable position on his/her side, the rescuer must be absolutely certain that the casualty is still breathing. The stable position on the side (see Figure 9.4.1) should only be used if the casualty is definitely still breathing; in cases of doubt commence resuscitation measures immediately (CPR, see Section 9.2, Page 102).
- Exercise common sense: a casualty should only be left in the position in which they fell if they are definitely breathing and if the organised rescue party will be arriving within a very short space of time – this justifiable period is dependent on the weather (cold, wind) and also the location (if the fall occurred quite close to a Swiss Alpine Club hut, for example). The most reliable way of assessing a casualty is when they are lying on their back, this is also the easiest way of keeping the airways clear.
- Ensuring that the airways are clear and safe is an absolute priority: care must be taken to ensure that the casualty is able to breathe without difficulty; if the position of the head is markedly bent forward as a result of the fall and the casualty's breathing is noisy ("rattling"), the neck must be carefully extended so as to extend the head and this position maintained until rescue arrives. It is also important to intervene quickly should any change to the casualty's condition become apparent (e.g. turning the casualty in the event of vomiting).
- If the casualty is alert and responsive, they will dictate the position which is the most comfortable for them. Always ask the casualty what he would like. Patients suffering from an attack of asthma, breathing difficulties at high altitude or where a heart attack is suspected may prefer, for example, a position with the upper part of the body raised. Patients with abdominal pain or injuries to the abdomen will automatically get to their feet to take the tension away from the abdominal wall (see Figure 9.4.2, Page 127).

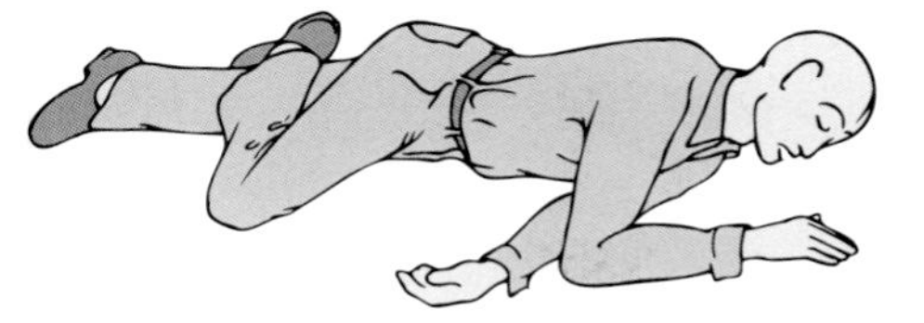

Figure 9.4.1: *Safe lateral positioning: Slightly elongate the neck to extend the head (the head may be placed on an underlying support such as a jacket). The face should be inclined downwards (lowest point). For any restrictions that may be indicated see text.*

Unconscious casualties: In unconscious casualties who are lying on their back, the safety of the airways is not guaranteed. If the tongue falls backwards it can block the airways and cause the casualty to choke. In the supine position the airways can be kept clear by applying slight tension to the chin and slightly tilting the head backwards. The easiest way of monitoring breathing is in this position and the start of resuscitation will not be delayed. Also, the primary survey as well as treatment for other injuries is also normally carried out in the supine position.
In cases of (repeated) vomiting, if blood or secretions are flowing into the throat and mouth or if it is not possible to monitor the casualty constantly, the casualty should be placed in a stable side position at an early opportunity.

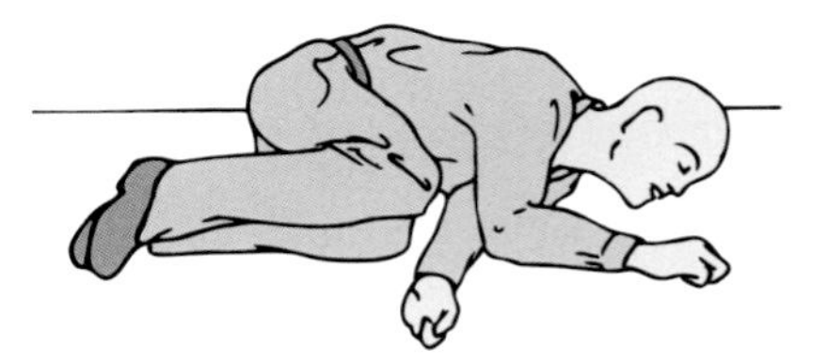

Figure 9.4.2: *Position for abdominal injuries: In straightforward cases it may also be possible for the casualty to lie in the supine position (upper part of body raised, legs bent). Drawing up the legs will relieve tension on the abdominal wall and thus reduce the pain.*

In the case of casualties who are suffering from shock (see Section 9.2, Page 101) and unconscious casualties, the blood flow to vital organs can be improved by placing a rucksack under the legs in the stable side position (modified shock position, for classic shock position see Figure 9.4.3). The slope of the land can also be utilized to position the legs slightly higher than the torso–around 10° will be sufficient.

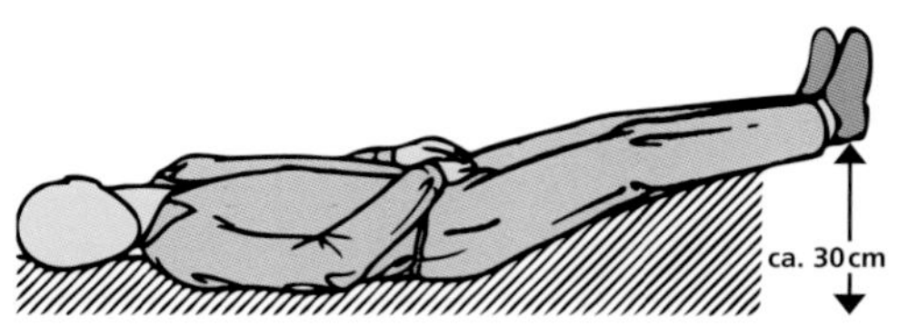

Figure 9.4.3: Classic shock position: *As a rule (where the causes of the state of shock are unknown), the casualty lies on his back, with the legs raised approx. 30°, with the upper part of the body and the head flat. In the case of shock casualties who are not unconscious but are experiencing difficulty in breathing, chest injury, injury to the skull or a heart attack, placing the upper part of the body in a raised position is indicated.*

⇨ Unconscious casualties who are breathing but who are feared may have an injury to the rib cage and/or the lung (coughing up blood, open wound above the rib cage) and who need to be positioned on their side because they are vomiting or need to be left alone should be placed on their **injured** side so as to ensure that blood or any secretions cannot flow into the healthy lung.

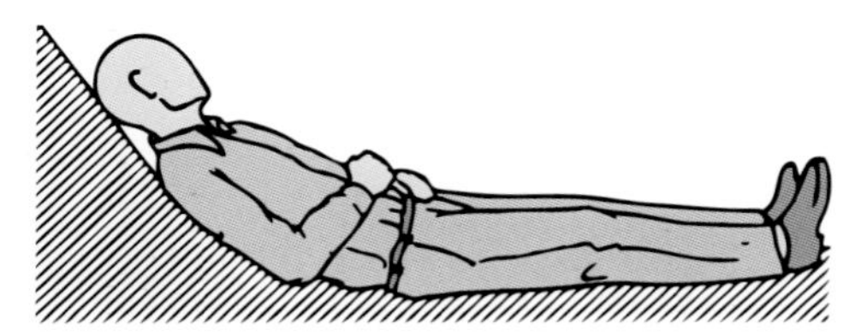

Figure 9.4.4: *Elevation of the upper body.*

Positioning in the event of injury to the spinal column: In and responsive casualties, any suspicion of injury to the spinal column will be based on descriptions of symptoms such as impaired sense of touch, paralysis and intense pain in the area of the spinal column. Patients must be positioned as safely as possible to avoid any further injuries. When repositioning in the supine position it is essential that torsional movements (twisting) of the spinal column are avoided ("en bloc" rotation) (see Figure 9.3.1, Page 115).

In unconscious casualties, the situation is much more difficult to assess. In a high energy accident (falling from a height of more than three meters, being struck on the helmet by a heavy stone etc.) injury to the spinal column must be assumed and the cervical spine must be consistently protected (see Page 140). Since the safety of the airways has absolute priority, an unconscious casualty, even with a verified back injury, must also be placed in the lateral position if he is vomiting or cannot be consistently monitored.

General Dressings/Bandages

Dressings/bandages may be used to cover wounds, to stem the flow of blood and also to protect an injury from further contamination. They can also be used for immobilizing limbs.
Some bandages/dressings are easy to improvise: we have all tied a hankie around an injured finger ... shoelaces, lengths of rope, belts, ski straps may double as valuable aids (see further below).
A dressing or bandage is not there to look "pretty," it's there to serve a purpose. This means going to painstaking lengths to ensure that the bandage is not restricting the circulation.

Wound dressings in the event of bleeding: A superficial injury to the skin that does not bleed heavily or for a long time can be covered with a dressing that is as clean as possible (gauze compress, clean handkerchief, start section of bandage) and held on to the wound using a bandage that is not too tight (e.g. triangular bandages see below). If getting the dressing to cling to the wound is likely to be problematic, it is possible to cover wounds of this nature very easily with a piece of clean plastic as described for blisters on the feet in (Section 16, Page 202).

It is possible to create some practical emergency dressings using a simple **triangular bandage.** Such dressings are especially suitable for covering a large scale wound area and protecting it from any further contamination.

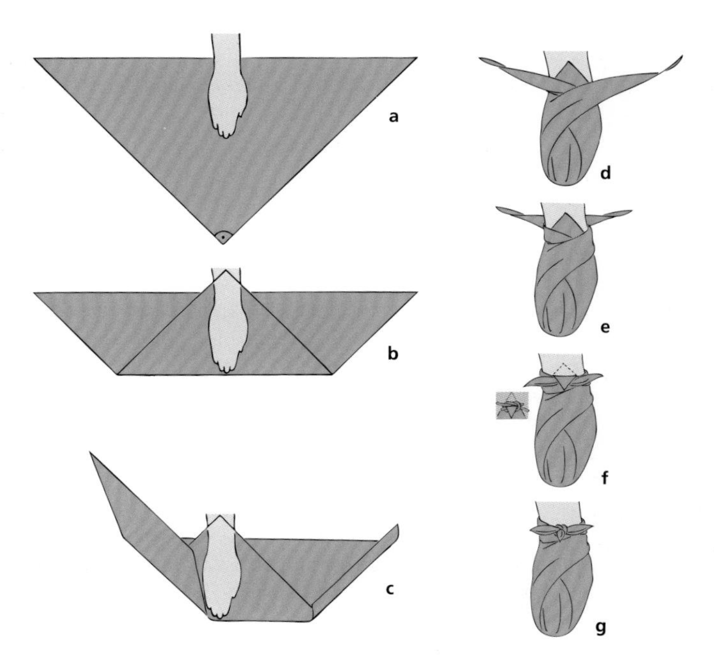

Figure 9.4.5: *Place the hand or foot on the cloth in such a way that the central point of the base is located a long way above the wrist or the heel (otherwise an open pocket will be formed). Turn over each tip of the cloth to face the joint and knot.*

⇨ Deep-seated injuries such as stabbing or cutting injuries (especially to the hand) should be examined as soon as possible by a specialist doctor (if possible within the first six hours).

In cases where there is **intense bleeding** the most important thing is to keep the loss of blood as low as possible–which means stemming the flow of blood as quickly as possible. Where the bleeding is substantial, use the fingers or the fist to press directly down on the wound and stem the bleeding. Bleeding from locations on the trunk (head, back, buttocks) are frequent in practice and stemming bleeding of this nature is more difficult than on the arms or legs. Luckily, bleeding from the trunk does not in the majority of cases relate to any of the larger blood vessels. With bleeding from the extremities, even faster control of the bleeding is possible by elevating the limb and if required, by applying pressure to the supplying artery on the upper arm or in the groin.

In instances involving injuries caused by cutting or rupturing, the edges of the wound may be compressed laterally. In the case of wounds below the scalp that are bleeding heavily, the bleeding can be stopped immediately by pressing on it with the flat of the hand. These initial measures can also be carried out by the casualty and must be kept up until the necessary dressing or bandaging material is ready.

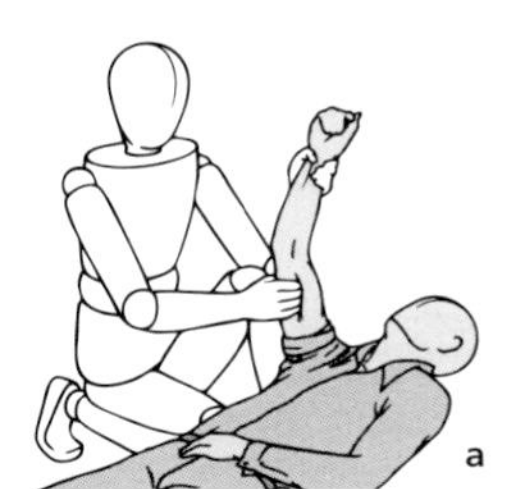

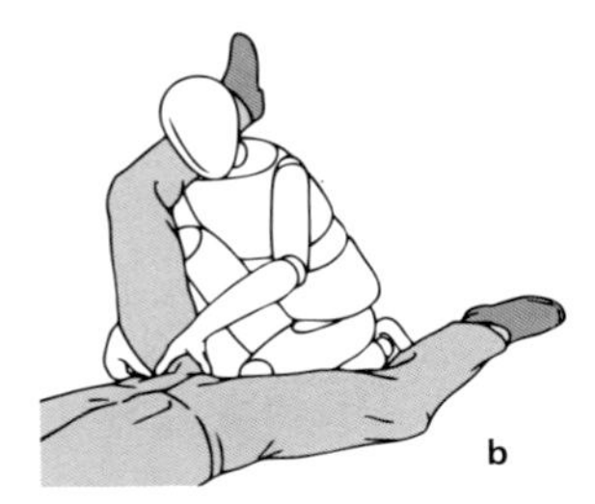

Figures 9.4.6 a–b: *Pressure points and elevated position: Using four fingers, push the artery of the upper arm on the inside (in the crease between the crook and the extensor muscles) against the bone. Using two fingers, press femur artery in the groin against the public bone.*

Following initial stoppage of bleeding, apply a pressure bandage to any wounds on limbs that may be bleeding heavily.

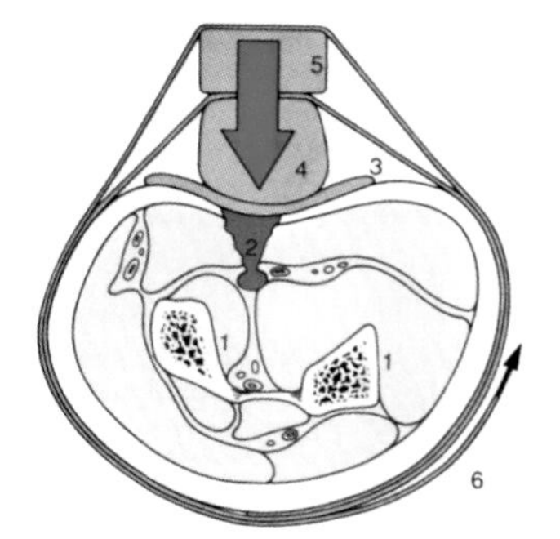

Figure 9.4.7: *Pressure bandage:*
1 Bone, 2 Area of wound, 3 Compress,
4 First pressure pad, 5 Second pressure pad,
6 Turns of bandage

Pressure bandage: Eine Place over the wound and follow with one or two tight turns of the bandage. Then lay a hard object (stone, Swiss Army knife, wristwatch ...) to suit the size of the wound over it and secure again with several tight turns of the bandage. Wherever possible ensure that pressure is only exerted on the wound and that is not under any circumstances allowed to completely stop the flow of blood in the limb: check for pulse (wrist, inside of the ankle, arch of foot, just below the medial malleolus and Achilles tendon–practice!) If you cannot be certain that you can feel a pulse or should dysaesthesia (pins and needles) develop, you should loosen the bandage slightly, avoiding having to undo the entire bandage. It is helpful to note the time when the bandage was applied.

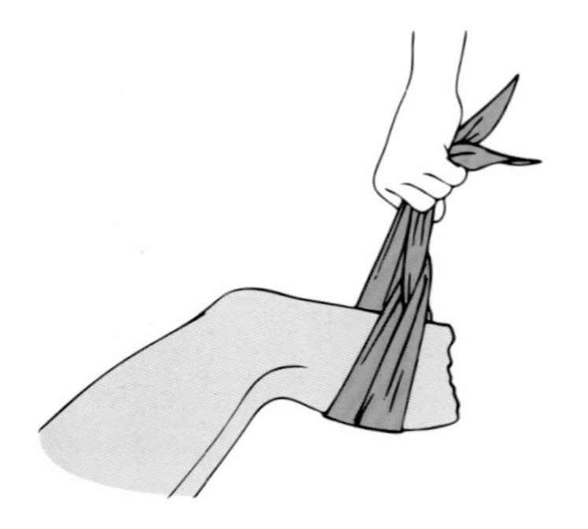

Where pressure bandages are concerned, it is crucial that blood should still be able to flow under the bandage so that the more distant part of the limb does not go numb or necrotise. However, in all cases, stemming the bleeding has priority, even if it is not possible to maintain the peripheral pulses.

Figure 9.4.8: *Tourniquet dressing: Wherever possible, the ligature should stay in position pending treatment by a doctor, whenever this Is possible but in any event for no longer than $1^1/_2$ hours. If possible, the ligature should be slowly and carefully loosened at intervals of 20–30 minutes. Often any continuous bleeding can be stemmed using a pressure bandage. If the bleeding is still too intense, retie the ligature. Note down time to the nearest minute.*

The application of a tourniquet (see Figure 9.4.8) to a limb is only indicated in the exceptional circumstance where bleeding cannot be stopped in any other way, for example, where a hand or a foot has been torn off **(amputation)** due to ropes becoming looped around limbs during a fall. Amputations, such as those occurring in road traffic or industrial accidents, are very rare in mountaineering. Here they are mostly associated with the effect of massive external forces and injury to tissue which, in most cases, makes successful reattachment impossible. However, a decision on this cannot be taken at the scene of the accident.

Treatment in cases of amputation: Should an amputation occur, stopping the bleeding is the most important factor. The tourniquet should be applied a good hand's width across the wound and care must be taken to ensure that no constricting materials (shoelaces, cords) are used so as to avoid any damage to tissue. An elastic bandage, a belt or, for example, a triangular cloth folded to a width of 4 to 5 cm can be used. With this it is possible, by monitoring the torque, to keep building up the pressure until the bleeding stops (or see Figure 9.4.8). If smaller parts of the body such as fingers, toes or ears are ripped off the bleeding is initially not nearly so intense and the casualty is usually able to keep the bleeding under control by firmly compressing the area where the amputation has occurred with the hand. This can also be carried on over a lengthy period of time and renders the application of a tourniquet (invariably awkward) superfluous.

Procedure: Note the time of the accident, provide the rescuers with the relevant information and, where possible, collect up any available body parts and, keeping them clean and dry, hand over in a clean cloth together with the casualty. The severed body part must be stored in the coolest possible conditions but not in conditions likely to produce frost damage. If the correct measures are deployed it will be possible to limit the damage to the tissue as a result of lack of oxygen and replantation will, in theory, be possible for up to six hours.

Under no circumstances must the amputated part be allowed to come into direct contact with snow or ice. If leakproof plastic bags and snow are available, the amputated part may be placed in a plastic bag which can in turn be placed in another bag half filled with water and half with lumps of ice or snow.

Disinfecting Wounds: If there is a disinfecting agent available the wound should be disinfected, especially on expeditions and treks; as a result of the reduced oxygen content in the tissues, wounds become infected more quickly at higher altitudes.

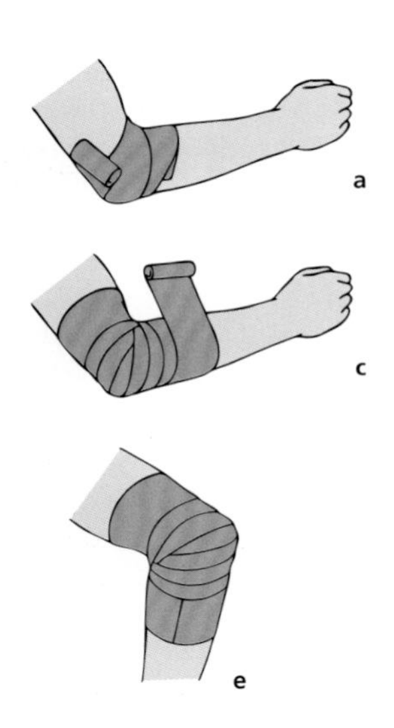

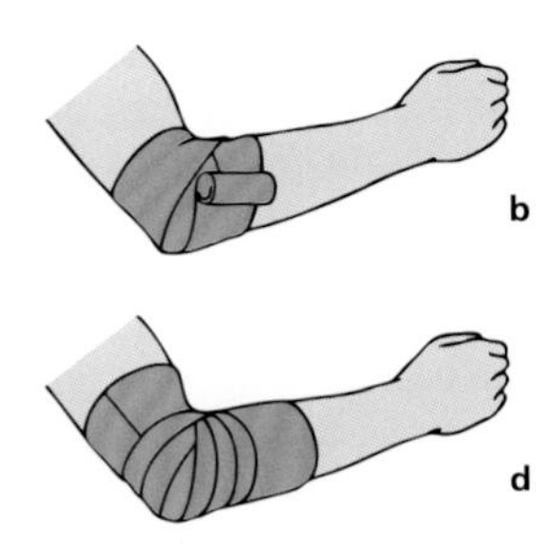

Figures 9.4.9 a–e: *Knee or elbow bandage: With elbow/knee semi-flexed, apply bandages in a fan shape so that they extend upwards and downwards from the elbow (or the knee). Commence bandaging with 2–3 turns around the elbow (knee) and finish with 2–3 turns on the upper arm (lower leg).*

Special Bandaging Techniques

Support bandage with **elastic bandage:** Strains and sprains are common in most mountain sports. For instance, wrenching and sprains to the knee joint or the thumb joint (skier's thumb) frequently affect participants in ski tours or simply when out piste-skiing. If the injury is considered to be not too bad and if the casualty can still walk and/or ski, the injured joint can be supported using elasticated tape or a straightforward elastic bandage so that in most cases it is still possible to go downhill without any pain. For this, the bandage is applied, to the area above and below the kneecap alternately, using tight turns, over the clothing, which also has a certain stabilizing effect.

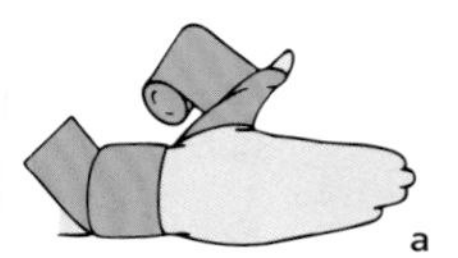

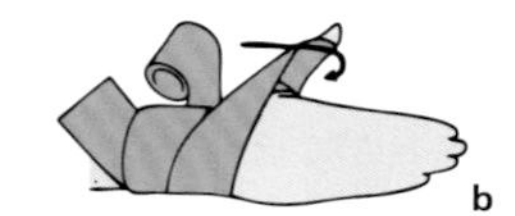

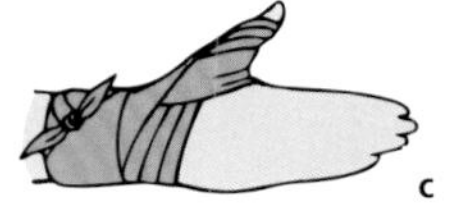

Figures 9.4.10 a–c:
Bandaging a case of skier's thumb: Starting at the wrist, 1–2 circular turns around the thumb, eight turns around the thumb and wrist (interspersed with circular turns), terminating on dorsal side of wrist.

Tape support bandage**:** Using nonelastic strapping tape such as Leukotape® it is possible to stabilize injured limbs and enable the injured party to keep going. It is also possible to use it to stabilize finger and toe fractures. The most suitable tape for this is a 3.75 cm wide tape. It is best if any hair on the skin is shaved and dried well before the dressing is applied. Before expeditions and treks it is a good idea to apply a test dressing to see whether you have a skin allergy to the adhesive.

Ankle: In most cases, it is the lateral malleolus that is wrenched or sprained. You start by fixing some of the adhesive strapping around the leg about 0–15 cm above the lateral malleolus. Be careful to ensure that you do not end up with circular adhesive strips that totally encircle the limb and which could disrupt the blood flow. Working outwards from this horizontal strip, attach strips crosswise to it that reach up higher so as to cover the ankle bone, the sole of the foot and the inside of the foot. At right angles to these, apply a few strips working toward the hind part of the foot from the arch up and over the ankle bone in the direction of the Achilles tendon. Carry on until several strips have been applied in a pattern similar to roof tiles.

This tape will stretch slightly during the first few steps and can hardly be felt once in place. Tape of this kind can be kept on for several days (subject to its continuing to stick) and if hygiene is not too important a factor.

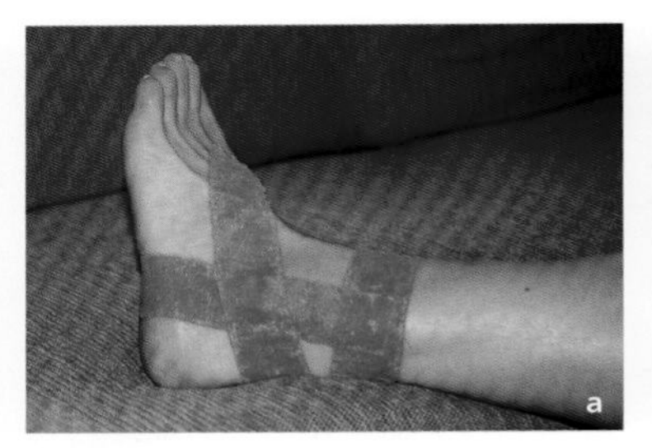

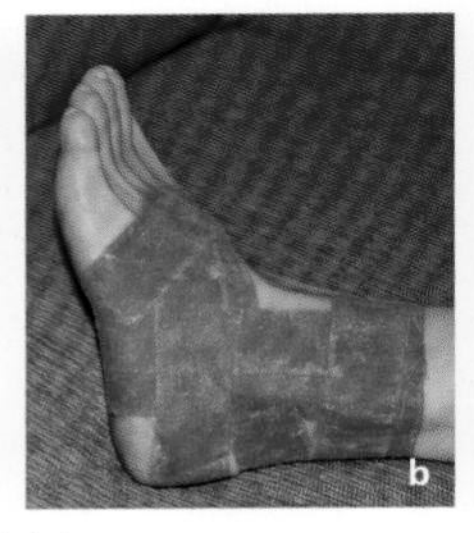

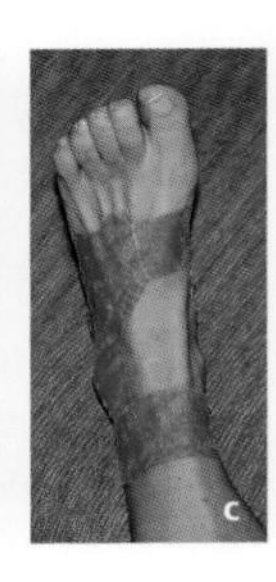

Figures 9.4.11 a–c: *Taping of the ankle joint.*

Fingers and Toes: Where possible an injured finger or toe is fixed using an adhesive strip between two intact digits. It is best if a piece of gauze or a scrap of cloth is placed between the fingers or the toes. The injured hand or foot can be washed without removing the tape and with no need to change the bandage until later.

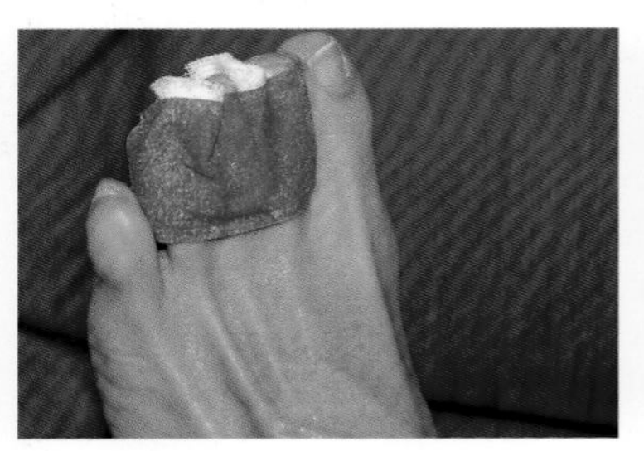

Figure 9.4.11 d: *Taping of the toes.*

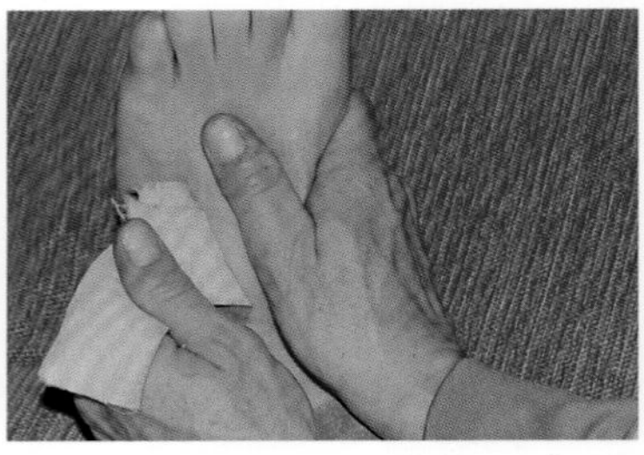

Figure 9.4.11 e: *Removal of tape plaster.*

The tape can be removed painlessly using one hand to pull on the dressing and the other to exert strong counter-pressure on the skin directly behind the tape dressing.

Immobilization and Fixation

The immobilisation and fixation of an injured body part is the most important measure to combat pain in an emergency situation.

Immobilisations

Correct fixation of broken bones will prevent any further injuries resulting from the sharp broken edges of the bones that may cut through nerves, blood vessels and muscles in the soft tissue mantle.

Collarbone: In order to make it possible to descend the valley, for example, such fractures (see Section 9.3, Page 123) may be temporarily immobilized very effectively using a rucksack bandage (see Figure 9.4.12).

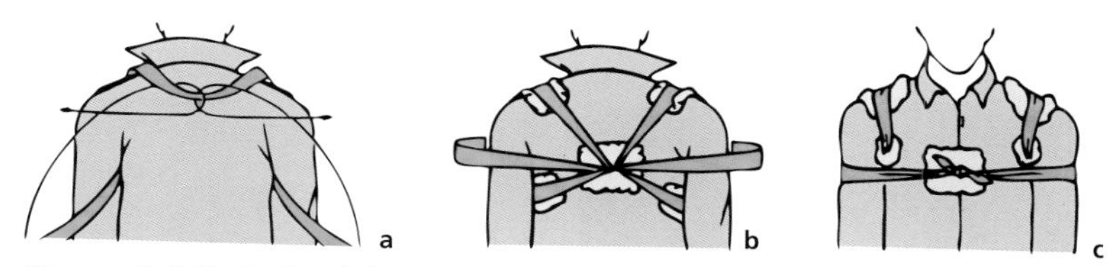

Figures 9.4.12: *Rucksack bandage: In order to relieve pressure on the fracture, both shoulders are pulled back applying equal tension. If slings are inclined to cut, use pads. The bandage will need to be checked/adjusted every day.*

Upper extremity (shoulder girdle, arm, hand): All these parts of the body can be immobilized quickly and efficiently using very simple methods so that the casualty is still able to walk down into the valley without excessivemovement of the injured limbs.

The easiest way of effecting an immobilization is with a T-shirt. The choice of this option means that it is important to pull the T-shirt up as far as possible over the shoulders on the injured side. A small item (stone, scrunched up handkerchief, watch) can be used to hold the T-shirt in place. This should be inserted above the chest on the injured side of the body and then secured in place using a piece of string (shoe laces).

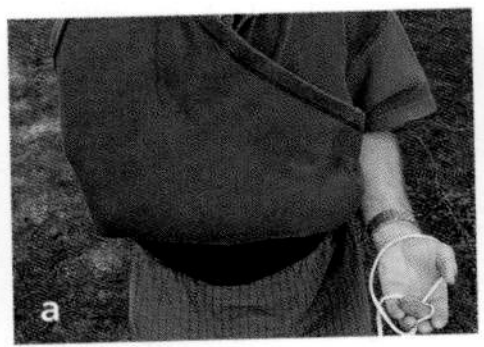
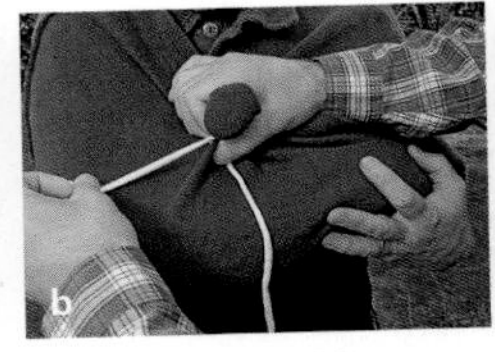
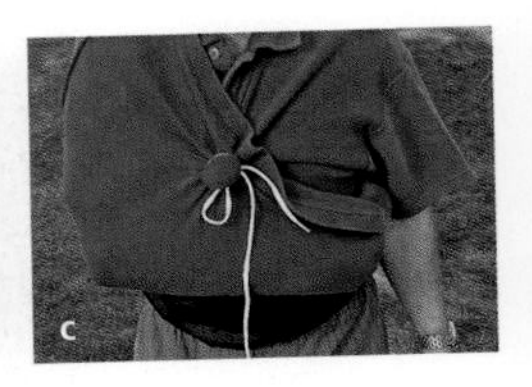

Figures 9.4.13 a–c: *Immobilization of shoulder.*

The entire "sling" must be taut so that the casualty is able to allow his arm to hang in the rectangular position without making any effort (see Figures 9.4.13 a–c).

Immobilisation using a jacket or an anorak (which is just as easy to do) has the advantage that the injured limb is so thoroughly immobilised that even slipping or a fall when walking in rough terrain will not entail any major displacement of the fractured part(s). Protection from the cold is also guaranteed.

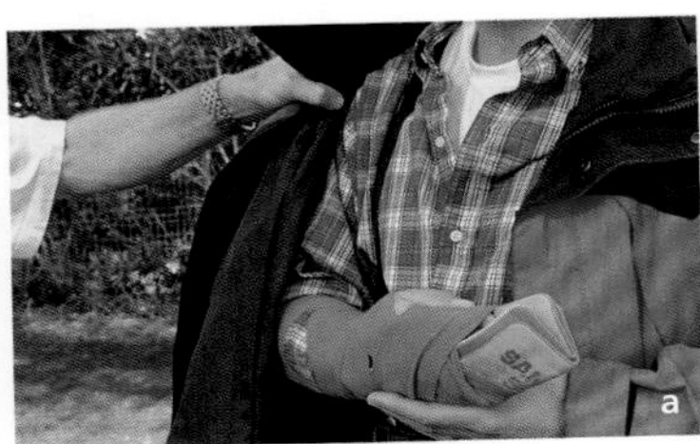
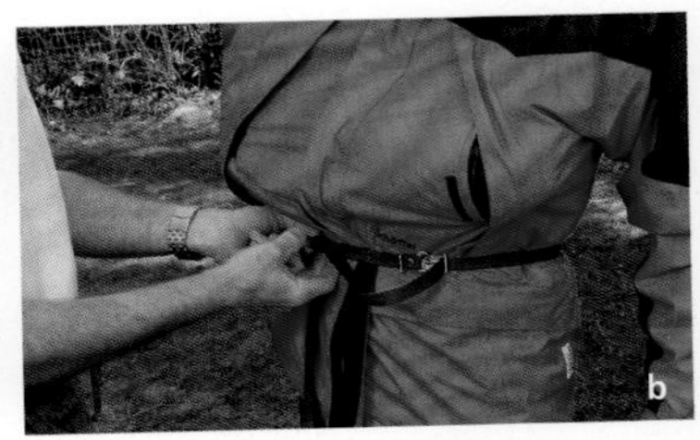

Figures 9.4.14 a–b: *Immobilization of an injured arm. In the picture the arm is already held in position with a SAM® splint (a) and prevented from moving by fastening the jacket tightly (b).*

The casualty uses his uninjured arm to slip on his jacket. It is best if the sleeve on the injured side can be pulled into the jacket so that it can act as a filling and additional padding. The jacket is fastened tightly above the hips using a belt, piece of cord etc. so that the injured arm can be rested on this without straining (see Figures 9.4.14 a–b). Another possible solution is to pull up the Windstopper (see Figures 9.4.15 a–b, Page 139).
Immobilizing the arm using slings or triangular bandages alone is time-consuming and also not as good as "clothing bandages" in terms of stability and pain control.

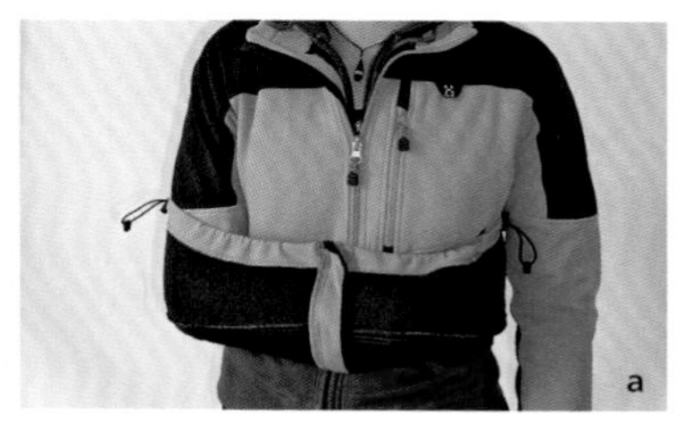

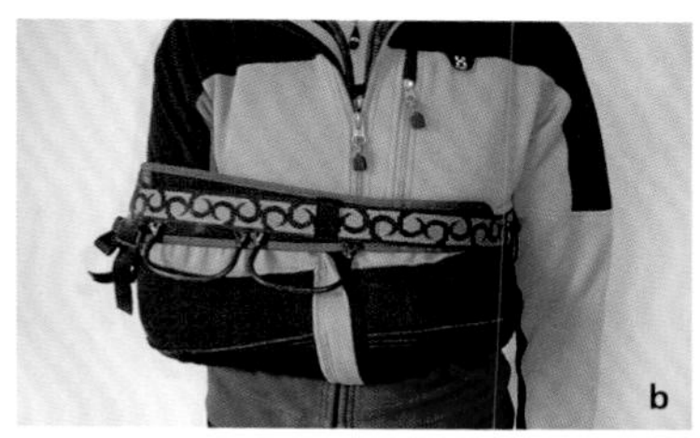

Figures 9.4.15 a–b: *Immobilization of an injured arm using a pulled up Windstopper. This method is suitable for injuries from the shoulder to the forearm. If the item of clothing is tight enough there will be no need to resort to any further means of fixation (a), otherwise the arm can be fixed in position using additional dressings or climbing equipment (b).*

Fixation

The SAM® Splint is highly suitable for fixing and stabilizing a range of injuries in the field.

The **SAM® Splint** was invented by Dr. Sam Scheinberg, an American orthopaedic surgeon, more than 30 years ago. It consists of a strip of soft aluminium, embedded in two layers of closed cell foam.

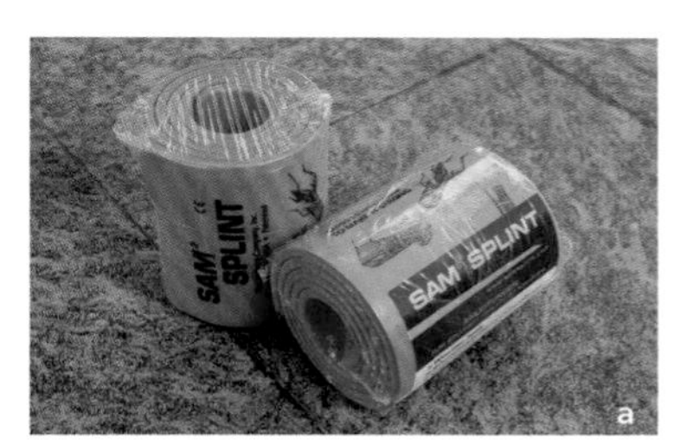

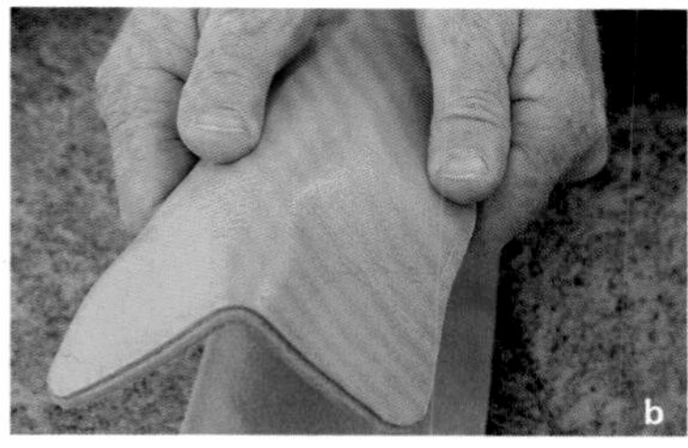

Figures 9.3.16 a–b: *SAM® Splint: Pre-bending the rail into a semi-tubular shape helps to ensure stability.*

Cervical Spine (CS): Until proved otherwise, routinely assume that any unconscious victim of an accident will have a fracture of the cervical spine (CS) (see Section 9.2, Page 108).

Correct immobilization of the cervical spine also helps to keep the airways open in an unconscious casualty.

The SAM® Splint enables rapid improvised immobilization of the CS. One rescuer stabilizes the head and the CS as shown in Figures 9.4.17 a–b. Heavier items of clothing are loosened slightly (or cut open)–long hair and thinner items of clothing can be incorporated without further ado in the SAM® Splint immobilization process.

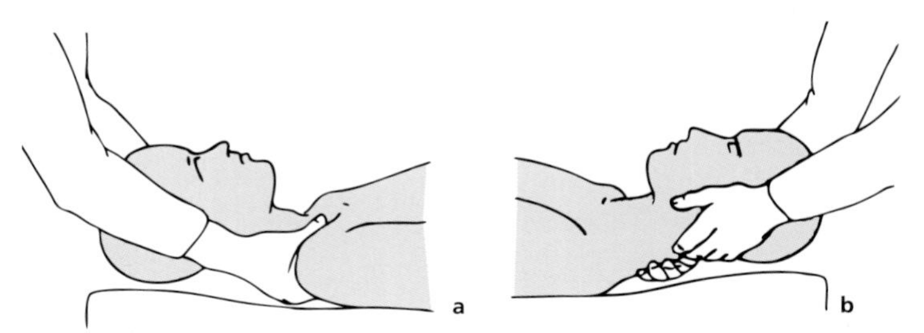

Figures 9.4.17 a–b: *This emergency grip is used if the casualty needs to be repositioned (for example, out of the prone position) before the cervical collar is fitted.*

With the casualty lying on their back (it is difficult in the side or prone position) push one end of the flattened SAM® Splint through under the neck and chin and, using one hand, gently draw up across the throat. At the same time the rescuer at the head must hold it to allow the orthosis to be applied to straighten the neck (do not use force to extend).

The rest of the SAM® Splint is wound gently round the neck and is best secured by means of adhesive or one turn of a bandage (see Figures 9.4.18 a–d).

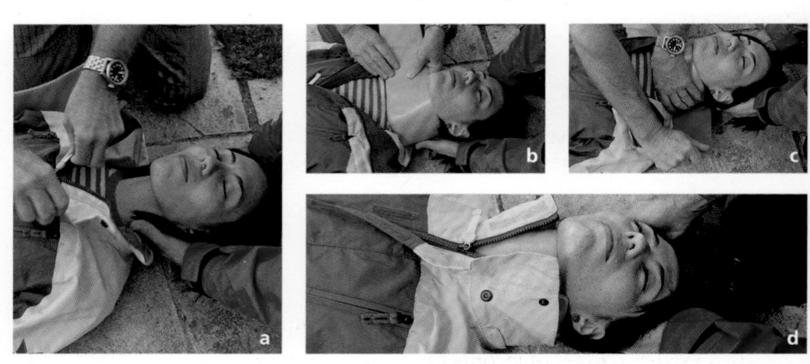

Figures 9.4.18 a–d: *CS fixation with a SAM® Splint. The edge underneath the chin can be bent outwards slightly if necessary.*

If a conscious casualty complains about being able to feel pressure at certain points, this can easily be remedied by bending the material outwards.

Straightening and Reduction of Fractures and Dislocations

When rapid rescue and medical treatment for a significantly displaced bone fracture are not possible (for example, aircraft unable to fly due to the weather, cannoning, caving), an attempt should be made at reduction. Here, continuous traction should be applied to the grotesquely bent limb to make it as straight as the corresponding healthy limb on the other side.

This is because it is possible for the blood vessels, skin, muscles and nerves to be so badly damaged as a result of flexion that a subsequent repair is no longer possible.

These procedures are not always as painful as one may imaginebut may be very painful if the fractured bones are impacted. Compound fractures should be cleansed superficially of coarser particles of dirt before any reduction. This will enable as clean a dressing as possible to be applied post-reduction. Any constriction or strangulation as a result of dressings/bandages must be avoided at all costs although, if there is bleeding, priority must be given to stemming the flow of blood. Before touching the casualty, the most experienced rescuer in the team should briefly think through the planned manœuvre step by step and issue clear instructions to the others. Immediately before reduction, the casualty must be informed about the action planned. Only when the necessary materials (bandages, pieces of cord, SAM® Splints etc.) are to hand can a start be made.
Any painkillers available should of course be administered to the casualty, but don't wait for them to take effect (waste of time–it takes 30–60 minutes for a painkiller to work).

It is important that any material used for fixation should always be adapted to the other (uninjured) limb and that steps are taken to ensure that it is not in contact with the injured limb: every instance of unnecessary contact with the affected part is a pain stimulus that will make the manœuvre more difficult.

In the event of a failure, a second attempt may be made, if feasible; however, under no circumstances should this be insisted on as further damage could be caused as a result of incorrect application of force.

Immobilisation: Any dislocated joint should be immobilised, even after successful reduction. In most cases several weeks of rest are required for the injured structures to regain stability. If we have to carry out a second reduction within short time, immobilisation was insufficient. Even after a successful reduction in the field, the casualty will still need to be checked over by a doctor.

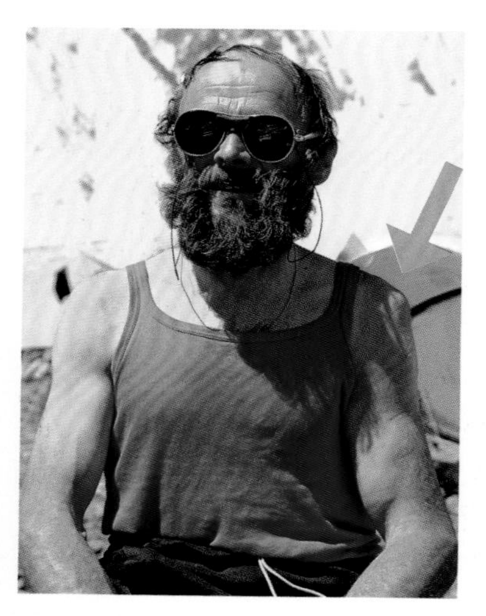

Dislocation of the Shoulder

Dislocation of the shoulder is a frequently occurring injury of the shoulder joint. Helpers in a wilderness environment should be as sure as they possibly can be that the injury is in fact a dislocation of the shoulder and not a fracture of the humerus in proximity to the shoulder (or, in cases involving children and young people, a fracture of the collar bone).

Figure 9.4.19:
Dislocation of the shoulder at the K2 Base Camp. The dislocated head of the left upper arm is readily visible and palpable: a comparison should always be made with the healthy side.

The following criterion has proved itself to be "sufficiently safe" in an emergency environment:

- In a casualty who has suffered a dislocated shoulder, complete adduction of the elbow to bring it closer to the median (sagittal) plane of the body will not be possible (test by applying gentle pressure to the elbow).
- If the casualty is able to press the elbow of the injured upper limb against the body (chest-flank) the injury is very probably not a dislocation of the shoulder joint and reduction must not be attempted. In such cases the arm must be fixed as it is.

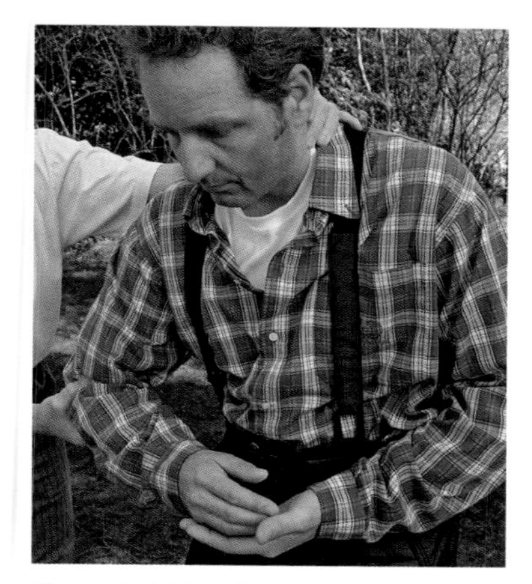

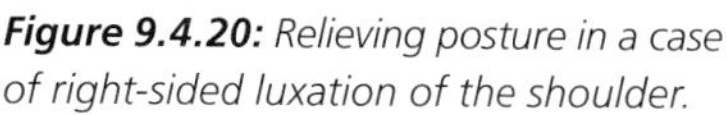

Figure 9.4.20: *Relieving posture in a case of right-sided luxation of the shoulder.*

In an emergency situation shoulder dislocations should only be reduced if no professional help is expected to arrive within the hour (except where the dislocation recurs frequently (this is also termed recurrent dislocation) and the casualty is familiar with the technique to be used). If a reduction is to be attempted it should take place in the first few minutes after the accident before the muscle tension caused by the pain becomes too intense.

Treatment: There are numerous methods for reducing a dislocated shoulder. The Medical Committee of the International Commission for Alpine Rescue (IKAR) recommends the method suggested by the Swiss Federal physician Rudi Campell (approx. 1920) because hardly any additional injuries occur with this method.

Reduction using the Campell Method: The rescuer uses his dominant hand to grip the elbow on the injured side and exerts slight axial tension in the direction away from the shoulder. In this way he attempts, as the casualty lies down, to maintain the angle in the shoulder joint that the casualty has spontaneously adopted as being the least painful.

The rescuer supports the casualty as he lies down by placing the other hand on the nape of his neck. The casualty lies down slowly and cautiously. Before he lies down the rescuer needs to ascertain the length ratios – if the casualty is clearly taller than the rescuer, searching out a location where the rescuer can stand on a boulder, rucksack or similar to ensure sufficient leverage is to be recommended.

Then the rescuer uses both arms to apply progressive traction to the casualty's wrist. The rescuer slowly straightens up, whilst continuing to maintain traction, until he is roughly perpendicular to the casualty's rib cage. If necessary, he may stand on a boulder. Traction is progressive, where possible using the legs and with the arms outstretched, and applied with a force that results in part of the casualty's chest being lifted from the ground.

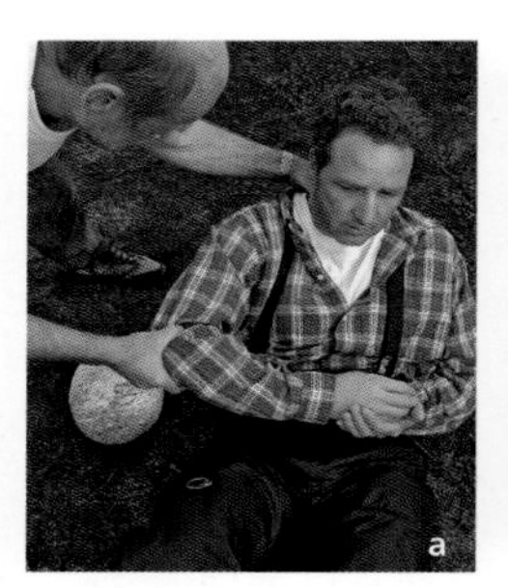
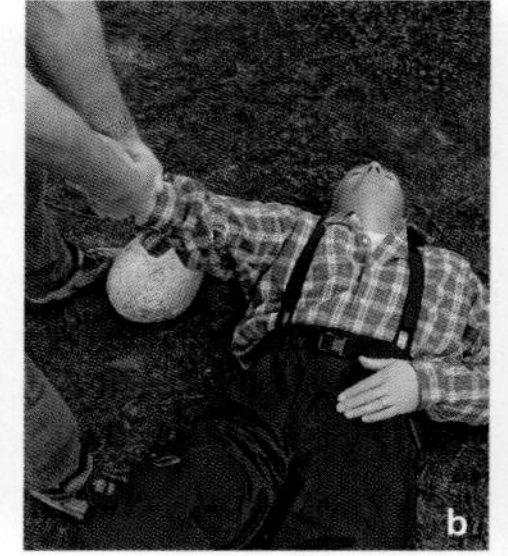
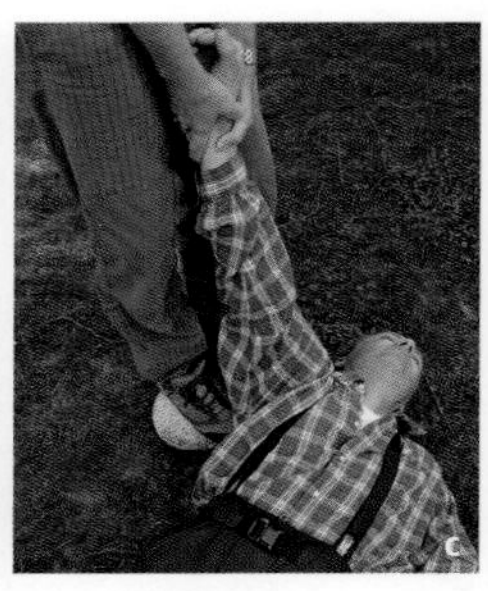

Figures 9.4.21 a–c: *Shoulder reduction using the Campell Method.*

The traction may potentially need to be kept up for several minutes. Wrapping a handkerchief (T-shirt etc.) around the casualty's wrist is recommended to ensure that you do not lose your grip.
The manœuvre must not be allowed to cause any additional pain (apart from the pain associated with lying down); by contrast, applying the traction will cause the pain in the shoulder to gradually diminish. However, gripping the wrist energetically may cause pain.

⇨ If, during the traction phase, there is a significant increase in the pain in the shoulder joint, the attempt must be halted (suspicion of trapped tendons, muscles or nerves).

It is important to **relax** the casualty. Often bystanders can help by distracting the casualty's attention or little tricks can be used, for instance, the rescuer may say to the casualty: "While we are working on your arm, make a fist and try to reach the sky" or "Try hitting me on the nose with your fist." Often an active movement in the shoulder joint on the part of the casualty will succeed in tricking the restraining muscles into a state of relaxation.
Even if the manœuvre is successful the characteristic "pop" when the head of the upper arm springs back into its socket is not always audible. After a few minutes of traction the rescuer will start to become tired and progressively decrease the traction. Sometimes the casualty may feel that the shoulder is "in," even if no sound has been heard. If successful, the pain will be considerably eased or may even have disappeared entirely.

⇨ If the manœuvre is not successful the shoulder will need to be immobilised using the anorak technique and professional assistance sought as quickly as possible (see Figures 9.4.14 a–b, Page 138).

Wrist and forearm: Displaced fractures can be easily reduced by means of traction. Immobilization is best carried out with a SAM® Splint (Figures 9.4.22 a–b) and then deploying a jacket or Windstopper as shown in Figures 9.4.14 and 9.4.15, Pages 138 and 139.

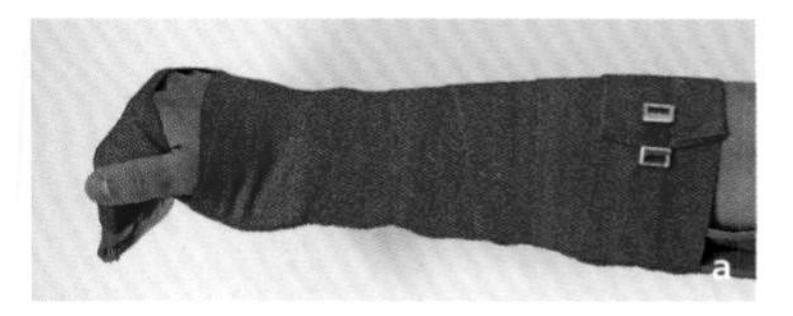

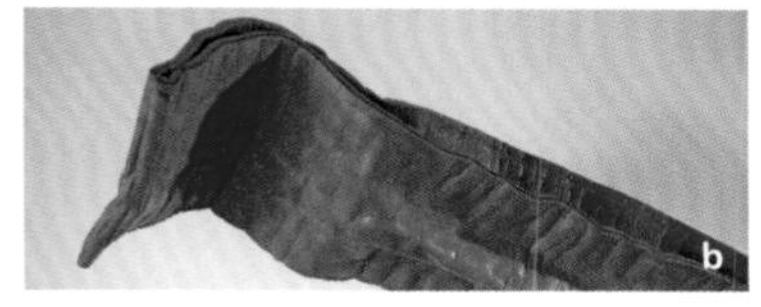

Figures 9.4.22 a–b: *Fixation of the lower arm with SAM® Splint.*

Finger dislocation: This is a not infrequent injury e.g. when cannoning (see Chapter 14, Page 189) and wherever possible, it is better to support oneself with the fist rather than the open hand on slippery rocks.

It is also important with a dislocation of this nature that a successful reduction is carried out as quickly as possible after the accident. As a rule the casualty can fix the dislocation himself by simply pulling on the finger. It will then be no problem to make a finger splint in a short space of time with a piece of SAM® Splint: cut off a piece with a knife or bend the material backwards and forwards a number of times until it breaks (see Figures 9.4.23 a–c).

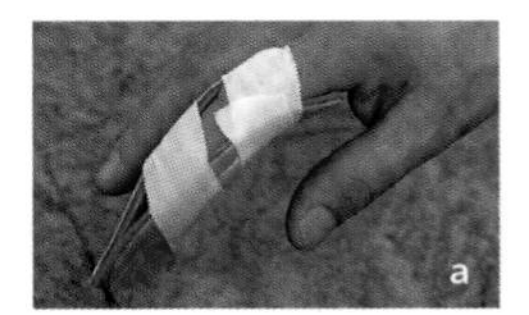

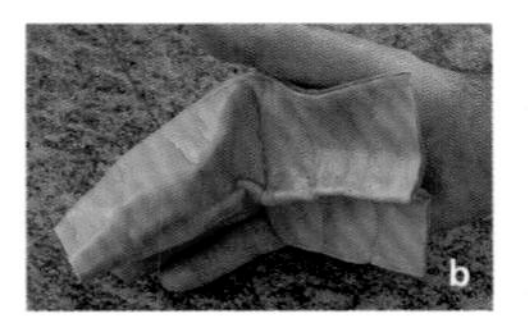

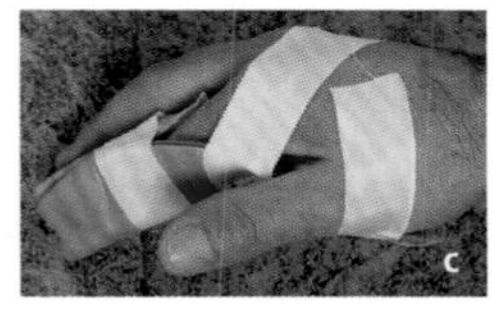

Figures 9.4.23 a–c: *Finger dislocation and fixation with SAM® Splint.*

Elbow, hip and knee dislocation: these are all serious injuries that are difficult for lay persons to reduce in a wilderness environment. Since a high level of force is required for a reduction, even in hospital it is normal practice for an anesthetic to be administered. Accompanying injuries are common. The best that can be done in the field is to fix the joint in the appropriate position in order to minimize the pain.

Dislocation of the upper ankle joint (talocrural region): this injury is generally associated with a fracture of the tibiofibular joint and should wherever possible be reduced in order to minimize any additional damage to soft tissues and for better pain control.

The shoes should, as a matter of principle, not be removed. If the shoe is felt to be too tight, carefully undo the straps or loosen the laces (even cut open if necessary). Even if there is blood visible in the shoe, removing it is not recommended. **Exception:** If the rescue is likely to take some time or if one is reliant on one's own resources, only remove the shoe once a safe place has been reached. The swelling can endanger the soft tissues and an assessment of the foot cannot be carried out while it is still in the shoe. Good insulation is very important where there is a risk of freezing to death, otherwise, raise the affected limb and keep it cool!

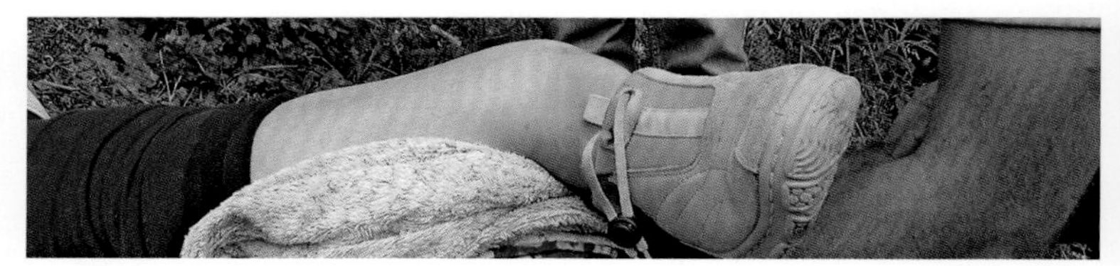

Figure 9.4.24: *Abnormal position of the ankle.*

The casualty is gripped by a rescuer in such a way that there is no risk of him pulling away when traction is applied to his leg and he also feels safe (see Figure 9.4.25 a). Without touching the injured leg, use the uninjured foot to size the SAM® Splint(s). Ensure that a bandage or a piece of cord (shoelace, belt etc.) is ready.

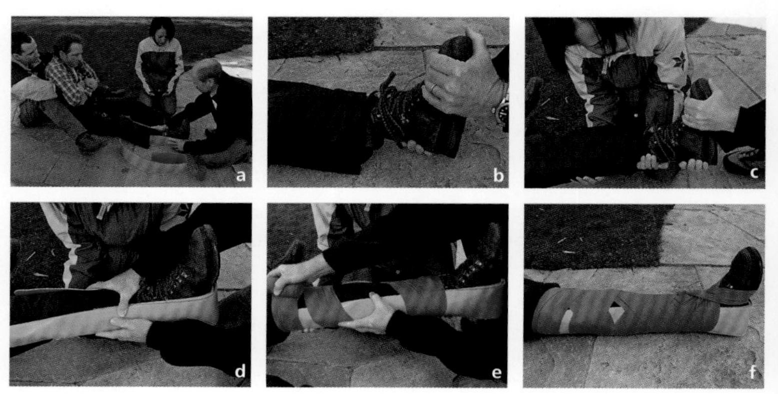

Figures 9.4.25 a–f: *Fixation of lower leg together with ankle.*

The planned procedure is explained to the casualty and the rescuers.

The rescuer grasps the heel and toe of the shoe with both hands and pulls progressively and hard (but not jerkily) in the direction of the long axis of the leg (see Figure 9.4.25 b, Page 146). With assistance from another rescuer, arrange one or two preformed SAM® Splints in a U shape above the ankle and bind firmly using a bandage or another material. The upper ends of the SAM® Splint should be covered wherever possible by the bandage material as the free ends are no longer capable of fulfilling a stabilizing function (see Figures 9.4.25 c–f, Page 146).

If there is no immediate success with realignment, a second attempt will usually be pointless because of muscular pain inhibition of the affected limb. The upper ankle joint will need to be splinted in the position it was in following the accident and evacuation organised as quickly as possible.

Preparations and Evacuation

Once the organized rescue service has been informed and is on its way, the preparations for evacuation are straightforward:

- Be as calm and positive as possible in all dealings with the casualty, find out who is to inform whom and when (parents, friends)
- Use clothing, aluminium foil and similar items to keep the casualty warm (even in summer!)
- Insulate the casualty from the ground (rucksack) if they can be moved
- If the casualty wishes, give them something to drink (best of all water or tea)
- If sufficient time is available, the doctors responsible will find a report helpful in which the time of the accident and the any change in condition are noted down (e.g. on an accident sheet)*

If transport cannot be organized through a professional organization, the most experienced rescuer will find himself confronted by a challenging job.

* e.g. Emergency Information Sheet Swiss Federal Office for Sport (BASPO) 2532 Magglingen

He must at all costs assume a clear **"position of leadership"** and analyse the situation as comprehensively as possible (take a little time for this!): Where are we going? How many rescuers are there? Is there any risk of making the casualty's situation worse by transporting them? Can we manage this or do we need to wait for a terrestrial rescue team to arrive?

In Switzerland it will often be possible to make contact by mobile phone with a mountain hut close by if the weather is poor and to request rescuers and transport materials (blankets, stretchers, sledges). All the points addressed above will also apply when it comes to making preparations for improvised transport. In addition, particular consideration must be given to preventing the casualty from becoming chilled. Patients who need to be transported lying in a supine position are best off wrapped in a sleeping bag.

Improvised Transport

During inclement weather in particular it may from time to time be preferable to carry the casualty to a safe place (house, hut, tent, vehicle) rather than wait in the rain for the organized rescue squad. This decision may be taken in collaboration with the emergency response center (Tel. 144) who can tell the rescuer how long a terrestrial rescue team would need to reach the point where the accident has occurred.

Single Rescuer Method (casualty with minor injuries – not unconscious)

Climbing rope: If there is a climbing rope available it will be possible to create a practical carrying structure in just a few minutes.

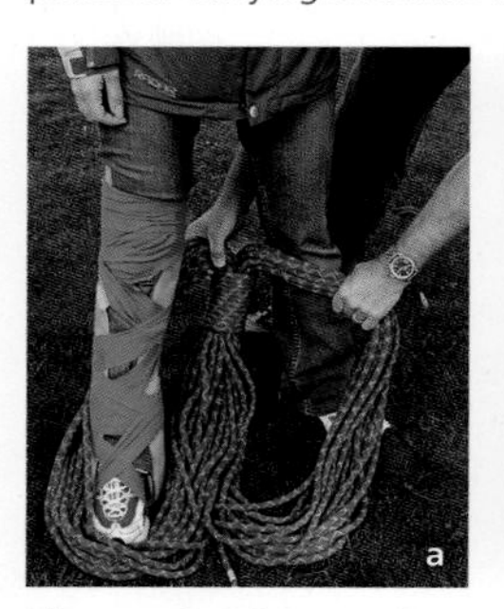

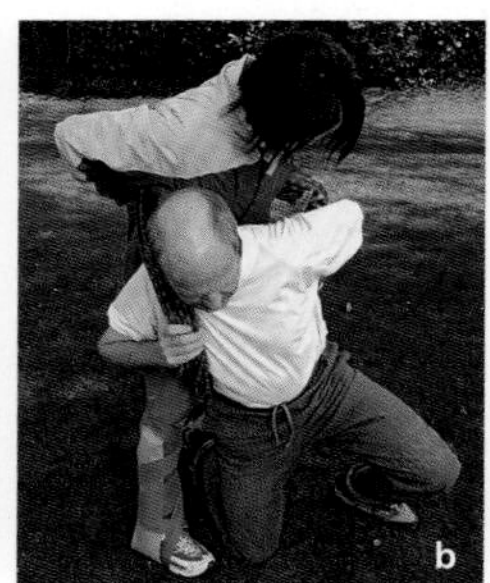

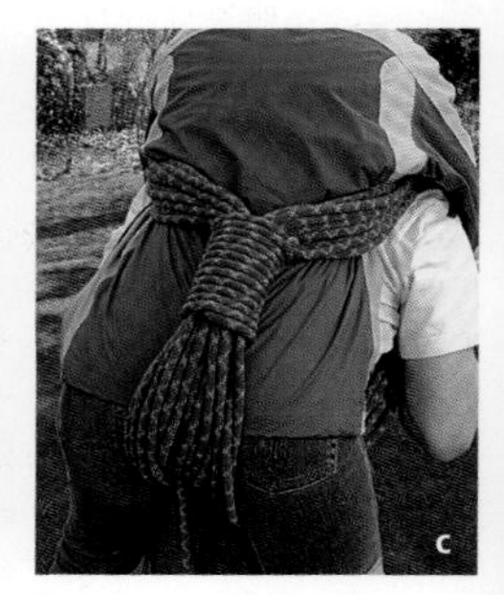

Figures 9.4.26 a–c: *Evacuation using a rope makeshift: The rope needs to be threaded through the ring. The size of the ring must be adapted so that it will accommodate the carrier's body and that of the casualty (experiment in advance!).*

Helped by the person who is to carry him, the casualty climbs into the rope ring. The casualty pulls the rope seat created up over his hips. The rescuer hoists up his "load" in a piggyback fashion. When straightening up with a heavy person, the rescuer is recommended to use a boulder, tree, hedge or similar to pull himself up so as to minimize the load on his knees.
The position of the knot in the rope is important: this must be located at belt height on the casualty's back.
Carrying someone over short distances in this way is not unduly strenuous. The disadvantage of this method lies in the fact that the casualty's legs hang down to a relatively low level; the casualty tends to catch his (injured…) feet when going downhill and only one rucksack/piggyback load (in this case, the casualty) can be carried at once.

Rucksack Technique: Select the rucksack with the longest straps. The rucksack can be kept full but should, for obvious reasons, not be too heavy… it is beneficial, before loading up, to have cushioning material (gloves, caps, handkerchiefs etc.) at the ready for the carrier's shoulders. The straps on the rucksack should be let out so that they are as long as possible and the casualty, assisted by the carrier, manœuvres himself into the straps of the rucksack.

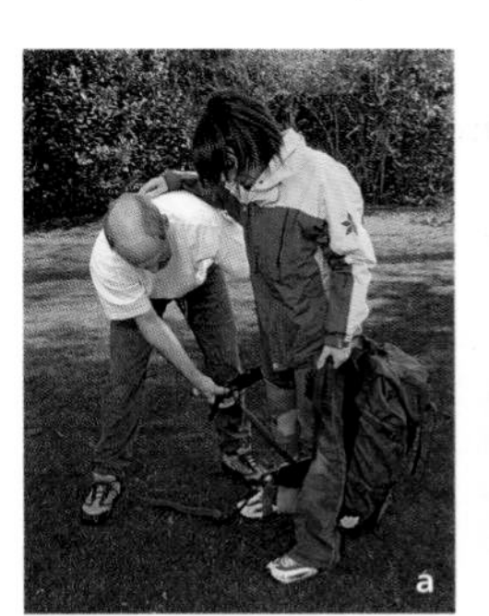

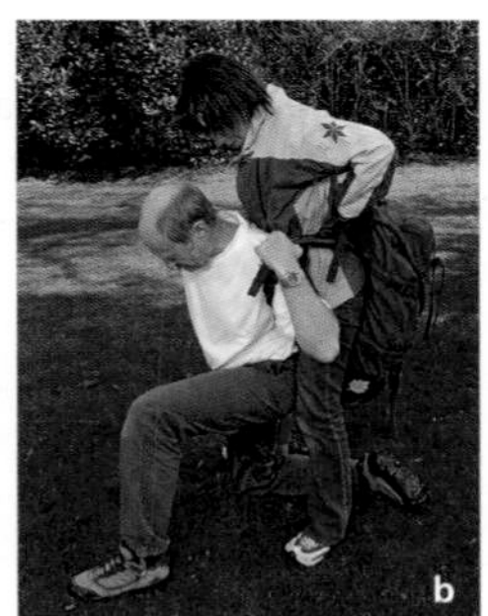

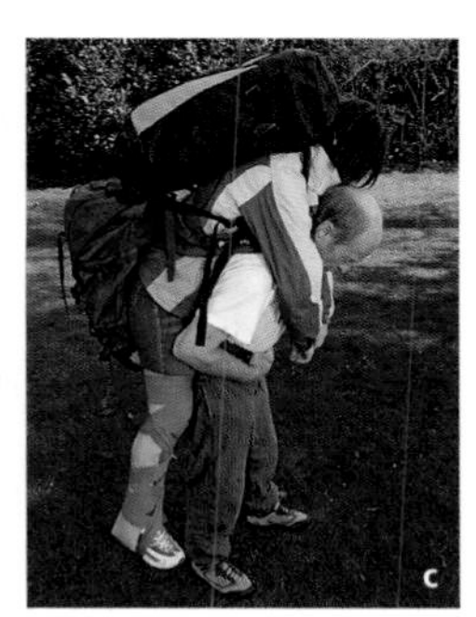

Figures 9.4.27 a–c: *Rucksack "Port-A-Casualty."*

The casualty then pulls the rucksack up as far as possible over his hips and the carrier slips into the straps, pads his shoulders and heaves the casualty aloft (supporting himself, if possible, on stones, trees etc.). At the same time the carrier needs to tell the casualty that he will finish up lying high up on the carrier's shoulders and that he could fall head first over the front.

If possible, the carrier should fasten the hip belt on the rucksack underneath the casualty's legs so that some of the weight is transferred to the hips.

The advantage of this method is that it is quick to set up, plus it means that the casualty tends to be positioned higher above the shoulders of the person carrying him and, in addition, that both rucksacks (the carrier's and the casualty's) can be taken along. This can be important on expeditions when material necessary for survival must not be left behind.

Multi-Rescuer Method

Repositioning: The methods shown in the following may be deployed to lie the casualty on a transportation structure or to transport him over short distances. As long as the casualty is being moved the CS must be protected, even once an improvised neck collar has been installed. The rescuer at the head is the one who issues the instructions.

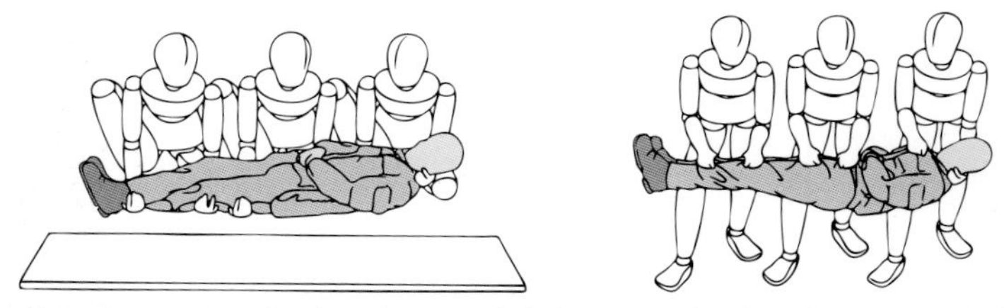

Figures 9.4.28 a–b: *Shovel grip and clothes grip: The shovel grip is particularly suitable for moving people on an Incline. The clothes grip is a very gentle way of handling people who are badly injured (including people with spinal injuries.*

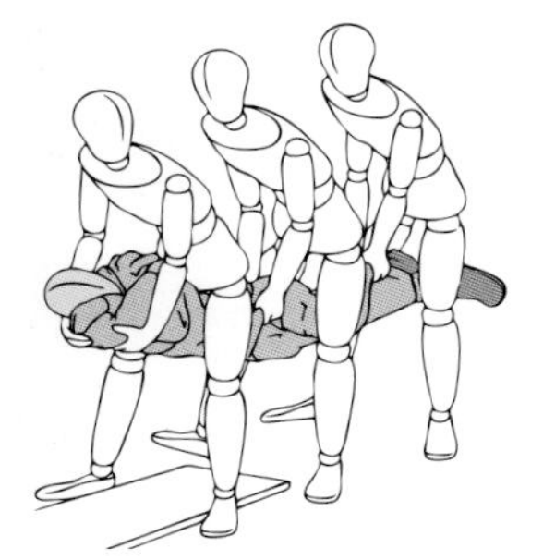

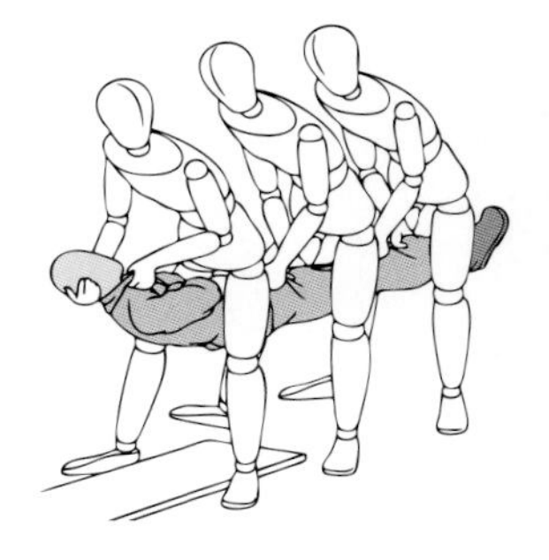

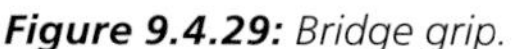

Figure 9.4.29: *Bridge grip.*

Rucksack stretcher: This makeshift stretcher is extraordinarily quick to cobble together (less than two minutes). The material required is no more than an individual would normally carry with them on a hike. It offers the opportunity to improvise a way of transporting even seriously injured and/or unconscious casualties as well as people with spinal injuries.

If there is any suspicion of spinal injuries, it is important to weigh up carefully whether the casualty should in fact be transported or not. However, there are situations where it is simply not reasonable to expect the patient to wait around for hours in the cold and wind.

If a fractured femur is suspected, secure the injured leg to the healthy one and transport the casualty on the stretcher.

Rucksack stretcher: depending on the casualty's height, you may need to select three or four rucksacks. It is best not to empty the rucksacks–they should all be more or less filled to bulging. Lay the rucksacks in a row on the ground and link up the carrying straps. In order to undo the straps you will need to cut open the seam at the end of the straps at strategic points. Leave the waist belts wide open, pull up the straps of the rucksack just as far as is necessary to ensure that, once the casualty has been placed on the stretcher, they are not underneath him.

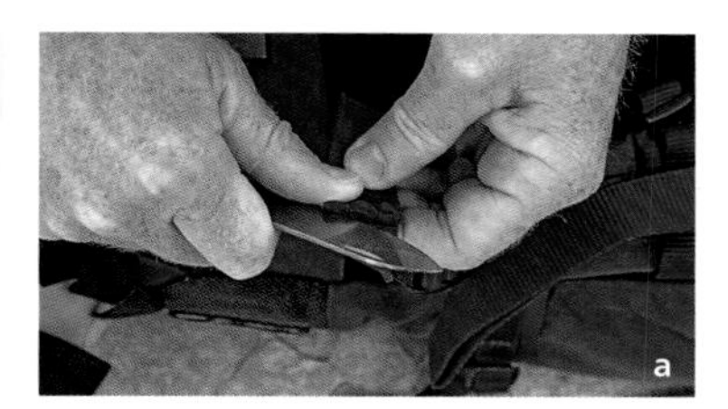

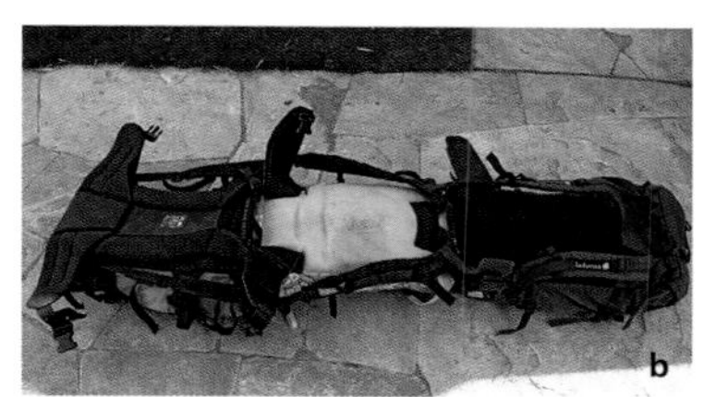

Figures 9.4.30 a–b: *Rucksack stretcher.*

The stretcher should be constructed as close as possible to the casualty or brought over so that it is lying close to him. Using either the shovel grip or the clothes grip technique, position the casualty on the stretcher, not forgetting to stabilize the CS and the head (SAM® Splint, in-line stabilization).
The casualty is then fastened securely to the stretcher using the hip belts on the rucksacks. The rucksack straps must now been tightened so that they are very taut in order to ensure that they are not torn off while the stretcher is being carried.

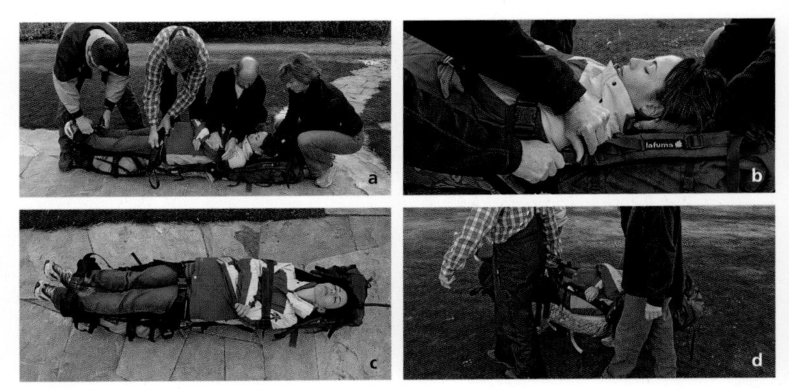

Figures 9.4.31 a–d: *Stabilization and Transport.*

Depending on the size of the casualty and the conditions under foot, the stretcher may be carried by four or six rescuers each using one hand each. This means that each will have one hand free to hold on with or to stabilize himself where necessary (in woodland etc.). It is important that the stretcher is carried only by the carrying straps of the rucksacks and not by any smaller straps that may also be affixed to the rucksacks.

With some imagination, further improvements can be made if the transportation exercise looks like taking longer (e.g. on expeditions). Attaching a carabiner and a rope sling to the straps of the rucksack, the whole of the body (via the shoulders) can be mobilised as part of the carrying exercise. Ski sticks can also be inserted into the rucksack straps and these will provide even more stability for the structure. In special cases the casualty may be wrapped in a sleeping bag before being placed on the stretcher.

Removal of finger rings in an emergency situation

Any injury to the hand (not only an injury to the ring finger) calls for any rings on the fingers to be removed as quickly as possible unless the swelling has become too pronounced.

One neat approach which works in most cases is to swaddle the finger using a thread (dental floss, core of a rope or bootlace, sewing thread ...).

Then insert one end of the thread under the ring and push the ring as close as possible to the middle joint of the finger. Having done this, the rescuer holds the end of the thread firmly with his finger and slowly and carefully starts to wrap the rest of the thread (which should be about 60 cm long) round the finger below the ring.

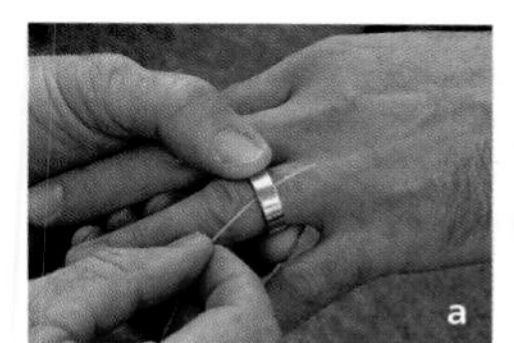

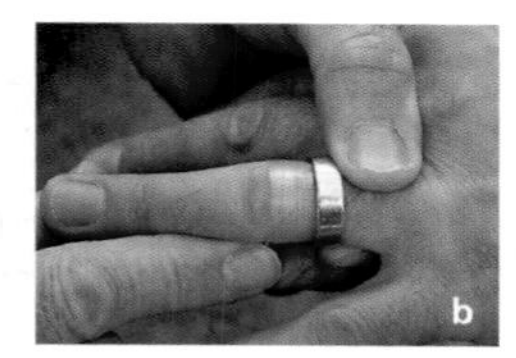

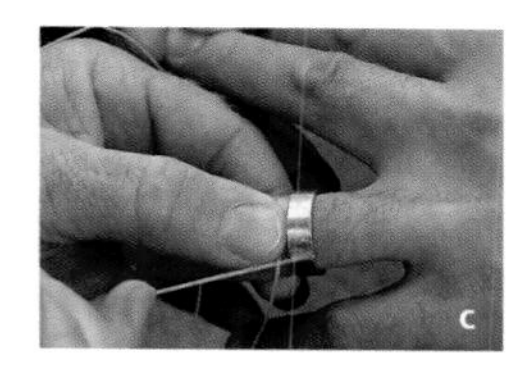

Figures 9.4.32 a–c: *Removing a ring.*

It is important to take your time over this procedure and to neatly wrap the thread around the finger turn by turn so that the thickened part of the middle joint is tightly covered. Then, holding the lower end of the thread firmly, pull slowly on the end over the ring on the hand side. As a result of the gradual pulling, the ring will usually slide over the middle joint and come off the finger shortly after that. The entire procedure may cause some pain–especially if the finger has already started to swell as a result of the injury.
In most instances it is not possible to remove a finger ring in a wilderness environment using knives, clippers etc.

Bivouacs-Basic Principles

Setting up an emergency bivouac is out of the scope of this medical book. If at all possible the following principles should be borne in mind:

- Give some thought to a bivouac in good time before the group becomes tired and cold.
- Wind, moisture and lack of water (dehydration) are the most important factors to be anticipated which will affect the ability to maintain body heat. For this reason, when constructing a bivouac, you should make sure that you do not overexert yourself to the extent that you end up sweating because this will mean that your clothes will be wet through and a great deal of heat will be lost from your body. If at all possible change your clothes as soon as the bivouac is completed.
- Ensure that you make every effort to insulate yourself against the ground (sit on your rucksack, rope slings, skis).
- Remember that, in a tightly sealed snow hole, the oxygen can be used up and/or there may be too much carbon dioxide in the air. This will initially lead to sleepiness, then to unconsciousness and finally to death. If you have a candle to hand you should let it burn. If it goes out on its own then that is the time to take urgent action to obtain fresh air! The same applies to high altitude army tents that get snowed in and thus inevitably become more and more airtight.

9.5 Triage in Situations involving Multiple Casualties

Accidents take place unexpectedly. If you are lucky you will find yourself reasonably well equipped and the accident victim to rescuer ratio will be good–with the majority of mountain accidents more than one person is available to tend to the needs of an injured party. In such situations there will be no need to give consideration to the question of triage or shortage of resources.

However, sometimes accidents occur when there is no first aid kit available. In a worst-case scenario an uninjured person may be required to look after a number of casualties, some of whom may even be seriously injured–here things may become critical and, under certain circumstances, one may even be forced to decide where one's skills can best be deployed.
Extreme situations of this kind are easier to overcome if one has already given some thought to this previously and if one is familiar with some of the principles of triage.

The term **triage** is derived from military jargon where they have been familiar with this problem ever since the first wartime confrontations–there were always too many wounded individuals and the resources had to be deployed constructively right from the start–i.e. as far as possible no resources were to be wasted on hopeless cases.

In the civil sector the important thing is to save all lives and determining the priorities depends on the degree of severity of the injuries. Decisions about the chances of survival and likely response to therapy do not usually belong at the scene of an accident–except, perhaps, in extreme situations with many people gravely injured casualties and only a few rescuers.
The following basic rules relating to triage may be helpful (see also Section 9.1, Page 91).

Safety–Look–Think–Act
Alert–Make Safe–Rescue

Only once the first two of these principles have been taken into account that you can start thinking about First Aid. Where there is a shortage of resources one does not have the luxury of meaningless actions and merely coasting along and, for this reason, a good overview and targeted actions are all the more important. Two further principles should therefore be borne in mind here:

Classification of Casualties in accordance with ABC

Before doing anything, each potential casualty should be assessed and roughly divided up into problem category A, B, or C (see also Section 9.2, Page 97). The assessment should not take more than 30 seconds. This is the actual triage process. Patients who are walking around, shouting and calling out are not likely to fit into the "A and B" problems category.

⇨ The problems of the injured parties can change at any time.

If you are present at the time an accident occurs (e.g. a hiking group is caught up in a fairly sizable rock fall) it can be assumed that even very badly injured persons will still be alive during the first few minutes, even though they may possibly have come away with fatal injuries. Even a professional rescuer cannot make a definitive decision at this point in time and we need to treat these casualties as a high priority, even though they may have poor chances of survival. It is only where death has obviously occurred instantly that a casualty can be assessed as no longer treatable in the early phase. Such a decision is, however, only possible as far as lay persons are concerned where the physical injuries are very serious and are not compatible with life (e.g. massive crushing, decapitation).

The next step in the triage sequence is:

Treatment of the Casualty on the basis of ABC

Essentially, the treatment of a number of injured parties (as is also the case when attending to just one injured person) must be conducted in accordance with the rules of the ABC. This means that a casualty with an A problem (e.g. unconscious and with airways obstructed by blood) must be treated before the casualty with a B or C problem. When faced with the dilemma of what to do when two A casualties are present at the same time, there is unfortunately no solution. Here any decision has to be taken on the basis of other criteria (for example, children/young persons before older people). In a tragic extreme situation, a rescuer may well have to decide in favor of one casualty, knowing that the other will not survive. Such situations, which are associated with major psychological strain, are fortunately extremely rarely.

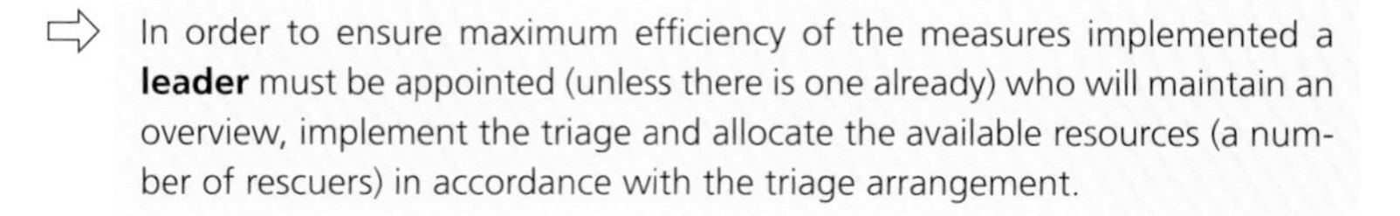

⇨ In order to ensure maximum efficiency of the measures implemented a **leader** must be appointed (unless there is one already) who will maintain an overview, implement the triage and allocate the available resources (a number of rescuers) in accordance with the triage arrangement.

10. Ski and High Alpine Tours

B. Durrer

Various hazards lie in wait in the snow-covered mountains. The most important of these are avalanches, cold and, in the high mountains, crevasses. By adopting the appropriate behavior it is possible to minimize all these risks.

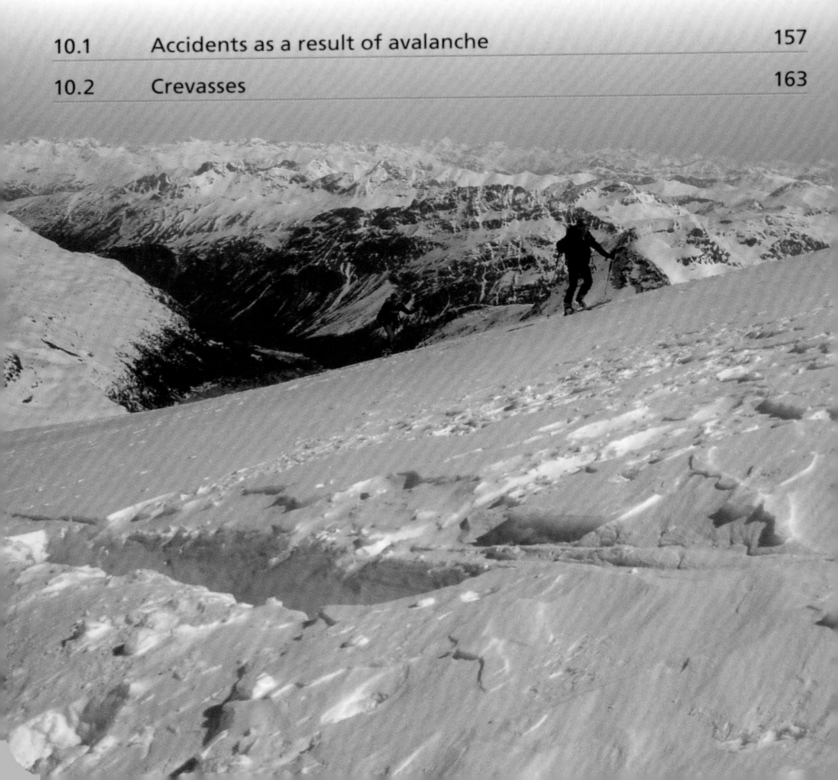

10.1 Accidents as a result of avalanche

Causes of Death and the Chances of Survival

The majority of victims of avalanche suffocate. This is why every second counts in an avalanche accident. Despite all the high-tech survival and orientation devices, being buried in an avalanche still represents the highest possible risk to life.
65–80 % of all persons buried will suffocate, 15–25 % will die from their injuries while only approx. 5 % will succumb to general hypothermia. In addition to the lack of oxygen, the increase in carbon dioxide (used air) in the air pocket also seems to play a negative role as far as survival is concerned.

The chances of surviving being buried completely will depend on the duration of burial. Within the first 15 minutes of burial the chance of survival is 92 %! Between 35 and 90 minutes it is around 30 %, after 130 minutes it is only 3 %.

The first 15 minutes are crucial!

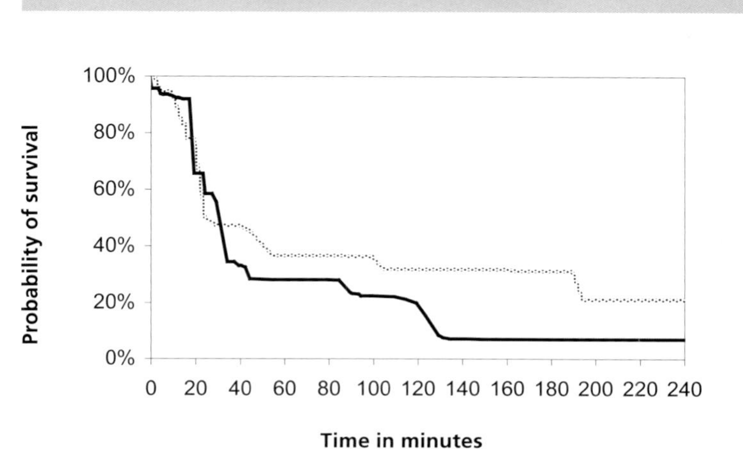

Figure 10.1: *Likelihood of survival–persons totally buried Switzerland 1981–1998 (n = 735) dependent on duration of burial (minutes) in the open air (black, n = 638) and in buildings, on traffic routes (gray, n = 97).*
Reprinted from: Brugger H., Durrer B., Adler-Kastner L., Falk M., Tschirky F. Field Management of Avalanche Victims. Resuscitation 2001; 51:7–15 with the kind permission of Elsevier Science.

Prevention

In Switzerland around 25 persons still die every year as a result of being buried by an avalanche. With the right preparation and information from local mountaineering professionals it should be possible to reduce this number. Achieving this calls for a precise study of the Avalanche Bulletin and the Weather Report as well as selecting ski tours correspondingly (exposure and inclination of the slope?). Experience, caution and the exercise of a skilled approach are the best protection against accidents as a result of avalanches. Ignorance and arrogance lead to accidents. The way to gain experience is to get out and about with mountain guides and to attend avalanche courses.

Technical aids that will help to prevent any risk of being buried (e.g. airbags), reduce the amount of time during which a person is buried (e.g. devices that are able to detect people who have been buried by avalanches [LVS], avalanche cord, avalanche ball) or which are designed to prolong the period of survival after a person has been buried (e.g. Avalung) can instill a **false sense of security.** An avalanche always represents a risk to life. So never ever risk being buried!

(See also "Safety in the Mountains," Pages 18–22). Should you, despite all the preparations and precautionary measures, be unlucky enough to encounter an avalanche, here are some guidelines on how to respond:

- Make every effort to get out of the area of the avalanche as quickly as possible.
- Release as quickly as possible your skis, poles and, if necessary, rucksack. Note: Binding straps are dangerous! Ski stoppers are better.
- Try to get your knee against your chest and hold your arms in a protective pose in front of your face so as to create a small hollow to enable you to breathe once the avalanche has come to a standstill.

Location and Excavation

When it comes to locating people buried by avalanches there are feature-independent (e.g. avalanche dogs) and feature-dependent (e.g. avalanche transceiver, Recco) search methods. In an ideal situation, a successful **Companion Rescue** (location, extrication and First Aid by the Group) will be mounted within the first 15 minutes to assist a victim of an avalanche. The organized rescue facility (helicopter and ARS/KWRO rescue squad or piste patrol) will as a rule take longer than 15 minutes to arrive at the location of the accident.

Companion Rescue

Taking into account the chances of survival, it is essential that a buried person is dug out of the snow within 15 minutes. Today, carrying an avalanche transceiver represents the gold standard on ski tours and is recommended as a precautionary measure, regardless of the avalanche risk. However, any device is only as good as the user's training and the amount of practice he or she has had. An avalanche transceiver offers no protection against avalanches but will enable a victim's companions to rapidly search a large area. The avalanche transceiver also includes an avalanche shovel and a probe pole.

In around a third of all ski tour accidents involving avalanches, a number of persons are buried. The latest avalanche transceiver digital instruments will indicate multiple burials and are sometimes fitted with an additional impulse detector. Where a number of people are buried this makes it possible, if need be, to triage on the avalanche field which locations need to be excavated as a priority. All alpine clubs and climbing schools offer practical avalanche transceiver courses. Preparations of this nature are absolutely necessary to help participants get to know their own equipment.

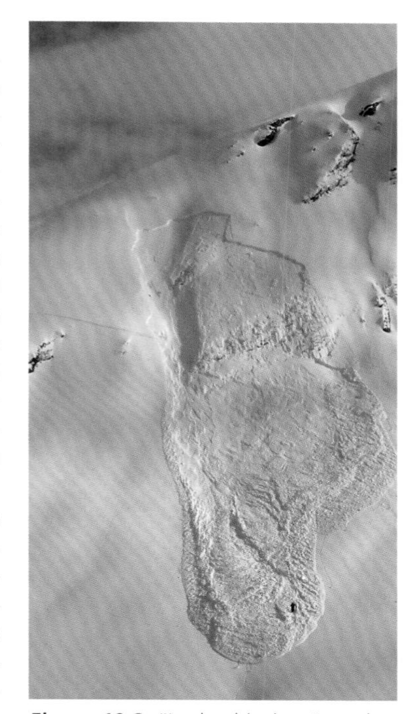

Figure 10.2: *"Lucky this time," partly buried off-piste skier is able to free himself and raise the alarm. No ava-* lanche transceiver *device with him. Preventive deployment in the Avers Region (D. Hunziker).*

Deployment Tactics

Following an accident involving an avalanche, finding the victims is the top priority. The **alarm can be raised** by cellphone or by radio without losing any time (see Section 9.1, Page 92). At the same time the search can be commenced without delay with all necessary helpers. If no cellphone reception, priority must be given to searching. Help must be called at the latest after 15 minutes of searching without success.

Organized Avalanche Rescue

As far as organized rescue is concerned, 90 minutes is regarded as the guide time for successful retrieval of those still alive who have managed to maintain a closed air pocket.

It is here that the avalanche dog is still the best means of location when it comes to a feature-independent search.

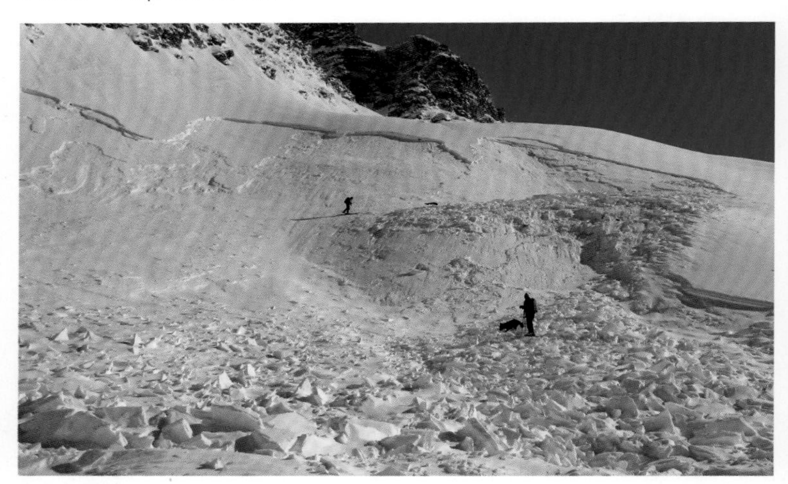

Figure 10.3: *Hunting for buried persons with avalanche dog. Skier on a tour is located with the help of an avalanche dog and retrieved dead. No avalanche transceiver device with him. Piz Lischana (W. Kuhn).*

First Aid on an Avalanche Field

If the head of the casualty is not buried under the mass of snow, we talk of "partial" as opposed to "complete burial."

With victims of complete burial the head must be uncovered as quickly as possible so that the ABC measures (see Section 9.2, Page 99) can be started.

⇨ Free airways (mouth and nose not blocked with snow) are one sign of an **air pocket.** i.e. that the person buried in the avalanche was still breathing.

The air pocket itself, which is defined as a free space regardless of how large it is, in front of mouth/nose is very difficult to assess on the avalanche field as it is frequently destroyed during the rescue. For further medical decisions (e.g. triage as arranged by the emergency doctor where there are several victims) the presence of an air pocket, given a period of burial in excess of 35 minutes, is of major importance: survival will not be possible without an air pocket.

The victim is completely dug out and carefully resuscitated. In addition, protecting them from any further chilling (hot drinks for conscious victims, protection from the wind, insulating blankets, thermal body bags, possibly warmth provided by companions) is crucial: in particular, ground insulation (conduction) and insulation against the wind (convection). Where there is a risk of potential heat loss due to the wind (convection), it may be necessary for the victim to remain in the snow cavity (duly protected) until he or she can be evacuated.

⇨ The post-rescue avalanche victim has the propensity to cool down twice as quickly as in the avalanche!

All victims must be taken to a place which is safe from avalanche. Persons who have been completely buried are best off being flown to hospital.

⇨ An avalanche victim can never be warmed up out of doors but at the most protected against further cooling.

Victims who are conscious:

- Protect against further cooling (including hot drinks)
- Evacuate under strict supervision (response capability, breathing, pulse)
- Where dulled awareness is a feature (hardly responding, motionless) a rescued person must never be forced into active movement (risk of post-rescue demise) (see also Section 18.2, Page 232).

Unconscious victim breathing normally:

- Lay carefully on his side, take into account risk of post-rescue demise (see also Section 9.4, Page 125)
- Provide protection from further chilling
- Strict monitoring of consciousness, breathing and pulse

Unconscious victim with no signs of life:

- Action to resuscitate as per Section 9.2, Page 99
- Protect from further cooling
- Resuscitation must be continued for as long as necessary until the casualty is handed over to the professional rescue services (see Section 9.2, Page 111)
- Death at the scene of the accident must be established by a doctor (and often not until after rewarming)

Case Study

A snowshoe trekker is buried by a snow slab on the Jungfraujoch one New Year's Eve at around 17.00 hrs just as it is getting dark. The alarm is raised by his colleagues during a snowstorm at night. Purely terrestrial response with the rescue team and the avalanche dog abseiling 150 m on to the avalanche cone. Unconscious, hypothermic accident victim (hypothermia HT III, core temperature 28 °C) is dug out after 3 hours 40 minutes from 1 m of snow. Careful rescue, protection against further chilling provided by means of insulation and thermal bags and buried person subsequently brought on to the Jungfraujoch using hoists and pulleys. Removal to hospital via the Jungfrau railway and the ambulance. On arrival the avalanche victim has become responsive with a body core temperature of 35.5 Grad.

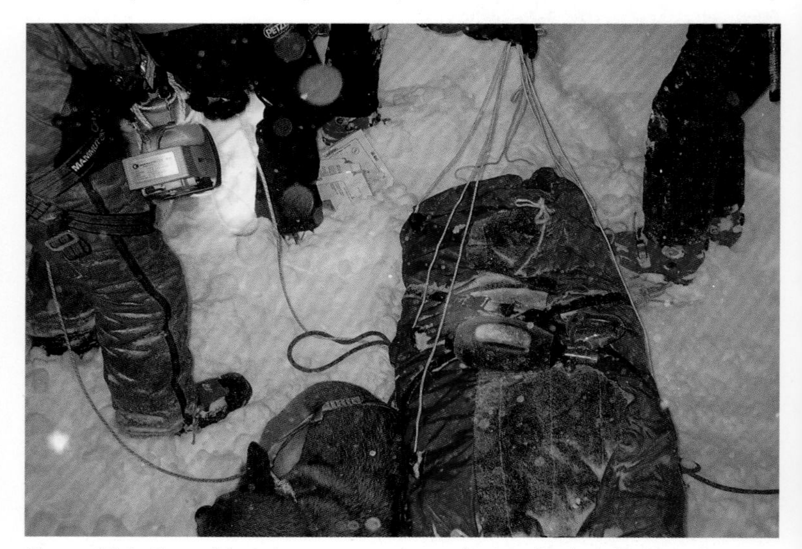

Figure 10.4: *Ground-based rescue attempt on the Jungfraujoch (B. Durrer).*

10.2 Crevasses

In the Swiss Alps each year, 40–50 crevasse accidents occur leaving 10–15 people dead. In addition to general hypothermia, injuries frequently play an important role.

Hazards

Following an accident involving becoming stuck in a crevasse, the victim undergoes rapid chilling and can develop life-threatening hypothermia within 1–2 hours. Suspension trauma may occur much faster as a result of the additional weight (heavy rucksack and skis on the feet). The know-how for a rapid companion rescue and support exercise is especially important in such situations (see Section 20.3, Page 265).

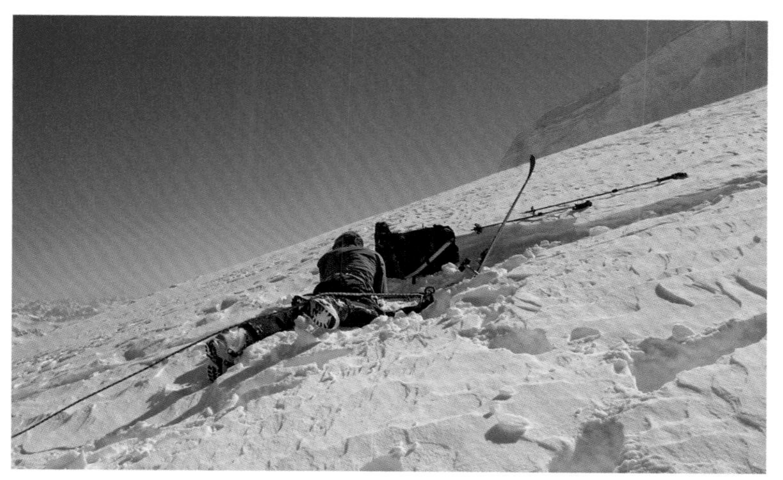

Figure 10.5: *Companion Rescue on glacier ski tour on the Sella Glacier–Bernina Group (D. Hunziker).*

Measures to be adopted

- Raise alarm immediately if the rescue of an uninjured person is not immediately possible using own resources.
- Prepare anchors (embed pickaxes, ski etc.)
- After the rescue give First Aid at the edge of the crevice with attention to injuries and the measures appropriate in the event of hypothermia (see Section 18.2, Page 232) and suspension trauma (Section 20.3, Page 265).

11. Sport Climbing

Ch. Schlegel, A. Schweizer, H.P. Bircher

Sport climbing and bouldering has been enjoying increasing popularity over the past decade. Already a high athletic level has been achieved across a wide swathe as a result of the availability of excellent indoor training facilities. This aspect and the optimized safety technology have seen the spread of injuries move from the lower extremity to the hand and the shoulder. This has also meant that new forms of injuries specific to climbing such as, for example, tearing of the ring ligament have made an appearance. The basic knowledge imparted here in regard to structured training, warming up, prophylactic and therapeutic measures is indispensable to enable participants to indulge in high-performance, injury-free climbing over lengthy periods of time.

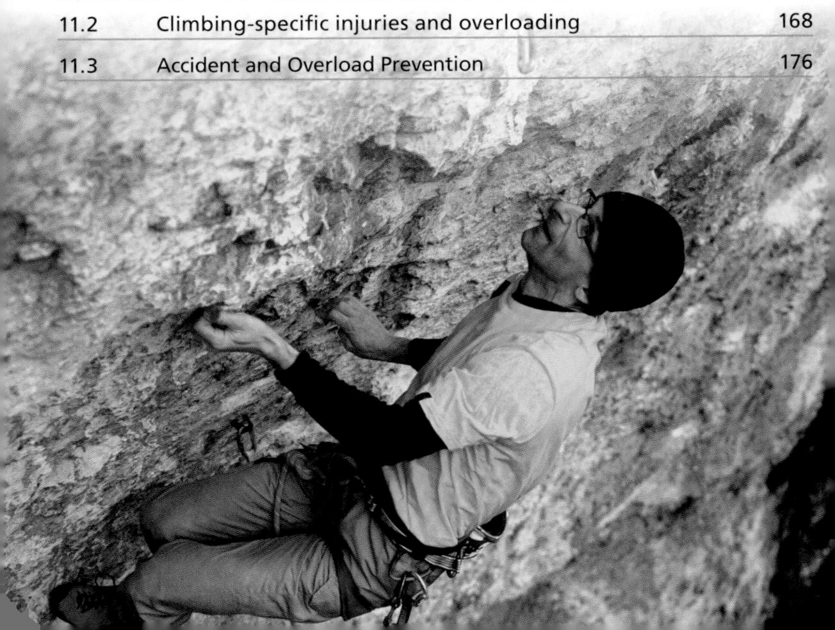

11.1 Training

As with any Alpine discipline, a solid foundation in endurance training is a precondition for sport climbing too. This should be climbing-specific and may take the form of walking/running, Nordic Walking, cross-country skiing, rowing or swimming as part of a general endurance training program. When it comes to climbing, the higher levels of difficulty can only be achieved through additional training which takes in all sporting factors. Assuming a central role here are primarily the strengthening of the finger flexor muscles (hand and forearm), the shoulder musculature (which is what enables the climber to make use of extensive manoeuvrability and ability to grip) as well as the muscles of the torso to promote stabilization of the body. However, the training must not be allowed to simply focus on rapidly measurable increases in strength, but should also take into account the carrier structures on the joints such as capsules, ligaments and tendons.

How the locomotive system adapts to major exertion and load

It is important to remember that, although climbing performance and, in particular, muscular strength can be enhanced very rapidly, the passive structures (such as tendons, ligaments, cartilage and bones) require significantly more time to adapt to high levels of exertion and load. Young climbers who are at the age where they are still growing are at particular risk from rapid increases in levels of exertion and load.

In order to avoid chronic overloading and premature wear phenomena on joints and tendons, specific training in climbing for beginners needs to be built up gradually in stages, taking into account regeneration times and the time needed for adaptation of the various tissues. Excessive loads resulting from training on climbing boards with additional weights, dynamic training on the climbing board as well as plyometric training (e.g. dropping down on climbing board and catching hold of the lower climbing holds) should be avoided in the first 3–5 years of training. In this time, assuming regular training, the strength of the various tissues will be built up significantly and training can then once again be increased.

Estimated adaptation times for the various tissues to high levels of load in sport:

Musculature: after 3 weeks of power training
Heart muscle: after 4 weeks of endurance training
Ligaments: 2 years

Tendons:	1–2 years
Cartilage:	3–5 years
Bones:	1 year

The passive structures require approx. 3 years' specific training for strength optimisation. This must at all costs be taken into account when planning training.

Climbing-specific power training

Sport-specific training is the most effective and this also applies to climbing. This means that actually doing some climbing is the best training for climbing. Bouldering in particular can probably be regarded as the most effective training of all when it comes to climbing. It can be readily adapted to the demands of lead climbing, Alpine sport climbing and sport climbing.
In order to achieve success, it is essential to take into account the basic principles enshrined in the training dogma. This primarily consists of a Training Plan with training divided up **over the year** into **2–4 macro-cycles,** each of 3–5 months, with corresponding rest phases in between. One macro-cycle incorporates a number of meso-cycles made up of strength build up, maximum strength and endurance phases.

The **power build up meso-cycle** as a rule incorporates a cycle of 4–6 weeks featuring medium to high levels of load such as, for example, boulder sequences or routes with 20–30 repeats up to the point of fatigue, these to be repeated 4 to 10 times (series).
There follows a **maximum power meso-cycle** with short, difficult transits consisting of 4–10 repeats (3–6 series with 4–10 repeats) for 2–4 weeks, after this an **endurance meso-cycle** incorporating 50 or more transits (3–4 series with 50+ repeats with low levels of load).

The third and final meso-cycle will naturally need to be adapted to the corresponding demands. If you go bouldering on holiday you are likely to stick to maximum-strength exercises in the final preparations phase; if you climb long Alpine routes you will find yourself placing more emphasis on endurance, at the same time combinations of endurance and maximum strength are particularly effective and come closest to sport climbing on the rock face.
Ideally, training sessions should take up 2 to 4 sessions a week (micro-cycle). Maximum power training demands lengthy recovery phases of 1–3 days; on the contrary,

when it comes to endurance training, there is no problem with training daily. What is important is to maintain maximum possible variability (types of hold, steepness, technology) but still to ensure a continuous increase in the degree of load (difficulty of repeats, additional weights, increasing the wall steepness at each training session). A supportive **climbing-orientated power training meso-cycle** twice a year will help to counteract any plateaus in strength increase. This may incorporate simple exercises such as pullups with the hands at different distances apart, bar dips, "hanging scales" and press-ups. Of particular importance is the function of the shoulder joint stabilizing musculature (rotator cuff) in preventing injury and for which training with elastic resistance exercise products such as Theraband is particularly appropriate. Polysportive training, such as, for example, slacklining, biking, football and cross-country running, helps to train balance, coordination and speed and to prevent injuries.

⇨ When it comes to climbing, the best training is actually go climbing (bouldering). Maintaining a high variability of climbing environments (steepness, type of holds, length of routes) will prevent you from becoming too used to them and stagnating.

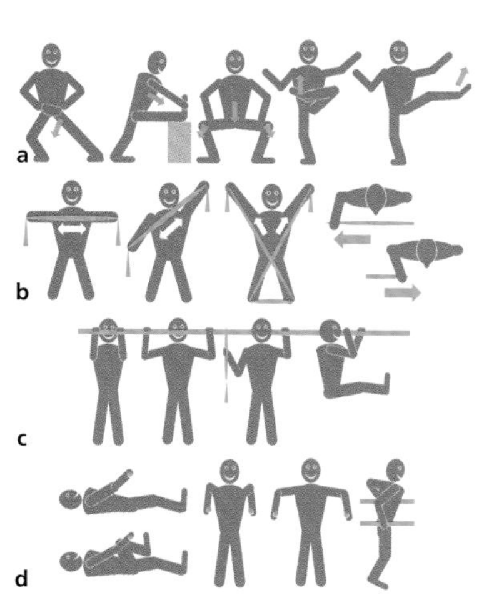

Figures 11.1: *Five simple stretching exercises (a) for the muscles of the hip & thigh. Of particular importance for climbing is active mobility (lifting a foot on to a high step) and this is what the two exercises on the right are for. Five exercises (b) to strengthen and balance the shoulder muscles with the Theraband; the two exercises on the right are especially important for strengthening the rotator cuff and improving shoulder centering. Pullups (c), "hanging scales" and bar dips (d) should be practiced using as many different variations as possible, to correspond to the situations that tend to be encountered during climbing activities (source: turntillburn.ch/verticalsecrets).*

Competitive Climbing

During the last 20 years we have seen an enormous increase in achievements where competitive climbing is concerned. A range of sub-disciplines is being embarked on, such as on-sight climbing, climbing after pre-practice (route can be rehearsed), speed climbing and bouldering. In on-sight, levels of difficulty of up to 8b+/8c may be encountered and surmounted. For those who wish to be able to participate in competitive sport at world cup level, the effort and outlay are enormous and well up with any other performance sport you may care to name. This calls for precision planning and excellent support for the athletes. The problems that have arisen due to increased performance are partly to do with the character of the routes (very steep routes, uniform difficulty in the strength endurance range) which, among other factors, favor a low body weight. This means that the best male athletes tend to weigh hardly any more than 60 kg. This can, especially where younger climbers, both males and females, are concerned, lead to undernourishment and nutritional deficits.
In addition, the fact that people are entering into competitive sports of this nature increasingly early is responsible for the fact that the growing skeleton is becoming overloaded (damage to developing joints, shoulder instability–see below). It is primarily the job of the trainer to point out the factors that cause such things (fingers in extreme positions, wholly relaxed shoulder muscles when shaking down, dynamic climbing) and to intervene at the appropriate time. With regards to accidents, a study has in fact shown that the increased risk associated with competition is only low grade, if it exists at all. To what extent there is any -long-term damage cannot yet be assessed at the current point in time.

11.2 Climbing-specific injuries and overloading

Basics of Treatment

With the majority of sporting injuries similar rules apply to treatment. The therapy is split into the acute phase, the healing phase and the build up phase.
In acute instances the **RICE Rule** applies, this means:

- **R**est
- **I**ce (ice compresses)
- **C**ompression (elastic bandage)
- **E**levation (above the level of the heart)

Ice should not be placed directly on to the skin; cool, wet compresses with small chunks of ice are better.
The injury is now assessed by the patient or a doctor and the subsequent treatment

determined (e.g. operation, splint, medications, bandages etc.). After this initial healing phase comes the build up of mobility and loading which is extremely important for the healing process. This build up phase consists of the following stages: mobility without load, increasing load up to the level of everyday exertion and load application and then sport-specific build up pending achievement of suitability for competition. The build up takes place using a staged protocol which is set by the physician or therapist, depending on the injury. As regards this staged protocol, the load/degree of exertion is increased every 2–3 days. Should pain develop as a result of the increased exertion/load and this does not disappear after 20 seconds, training is continued 24 hours later at the next lower level.

When does a doctor need to be consulted?

- More than two weeks of continuous and constant pain in relation to joint sprains
- Pains, swelling or restricted mobility in the finger joints affecting young people (risk of permanent displacement of a joint as a result of fracture of the growth zones)
- Pains in the knee and hip affecting young people (risk of irretrievable damage to joints)
- Extremities out of position after injury

In the event of an injury, initial treatment should be undertaken in accordance with the RICE rule. After initial treatment and assessment, a gradual step by step build-up to increase the load applied (load stages ladder) is an important part of therapy. Young people with pains in the finger, knee and hip joints should consult a doctor as a matter of urgency and ensure that any problems are sorted out.

Injuries and overloading to hand and forearm

Corresponding to the load level, sport climbing injuries and overloading tend to occur most frequently in relation to the hand, elbow and shoulder. They are not usually caused by a fault but when carrying out a difficult manoeuvre and predominantly feature soft-tissue injuries such as pulled muscles and torn ligaments.

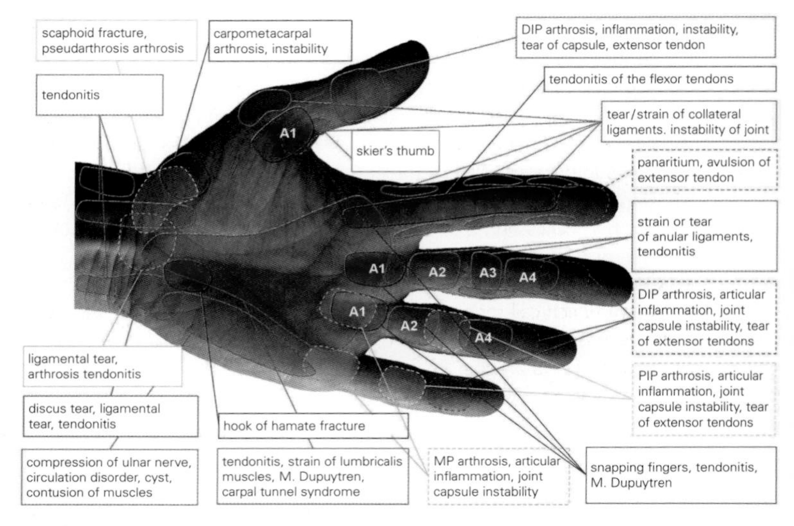

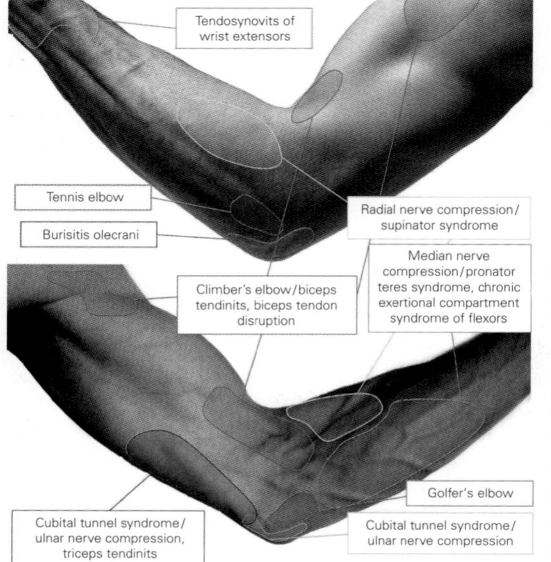

Figure 11.2: *The most frequent injuries sustained during sport climbing affect the upper extremity and, in turn, the hand. Different diagnoses may be made in relation to the painful areas and are intended to serve solely as an aid to orientation. The hatched areas signify that these can be found on the back of the hand (source and further information on the diagnoses: turntillburn.ch).*

Fingers: The most frequent injury sustained during climbing is the tearing of a pulley annular ligament (holds the flexor tendon to the bone) at the proximal or middle phalanx of the finger, something which is mostly caused by the rapid application of a high load in the overstretched position of the distal interphalangeal joint (crimp-grip-position). A clicking noise is followed by pain and swelling on the finger flexor side. Following diagnosis by means of ultrasound, the majority of injuries can be successfully treated with a special pulley protecting ring within 2–4 months. Only rarely is an operation necessary.

Sprains and twisting of the finger joints can lead to tears in the joint capsule and collateral ligament which call for special examinations (X-ray, ultrasound) and treatment (specifically, protective splint, taping) for 2–3 months.
When holding on to 1 and 2 finger depressions, it is possible for **strains** to occur in the metacarpal muscles (Lumbricalis musculature) and these need to be treated with special stretching exercises so as to avoid any scarring and/or movement restrictions. **Chronic overloading** of the ring ligaments and flexor tendons, occasionally also the extensor tendons, leading to inflammation of the tendon sheaths are treated functionally on the basis of the RICE rule. In the case of juvenile climbers, the crimp-grip-position can also lead to overloading in the middle phalanx of the finger and **injuries to the epiphyseal plates.** This joint must at all costs be treated with a consistent reduction in load and avoidance of the cocked position so as to avoid any long-term damage such as early-onset arthritis.
On the other hand, generally-speaking the wear phenomena that occur in the finger joints after 10–20 years of intensive climbing are less painful, but can also be reduced by avoiding the crimp-grip-position.

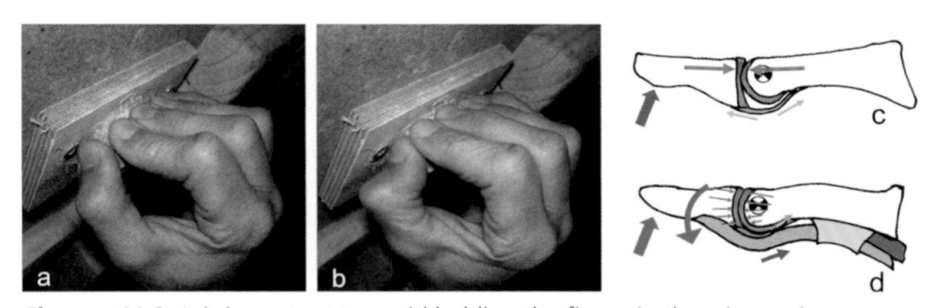

Figures 11.3: *It is important to avoid holding the finger in the crimp-grip-position (a, c). Significantly fewer major loads attributable to a more level distribution of pressure are exerted if the distal joints are stabilized 10–15° before reaching their final overstretched (cocked) position and the middle joint is not bent beyond 90°(b, d): from Vertical Secrets, 2009.*

Wrist joint: Due to the increased popularity of bouldering with frequent falls on to the hand, injuries in the area of the wrist joint have shown a significant increase. Because injuries to ligaments and broken bones (e.g. the scaphoid bone) cause only a few moderately serious symptoms, often only a few people bother to consult a doctor. After a few months, long term damage may occur and this can be very difficult to treat and the subsequent prognosis may be poor. Pains in the wrist joint after a fall which show no significant improvement after two weeks must at all costs be investigated. Tears to the ligament mostly need to be treated by means of an operation, whilst broken bones often have to be treated by resorting to an operation.
A chronic inflammation of the flexor tendon in the carpal tunnel may well be painful but can lead to **pressure damage to the median nerve** with initial, followed by permanent numbness and tingling of fingers 1–4. This so-called **carpal tunnel syndrome** occasionally has to be addressed by resorting to carpal tunnel release surgery.

During sport climbing, injuries to hands and fingers most often occur in the shape of a tear to the ring ligament or a capsular ligament sprain. These can mostly be treated functionally with a splint or tape but do not, however, call for prior consultation with a doctor. Among other causes, the cocked position is deemed to be responsible. In the case of juvenile climbers this should only be used to a moderate extent so as to avoid any injury to epiphyseal cartilage.

Pain in the elbow and forearm

The most frequently occurring phenomenon to affect the climber is **Golfer's Elbow** (Epicondylitis medialis). This relates to a chronic overloading of the tendon inserts of the superficial finger flexors and the underarm pronator at the medial epicondylus (inside of the elbow). The cause in most cases is a rapid unilateral increase in training or an overload over several months as a result of which the tendons have had too little time to make the necessary adaptation.
From a therapeutic point of view the focus therefore lies on targeted structuring and stretching of the corresponding muscles and a gradual increase in load when climbing. It is only in this way that the resistance capability of the tendon tissue can be improved. The following therapies may then be used at the same time: physiotherapy, bandages, anti-inflammatory drugs, ultrasound, extracorporeal shock wave therapy and local injections.

In the case of **Tennis Elbow** (Epicondylitis lateralis), pain develops on the outside of the elbow due to chronic overloading of the finger and wrist joint extensors. The applicable therapies are similar to Golfer's Elbow. For both sets of clinical characteristics, the prognosis is very good (patience).

Rarely, the causes of pain at the elbow and forearm may include **finger flexor compartment syndrome** and **nerve constrictions** resulting from chronic load or thickened tendon sheaths and muscles. In the case of the former, as a result of the increase in muscle volume contingent on load, an abnormal increase in pressure inside the muscle fasciae with reduced blood flow and corresponding pain may develop. Typically, these pains only occur after a certain period over which load is applied and can persist for a period of anything from half an hour to more than a day.
Where the nerves are constricted, tingling and loss of feeling in the hands may develop after extensive exertion/load application, especially at night.

Tennis and Golfer's Elbow can be to a major extent avoided by means of well-planned and regular training sessions as well as by ensuring the correct warming up routine. The crucial factor is an adequate period of regeneration after rigorous exertion (bouldering) and specific training of the muscles involved in the forearm.

Injuries and overloading at the shoulder joint

The shoulder joint features the greatest mobility of all the joints in the human body. Frequently it is pain on movement with the arms above the head that alerts us to this extraordinary flexibility and at the same time enables us to recognize the central role that the shoulder joint plays in climbing. In addition to mobility, however, the application of force with arm stabilization, not to mention the incorporation of body stabilization in a very wide range of holding positions, is essential to enable us to keep moving.
Depending on the age of the climber and/or duration of the climbing activity, in practical terms three problem areas may be identified in relation to the shoulder:

- Instability of the shoulder joint
- Problems with impingement in relation to shoulder movements with or without loss of strength
- Wear on the shoulder joint

Instability of the shoulder joint

The clinical picture is one of a dislocated shoulder. This situation calls for gentle reinstatement of the joint. Dislocations of the shoulder while climbing may occur

either as a result of falling with the arm abducted during a previous bouldering session or (and more rarely) due to the application of maximum force in critical arm positions. Depending on the circumstances that have led to the dislocation and the age of the climber, it is possible, by conducting extensive investigations, to estimate the likelihood of a major recurrence should the sporting activity be continued at the same level. Operating to stabilize the shoulder must be discussed after the second occurrence of a dislocation at the latest.
For a climber, a dislocated shoulder in the mountains may lead to difficult situations e.g. s/he may need to be rescued from an Alpine rock face.

Impingement problems in relation to shoulder movements, with or without loss of strength: the clinical picture consists of a painful weak shoulder which often feels as though it is paralyzed. Pronounced bruising to the shoulder, with or without a fall, the occurrence of a tear in the shoulder during climbing or sustained overloading of the shoulder during training or climbing are the most frequent causes of this. With repeated examinations of the joints and X-ray pictures, as well as targeted training under the supervision of a physiotherapist, it is possible to plan the right operative treatment (if necessary) within an orthopedic consultation.
Wear on the joint: The clinical picture of this ailment presents as a painful shoulder which is limited when it comes to extreme movements and which is also associated with creaking of the joint. A number of reasons, the details of which may not be known, may culminate in this clinical picture. In the case of the sportsmen, heavy loads, with or without stabilization or power deficits, may speed up wear and tear on the joint as a result of possible pathological loads. The aim of treatment should be to achieve a shoulder free of pain, with recovery of or slight improvement to mobility and strength ratios. The primary intention is to achieve this using methods to maintain the joint. Such methods may include physiotherapy, painkilling drugs and/or injections into the joint. Once these methods are exhausted, it will be time to consider an operation to irrigate the joint or, if an advanced stage has been reached, an artificial joint.

In the sequence of injuries sustained by the upper extremities, injuries to the shoulder joints take second place after finger and hand injuries. Should sudden dislocations or insidious pains occur when a load is applied, examination by a specialist is indicated.

Injuries and overloading of the lower limbs

Problems in relation to the lower limbs are only touched on in this section because we are not dealing with specific sport climbing injuries (see Section 9.3, Page 124). With increasing specialization in relation to climbing techniques, the lower limbs, especially the hip and knee joints, are also coming under definite strain. In particular, maximum bending angles linked with rotations (leg turned inwards, "Egyptian") will lead to overload on the knee and hip joints. As a result it is possible to injure the menisci, and more rarely even the ligaments, at the knee joint.
Arthroses and malformations of the hip joint which may be either congenital or acquired during the growing phase can restrict mobility and intensify wear in the hip joint in extreme positions (maximum bending and rotation).

Luckily, the lower extremities are seldom affected by overload phenomena. Injury to the menisci, however, occur repeatedly as a result of turning inwards and bending the knee joints to their maximum extent.

Injuries and overloading at the spine

The most frequent cause of problems in the area of the cervical spine and the neck are the hardening and shortening (myogeloses) of the muscles of the neck, in most cases triggered by the adoption of maximum positions of the vertebral joints during climbing and belaying in overhanging terrain. This can lead to irritation of these joints and pain and, last but not least, these joints may suffer damage themselves. By consciously activating the throat and neck muscles, avoiding tilting the head back to the absolute limit and frequent position changes, corresponding discomfort can be avoided.

Where prominent overhangs are a feature, the person doing the belaying is best placing himself with his back to the wall, so as to avoid stretching the cervical spine any more than is absolutely necessary. In addition, so-called prism glasses may be used where the direction of view is rerouted to the vertical via the glasses.

In climbing, holding on to low-lying undergrips (in particular) with the spine bent has the effect of putting strain on the spinal discs in the lumbar spine. This effect is further intensified by the fact that, in a climber, the back extensor musculature which controls this position tends to be poorly trained. Pains in the area of the lumbar spine (low back pain, lumbago) are mostly caused by blockades, irritation of the small vertebral joints or the sacroiliac joint (ISG) or small prolapses of invertebral discs (disc

hernias), which provoke muscle spasms and movement restrictions. More extensive disc hernias or spondylolisthesis can also narrow nerve routes and result in pain, loss of feeling and paralysis phenomena in the leg (lumboischalgia) (indication for a medical consultation, see Section 21.1, Page 270).
By strengthening the torso stabilizing muscles (straight and crosswise abdominal muscles, back extensors, deep stabilizing torso muscles), building up good body tension during training and preventing extreme positions with poor muscular control, loads on the cervical spine can be reduced.
Both the muscles in the lower part of the torso and the neck muscles can be specifically trained and stretched.

11.3 Accident and Overload Prevention

Remember that there is no institution that goes about checking climbing areas and routes! The hooks or the krabs at the top may often be in poor condition. It is up to each individual to take responsibility for checking, which requires pre-existing experience.
It is essential to practice safe falling into the rope and the proper way to belay a fall (dynamic belaying if there is enough space).
If there is any risk of suspension on the rope over a lengthy period, Prusik slings should be taken along and the technique of self-rescue mastered. Being suspended on the rope over a lengthy period carries with it the risk of death soon after rescue as a result of the reduced blood flow to the legs (see Section 20.3, Page 265).
When bouldering, it is essential that special boulder mats (crash pads) are used. When pushing off, the partner should not catch the fall but check that wherever possible the climber lands on his feet. As in parachuting, it is important to practice how to land correctly when pushing off.

When indulging his sport, the climber has great personal responsibility because there is no institution that checks outdoor climbing areas (climbing parks, Alpine routes). It is important to practise fall technique, belaying and spotting with bouldering.

Prevention of overload and wear

When it comes to preventing injury, a proper warm up is probably one of the most important things to remember. repeated, escalating muscle activity ensures an adequate flow of blood (duration 5–10 minutes) and nervous activity to the muscles. It is only in this way that corresponding peak performance can be achieved.
Activating the **cardiovascular system** and the metabolism (of the liver) will also ensure the provision of energy and the removal of waste products from the muscles. In order to stimulate these processes, the pulse must be increased to more than 120 beats per minute for 5–10 minutes. This can, for example, be achieved by means of a fast ascent to the climbing area. The preparation of the **structures of the passive locomotive system,** such as ligaments and tendons (fluid content, alignment of fibers) should also not be neglected. This is the procedure which, out of all the warming up processes, takes the most time. In climbing, 100–200 clips (approx. three sport climbing routes) are necessary, at the same time slowly increasing load levels, including the cocked position, in order to achieve the maximum load capability on the tissues and hence also ensure minimal susceptibility to injury. Whether **stretching the muscles** before training can reduce the risk of injury is a point that tends to be disputed. Nevertheless, when climbing, any stretching of the hip and upper thigh muscles is very beneficial from the point of view of mobility. This means that the center of gravity of the body can be brought significantly closer to the rock face, thereby reducing the load on the fingers and at the same time reducing the risk of injury.

Special attention must be paid to those routes with 1 or 2 finger holds. The muscles of the hand and forearm must be prepared in advance with a corresponding build up of load at single finger holds so as to prevent shear fractures in the palm of the hand. It is also important to note that, in the crimp-grip-position, full loads should never be applied to small ligaments in the finger joints in their end positions (the middle phalanx of the finger should never be bent more than 90°, the finger end phalanx is to be extended 5–10° less than the maximum so as to avoid damaging cartilage and degenerative joint disease).
Crucial importance is assigned to the mechanics of the shoulder joints, namely the optimum centering of the humeral head in the glenoid cavity. At the same time, the deep-seated musculature bordering the shoulder blade should be given equal consideration as the superficial muscles. This means that the shoulder must always be kept low, the shoulder muscles must remain active, even in maximum stretching when negotiating further sections is a factor, they must never be permitted to be fully extended and, in particular, when recovering and shaking down in overhanging terrain, the joint must never be left hanging into the ligaments alone.

The **epidermis** and the **subcutaneous tissue** require special preparation. This is the only way they can withstand the shear forces i.e. with pre-stretching and the fluid content at an optimum level. In addition, in the interests of friction optimization, the skin needs to be as free of grease (sun cream) as possible.

12. Mountain Biking: Accidents and Injuries due to Overexertion

U. Hefti

Mountain bikers and cyclists account for a quarter of all traffic accidents. This means that almost 20 000 persons fall victim to accidents each year in Switzerland. Up to 85 % of aspiring mountain bikers injure themselves once a year, whilst up to 90 % suffer one acute injury during the course of their mountain biking lives.

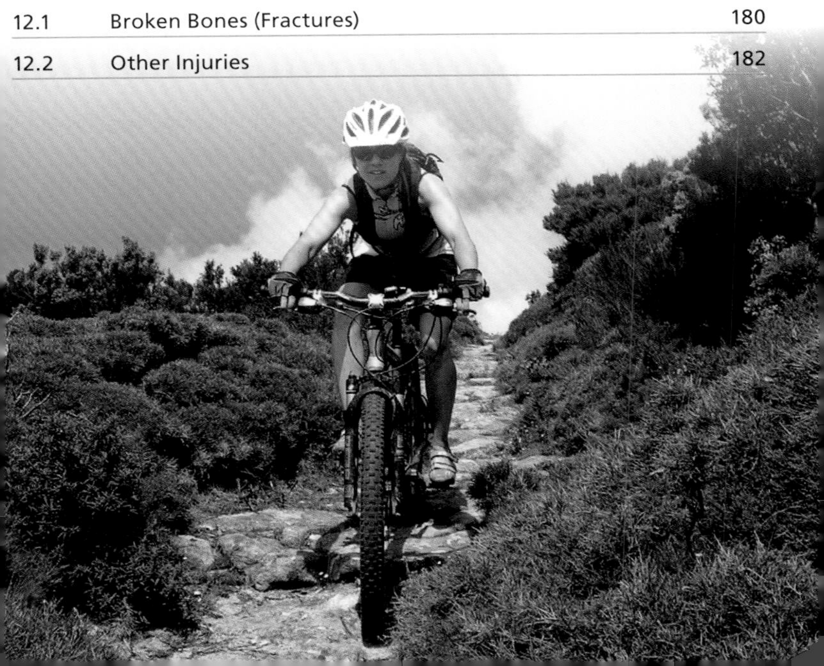

The majority of injuries relate to the upper extremity i.e. collar bone, acromio-clavicular joint and forearm. Bikers are still sustaining serious head injuries far too often. Injuries due to strain and overexertion understandably affect the area of the buttocks, the wrists and the knee. Adopting the correct seating position on a mountain bike is essential if injuries of this nature are to be avoided. It makes sense to obtain professional advice from a specialist dealer.
The correct equipment as well as general fitness training and training specific to mountain biking are essential when it comes to preventing injuries.

⇨ Wearing a helmet is compulsory. There is absolutely no excuse for not wearing one.

12.1 Broken Bones (Fractures)

Broken collar bone

This is the injury most frequently sustained when falling off a bicycle. In most cases the casualty will immediately hear and feel that something is broken. In addition, there is no problem in identifying or feeling an abnormal position of the collar bone. A bruise will quickly form in the area of the fracture. Very rarely bone fragments may pierce the skin. A fracture of the collar bone is generally a less serious injury and will heal in one way or another. This is why until recently almost all fractures were treated conservatively, i.e. by resorting to immobilization and the administration of pain killers. The results of more recent investigations have, however, shown that, where sports enthusiasts and active people are concerned, it makes sense to proceed with an operation and thus a correct reinstatement of the shape of the collar bone. However, this is not something that calls for emergency surgery and there is no problem if it is carried out even days after the fall.
First Aid on the bike tour is simple. As is the case with all injuries, the *RICE* principle applies. Relieve pressure as far as possible, (see Section 9.4, Page 137) and elevate. Take pain killers if necessary. It is not essential to consult a doctor straight away.

⇨ If the skin is damaged, a doctor must be consulted because there is a major risk of infection and an appropriate professional assessment will be necessary.

Injury to the acromio-clavicular joint

From the point of view of seriousness, this injury is the equivalent of a fracture of the collar bone but it is important to be able to distinguish between them. The injury can be recognized by the fact that the collar bone is elevated at the junction with the acromio-clavicular joint. Depending on how pronounced this is, the doctor will divide up the injury into different degrees of severity. It will be possible to press on the collar bone and to push it downwards by one to two centimeters, without any problems and with minimal pain for the patient. This phenomenon is known as the 'piano key phenomenon' and is typical of this injury. The initial therapy is similar to that used for a collar bone fracture. Depending on the degree of severity and the individual's sporting ambitions, an operation may be recommended.

Head of the radius

At the elbow the radius is thin and incorporates a head so as to enable turning movements to be made without any problems. This head may be fractured as a result of a fall on to the extended arm (fracture of the head of the radius). From a purely external point of view there is hardly anything to be seen. Nevertheless, severe pain will be experienced if there is any attempt to lean on the arm or if turning movements of the forearm are attempted. Such movements may also be restricted, either because of pain or sometimes also because the break represents a mechanical impediment. As regards to initial therapy, the RICE rule applies as always. It is only when an X-ray picture is to hand that it will be possible to state whether an operation is necessary or not. However, this injury is not life-threatening.

Ribs

Frequently, the rib cage sustains bruising during a fall. In most cases the biker "is winded for a short time." A sharp additional pain, especially one which makes it troublesome to breathe, may often indicate a fracture of one or more ribs.
The diagnosis can be made by exerting gentle pressure on the rib cage, with the investigator standing to the side of the patient and keeping one hand on the breastbone and the other on the thoracic spine and applying pressure. If the patient indicates somewhat diffused pains in the area of the breastbone but not precisely where the pressure was applied, this is a good reason to suspect a fractured rib.

It is important that the patient should lose no time in taking pain killers and so at least be able to breathe moderately well. Since the lung underneath the ribs may also be bruised and especially as pain killers on their own may not be sufficient, it may be sensible to **consult a doctor.**

Should the pains be too severe and if the patient is not taking sufficiently deep breaths, pneumonia may develop after a few days. The rib fractures do not necessarily have to be identified by means of an X-ray. However, pain can be expected to last for a matter of weeks; there is no need for a bandage or an operation.

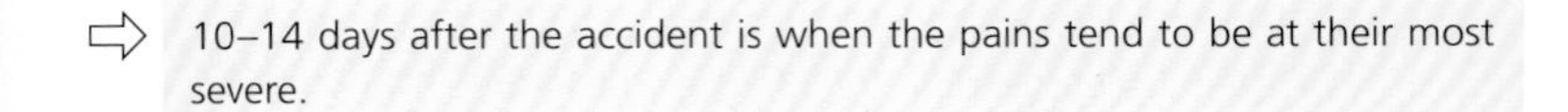

⇨ 10–14 days after the accident is when the pains tend to be at their most severe.

Traumas of the skull or brain, back injuries, ankle injuries and fixations see Sections 9.3 and 9.4, Pages 113 and 125.

12.2 Other Injuries

Ruptured Spleen

An injury to the spleen is a rare but nonetheless life-threatening injury. The spleen lies on the left hand side of the body, at the level of the upper abdomen, facing towards the back. In most cases the casualty falls with his abdomen impacting on the handlebars. In so doing he may sustain straightforward bruising or, at the other end of the scale, a laceration of the organ. As the spleen is copiously supplied with blood, a major loss of blood may occur in the abdominal cavity with subsequent circulatory problems.

Treatment in hospital, and sometimes even an emergency operation, is required. Professional help must be organized without delay if an injury of this nature is suspected. Raise the alarm early!

⇨ Initially the pain may not be so intense or it may subside again. If abdominal pain increases or the casualty starts to acquire a pallor, consideration must be given to this injury. NB: It is possible to die from an injury to the spleen.

It is practically impossible to administer therapy while on tour; in the event of circulatory problems (see Section 9.2, Page 101) the recovery position is recommended, if necessary with legs bent (positioning of persons with abdominal injuries) (see Section 9.4, Page 127).

Chafing of the skin

The skin is often damaged when biking. In most cases it is a matter of superficial chafing and therefore only minor injuries. In order to be able to estimate the extent of the injury, the wound needs to be cleansed (the easiest way to do this is to irrigate it–e.g. at a spring) or flushed with water. This initial preliminary cleansing of the wound also represents the most important initial treatment. Any further treatment will depend on the depth of the injury.

If the wound is very dirty and it is impossible to cleanse it properly or if it is very deep, it is essential to obtain a medical assessment and have the wound cleaned and, where necessary, have a stitch inserted.

It is possible to adequately dress small wounds using special, so-called **hydrocolloidal bandages.** Deep or seriously contaminated wounds must also be checked following correct initial treatment as an infection is still possible, even after a few days.

Infections can be recognised by reddening (rubor) and heat (calor) around the wound, throbbing pains, inflamed lymph glands and, in serious cases, fever. A doctor should be consulted by this stage at the latest.

Bruising

Painful bruises are an everyday occurrence in the life of a mountain biker. The best therapy is to take a break, cool down and have patience. Should a large hematoma form, this may be sufficiently troublesome and painful on occasions to merit removal by the doctor.

Overloading

Overloads are mostly loads that are wrongly distributed due to an incorrect seating position on the bike or excessive loads during "tramping," i.e. traveling in too high a gear at too low a cadence.

The ideal pedalling frequency is around 90 per minute.

Painful **tensions** may develop in the area of the cervical spine due to too low a seating position and the consequent need to overextend the cervical spine while traveling, the same of course applies to the lumbar spine.
Feelings of numbness in the area of the buttocks are caused by a compression of a vasomotor nerve (Nervus pudendum).

Ensure that you wear good quality biking trousers with padding.

Of course, the position of the seat should be changed by adjusting the seat in all planes. Sometimes it will be necessary to reconsider and redetermine the position of the seat on the bike, but it is essential that this is carried out with assistance from a qualified dealer or biker. In addition to the feeling of numbness, skin irritations, particularly at the start of the season, as well as even boils can make a biker's life more difficult. If need be, aliphatic salves can help.

An overload injury that is tiresome to treat is **"Biker's Knee,"** i.e. vague pains in the knee. This overload/over-exertion injury should be shown to an experienced sports medicine practitioner because there are many possible causes – irritation of the cartilage behind the kneecap, inflammation of tendons at their insertions, a painful mucosal fold in the knee, incipient arthrosis of a joint, other causes.

In the hand, tingling or feelings of numbness may develop in the fingers as a result of overextending the wrist and thus compressing the nerves of the hand (Median or ulnar nerves).

Preventing accidents means having good equipment. The following items should be kept to hand: an approved helmet, unbreakable spectacles, gloves, luminous functional clothing, a rucksack, back, shin and joint protectors in challenging terrain. Regular checks on the bike by a specialist dealer are also part and parcel of looking after one's equipment.

Adjust your selection of tours to what you know you can do; start in the spring with a tour that is easy both in terms of technique and condition. Take spare materials, a small first aid kit and a mobile with you in your rucksack.

13. Paragliding

Y. Villiger

Paragliding is a sport that has seen very rapid development since the 1980s. The first documented paragliding flights were carried out in Mieussy in France by the three parachute jumpers, Jean-Claude Bétemps, André Bohn and Gérard Bossonavec using ordinary parachutes. Parallel to its success there has also been a marked increase in the number of accidents in this new type of sport…

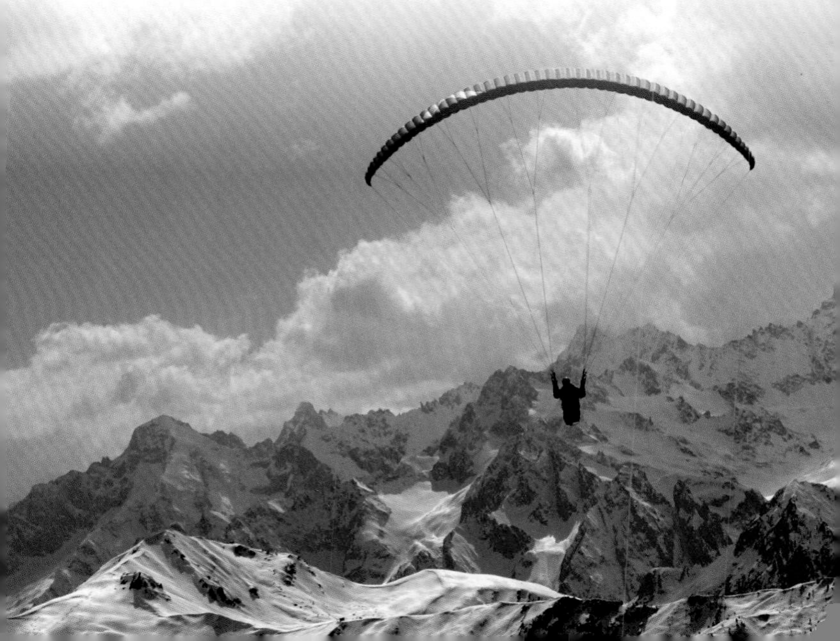

The majority of the accidents occur on launch and landing.
The high speeds attained in this sport lead to injuries similar to those that might be anticipated in the case of **high energy accidents**–comparable with motor cycle accidents. In addition, special injuries tend to occur which are predominantly dependent on the seating position of the pilot and the combination of horizontal and vertical speeds.

13.1 Statistics

The majority of accidents (60 to 90 %) occur in the phases when the pilot is close to the ground (on launch and landing) whereas only 10 % to 35 % happen during flight. The majority can be traced back to miscalculation of the weather conditions and pilot error i.e. they are caused by human error.[1] Material faults are a decidedly rare occurrence. In his study of 218 paragliding accidents, Krüger-Franke shows that the average age of pilots involved in accidents is 29.7 years.[2] 73 % of casualties suffer a single injury, while 27 % have multiple injuries.[3]

13.2 Specific Aspects

Paragliding in the high mountains chiefly entails two risks,[1] namely, the risk presented by the alpine terrain and the risk inherent in flying. In para-alpinism it is important to keep the equipment as light as possible. From time to time the pilot will need to leave his rescue chute behind, together with the heavy and cumbersome seats with their back protectors. This means that the paraglider pilot in the mountains is frequently less well protected than would be the case in a normal flight. The other side of the coin is that the lighter equipment will mean increased safety as he climbs because it is less voluminous and heavy than that used on classic flights.

⇨ The greatest risks when it comes to flying in the mountains are the terrain and the weather. This means that any medical problem that presents itself in the case of paragliding accidents in the mountains is likely to be compounded by very difficult terrain and rapidly changing weather conditions.

Accidents of this nature need to be tackled quickly and efficiently, because time spent at altitude is particularly damaging for someone who is badly injured. From the point of view of trauma, injuries sustained while flying in the mountains are comparable with injuries sustained during classic flights. In addition, there is of course the risk of rapid hypothermia as well as the damaging effect of the **lack of oxygen** at altitude. The objective dangers of the high mountains (cold, rockfalls, ice falls, avalanches) also make rescuing and looking after an injured person more difficult.

13.3 Injuries

There are some injuries that are typical of paragliding. They can be divided up as shown in Figure 13.1. In the spine, by far and away the most frequent injury is the fracture of the first lumbar vertebral body (37 %).[4]

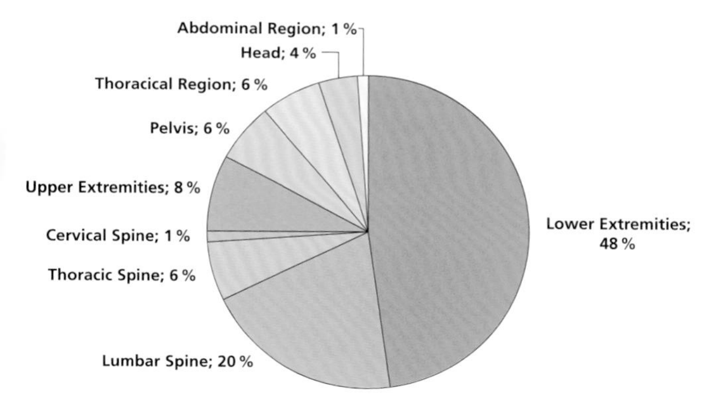

Figure 13.1: *Reproduced by kind permission of Christey G. R. 2005 Serious para-sport injuries in Auckland, New Zealand. Emerg Med Australas 17:163–166*

13.4 Rescue and Treatment

A characteristic of paragliding accidents in the mountains is that they tend to happen in the open country and normally not in proximity to an ascent or descent route. Frequently it is difficult, due to walls of rock, glaciers, glacial ice avalanches or water courses, to get to the scene of the accident and to save those injured. The paraglider may be caught up by the wind at any time which may drag the victim along with it. On the other hand, the paraglider often gets entangled in the terrain and the victim of the accident may be caught up with it. Caution must be exercised in approaching the victim. Otherwise the guidelines are the same as for other accidents. The safety of the rescuers is paramount, keep a record of the time. Determine the exact position and then raise the alarm, pointing out that this is a paragliding accident.

The management of a case of this nature from a medical point of view is the same as for a **person with multiple injuries.** Special notice must be taken of the fact that there is a high likelihood of a back injury and that, for this reason, the head/neck/trunk axis is in need of particular protection. The fractures of long bones (frequently observed) as well as the pelvis can very quickly lead to a haemorrhagic shock.

Where the circulation is unstable and a pelvic injury is suspected, compression of the pelvis using a sling, belt, climbing harness or other improvised means is the only effective and suitable course of action (see Section 9.3, Page 122).
Finally, the paraglider will need to be secured before the helicopter arrives in case the casualty needs to be flown out. A paraglider caught by the draught from the helicopter rotors can spell danger not only for the casualty but also for the rescuers.

Literature:
1) Foray J, Abrassart S, Femmy T, and Aldilli M, 1991. (Hang-gliding accidents in high mountains. Apropos of 200 cases). Chirurgie 117:613–617.
2) Krüger-Franke M, Siebert C.H, and Pförringer W, 1991. Paragliding injuries. Br J Sports Med 25:98–101. Christey G. R. 2005. Serious parasport injuries in Auckland, New Zealand. Emerg Med Australas 17:163–166.
3) Bohnsack M, and Schröter E. 2005. (Injury patterns and typical stress situations in paragliding). Orthopade 34:411–418.
4) Gauler R, Moulin P, Koch H. G, Wick L, Sauter B, Michel D, and Knecht H, 2006. Paragliding accidents with spinal cord injury: 10 years' experience at a single institution. Spine 31:1125–1130.

14. Canyoning

M. Walliser

Canyoning is a sporting genre that has developed over the last 15–20 years. Mastering gorges is technically challenging, the combination of rope technique and water in particular holds a certain charm. The following is a description of some typical accidents and injuries.

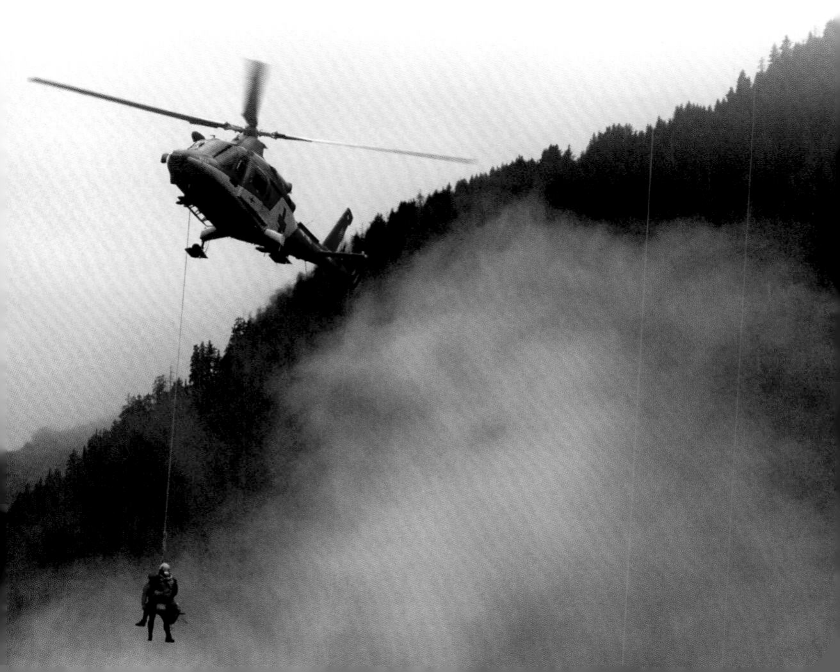

It is the aquatic part of canyoning that is principally responsible for the specific accidents and injuries. In addition, rescuers tend to find that access to gorges is difficult. Victims of accidents can frequently not be evacuated at all or only with difficulty (by resorting to long line techniques). Terrestrial rescues are often necessary and conditions may be similar to those encountered in cave rescues.

14.1 Hypothermia

Although neoprene wet suits offer a certain amount of protection from the cold, hypothermia often develops. In Alpine countries low water temperatures predominate. In the case of aquaseiling (abseiling down waterfalls) or where individuals are in the water for a lengthy period of time, cooling can progress very rapidly and compound existing injuries.
The diagnosis and treatment of hypothermia is described in detail in Section 18.2, Page 232. Essentially, the same guidelines apply, though it should be noted that cooling is faster in water than in the snow, particularly where there is insufficient protection for the body.

14.2 Drowning

Contact with fast moving water (currents, eddies, white water and undercurrents) and overcoming natural obstacles by water jumps or slides can be dangerous. In the event of an uncontrolled landing, hitting the head, whether wearing a helmet or not, may lead to unconsciousness, whilst misjudging the currents or the buoyancy of the water can lead to entrapment under water or in a waterfall and, ultimately, drowning.

Laryngospasm may be a precursor to drowning. When diving or swimming, a foreign body (in most cases a drop of water) may penetrate the upper airways during inhalation and irritate the vocal cords, which can trigger reflex closure of the glottis. This is to prevent the ingress of water into the lower airway, but blocks inhalation leading to depletion of oxygen reserves and loss of consciousness. If the individual is still in the water, they will subsequently sink. At this point the lungs are not yet filled with water.

If rescue arrives quickly, it will be possible to revive the casualty by means of artificial respiration (see also Section 9.2, Page 103). In young and otherwise fit patients, the heart may continue to beat for several minutes after cessation of breathing.

Immersion and genuine drowning: when entrapment occurs under water, drowning frequently results. Unless a spasm of the glottis is protecting the lower airways, the airways and lungs will be filled with water as a result of forced inhalation. Oxygen can no longer be transported and loss of consciousness will ensue after a few minutes – here too, cardiac activity can outlast loss of consciousness by several minutes. Subsequently the heart muscle will also cease beating due to lack of oxygen.

A timely rescue frequently means that the victim can be revived. Following successful resuscitation after drowning in fresh water, there is a high risk that pulmonary (o)edema may develop due to a biochemical process (osmosis).
Where drowning occurs in salt water, the same phenomena occur initially. The lack of oxygen and its consequences will determine the sequence. Because of the higher salt content, however, a range of different biochemical processes will subsequently come into play.

14.3 Injuries Specific to Canyoning

Shoulder dislocations often occur while canyoning, in particular when climbing and jumping into the water. The most common shoulder dislocation downwards and to the front tends to be the most frequent in this activity also (see Section 9.4, Page 142). A form of shoulder dislocation called **Luxatio erecta** is also worth mentioning. In this presentation the dislocated arm incorporates an upward component. This form of dislocation, which is visible on both sides, occurs exclusively when jumping from a considerable height when the arms are not flat against the body and are pulled outwards and upwards on impact. Reduction of this form of dislocation differs to some extent from the classic dislocation; occasionally, the abnormal position first has to be converted into a lower front dislocation before the maneuver is successful.

Joint dislocations affecting the finger or the hand (see Section 9.4, Page 144) also frequently occur during canyoning, favored by supporting oneself on rocks with the fingers outstretched, rather than with the fist.

Bruising of the testicles has also been observed, resulting from jumping from considerable height and adopting a less than ideal posture to enter the water. These injuries can be extremely painful but in most instances have no serious consequences. Other than cooling and painkillers, no further treatment is usually required.

A helmet should always be worn when canyoning. Injuries due to helmets may be sustained when jumping or becoming caught in slide passages if the helmet is subjected to mechanical strain. This can result in some nasty **injuries to the ear.** It is possible to avoid injuries of this nature if attention is paid to optimum fit and tensioning of the retaining straps.

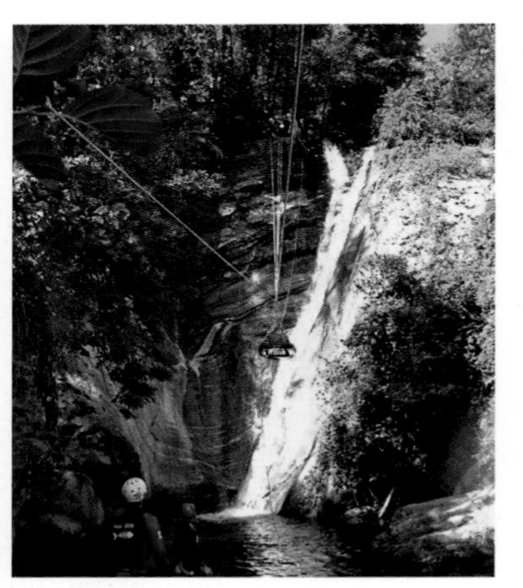

Figure 14.1: *Complex rescue attempt incorporating manœuvres with ropes during canyoning (P. Koster).*

Whilst canyoning in tropical regions **inflammation of the conjunctiva** (see Section 19.1, Page 245) and **inflammation of the external ear canal** have both been observed, particularly after prolonged water exposure. It is likely that, due to the higher water temperatures in tropical regions, the content of bacteria and other pathogens is higher than in our cooler alpine waters. The best way to deal with these problems is to take a day's break; treatment with topical antibiotics may occasionally be necessary.

15. Caving (Speleology)

M. Walliser

The exploration of natural caves is probably the oldest known type of sport–this was something that even the Neanderthals went in for in a big way. Cave rescues are characterized by particular problems: considerably more difficult access, lack of space and unique safety considerations make any cave rescue a significant undertaking–often a real battle between rescuers and the environment–fraught with many a risk for casualties and rescuers.

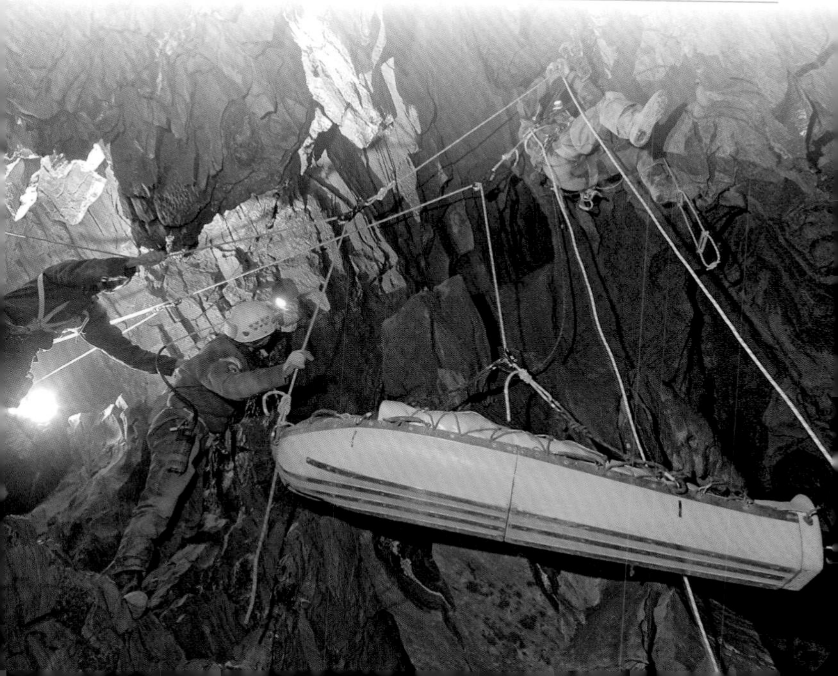

The most important aspects of cave rescue are restricted **communication** and **orientation:** it is possible for an accident to take place only a few meters away from a group and for an injured person to be left behind without being noticed. Acoustic communication tends to be more difficult, particularly in caves with moving water. In addition, because electronic forms of communication do not function underground (unless special technological equipment is deployed), raising the alarm is a matter of first getting to the mouth of the cave on foot. This may lead to delays in the rescue process, especially when an accident takes place some distance from the entrance. Darkness also makes the situation more difficult, and even with the very best equipment visibility is in most cases limited. The casualty may have lost his headlight during the accident, he may not therefore be able to look after himself very well or find himself a safe spot.

In speleology, prevention is even more important than in other disciplines. An accident must be avoided at all costs. Optimum training, the very best equipment and risk adverse behaviour are all absolutely essential.

15.1 Typical Injuries and Patterns of Injuries

Because of the environment, injuries typical in caving are very similar to the injuries sustained during cannoning (see Section 14, Page 190). In caves with water, water-related accidents are similar to those in gorges except that, in a cave, the search, rescue and treatment of a person who has sustained an accident in the water is significantly more difficult.
Otherwise injuries often occur as a result of falls, particularly in confined spaces/narrow gaps, occasionally where the victim becomes wedged in. First Aid for such injuries is equivalent to that which would be given in daylight, although darkness and lack of space complicate the situation.

15.2 Stress Reactions, Anxiety Reactions, Hyperventilation

Due to the conditions underground, increased stress and anxiety reactions may be observed resulting in hyperventilation, especially in novice and inexperienced cavers. If the first signs of stress are recognized early it will, in the majority of cases, be possible to address this and keep the situation under control. Talking reassuringly to the casualty is usually sufficient (see Section 21.5, Page 286). However, the trigger for the panic attack will still need to be addressed.

16. Trekking and Expeditions

U. Wiget

During a trek or an expedition it is primarily altitude that poses problems (see Chapter 17, Page 205). However, a range of other medical problems may occur – including traveler's diarrhea – which in most cases can be solved with a modicum of medical knowledge and a healthy dose of common sense.
In this chapter you will find plenty of practical tips on preparation, equipment and solving of the most frequent health-related problems encountered on a trek or expedition.

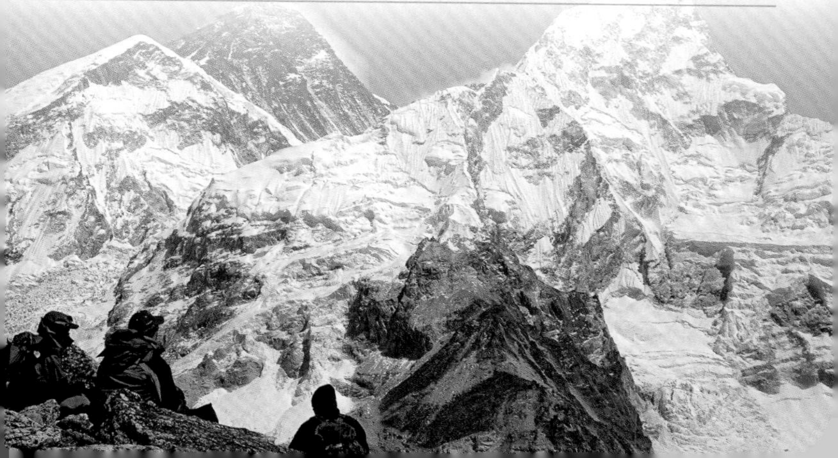

16.1 Introduction

Mountaineering expeditions and treks can take us both to great heights, and to tropical or subtropical regions. On expeditions one has plenty of time after arrival to get oneself organized and often has very little contact with the local population. A trek usually involves moving on to a different place every day, with plenty of contact with local people. This provides different medical challenges.
The preparatory period forms the basis for the success of the venture. On the trip there are several simple principles to observe when it comes to travel medicine.
We strongly recommend that you seek out an experienced specialist in mountain medicine to help with preparations for your trip. S/he may be prepared to meet the group leaders or team with a few important medical elements before the journey: prevention, indications and treatment of any altitude problems, comprehensive First Aid in the event of sickness and accidents distant from medical help.

16.2 Preparations at Home

These will depend to a major extent on the **aim** of the expedition/trek and the **style** of the expedition.

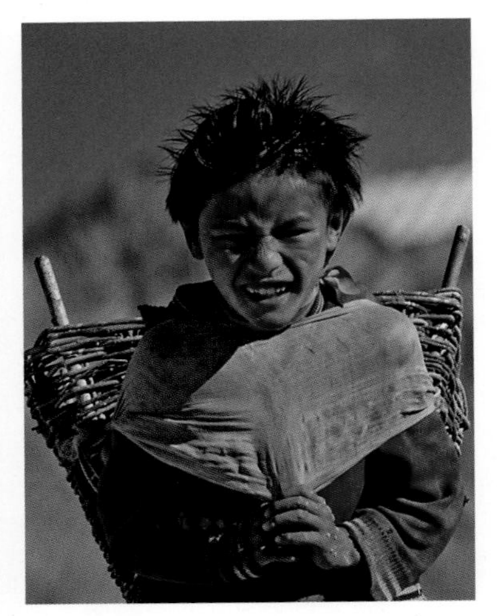

Figure 16.1: *Wayside encounters in the Khumbu Valley Nepal (U. Wiget).*

On an expedition to Tibet, where it is possible to drive as far as base camp, participants will have very little contact with the local population and have only the medical problems of their own team to contend with. On the other hand, in the Baltoro area of Pakistan, it is possible to have a large number of porters around over a period of 5–10 days, all of whom may lay claim to medical help. People embarking on a major expedition to an 8000 m high mountain will probably be more likely to take a doctor with them than a very small expedition made up of two or three friends, who will be dependent on each other for medical care.
Medical preparations at home will include pre-trip checkups and treatment of any pre-existing illnesses.

It will be up to the **GP** to decide whether any specialist check-ups are necessary regarding the heart or circulation. A **visit to the dentist** can prove invaluable in identifying any loose fillings or air bubbles, which may expand during the ascent and cause serious toothache (see also Chapter 7 and Section 21.2, Pages 75 and 274).

That the team must be physically fit goes without saying. However, experience shows that, especially on major treks, persons may be encountered, who should not be there: they have neither the necessary physical endurance nor are they safe on their feet.
The team must also be properly **insured for the country they are visiting:** return/repatriation insurance, insurance against both sickness and accidents. It is best if each participant organizes his own insurance. The majority of insurance policies today include mountaineering expeditions and trekking in the insured risks.

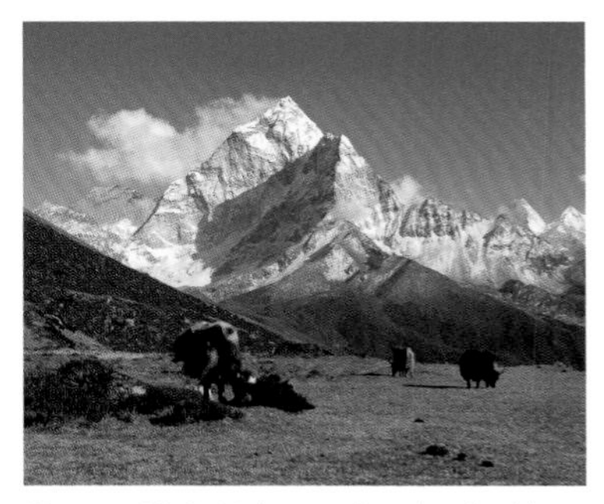

Figure 16.2: *Yak meadow backed by Ama Dablam 6856m, Khumbu/Nepal (U. Wiget).*

It is possible to obtain information on existing **rescue facilities** by referring to the relevant literature (travel guide) and/or people familiar with the target region. In a number of classic trekking and expedition areas helicopter rescues are possible, provided you can pay for them upfront. For example, a helicopter rescue in the Khumbu region of Nepal will set you back between 4000 and 5000 US dollars. Unless you have deposited this amount already with the trekking organization, it is advisable to take a **credit card** with you as this is accepted in many places.

In our opinion, taking time out to read the relevant literature on customs and habits in the respective region should also form part of the preparations. In conjunction with this we would also like to point out that, in certain trekking areas, there is a major risk of sexually transmitted diseases (HIV, hepatitis B etc.) and it is essential to follow the corresponding advice (such as practicing safe sex).

Vaccination advice should be obtained from an information office for travel medicine as the situation regarding infections is constantly changing. For an initial indication see web site **www.safetravel.ch.**

If you employ a local team you will also be responsible for these individuals and will need to take care of their technical and medical equipment. A reputable local travel agency should be able to arrange insurance for your local team, and such cover should be considered mandatory (see also **www.ippg.net).**

The **First Aid kit for the trek/expedition** in essence depends on the expedition objectives, the size of the team and the level of knowledge of the individuals. As a matter of basic principle, each participant should take with them their own regular medications. It is also a good idea to put together a small First Aid kit that will not take up too much room in the leader's day pack on the initial climb or during the trek.

On expeditions and treks with a large number of participants it has proved a good idea to split the "big" **basic First Aid kit** into at least two identical loads, as occasionally a yak manages to lose the very load containing the First Aid kit…

On expeditions, a small First Aid kit for the **high altitude camps** can also be made up. Here an experienced doctor or pharmacist will be of great help – the lists given here are merely food for thought.

It is also essential to follow the manufacturer's instructions on the medication leaflets. This information must be taken along for all medications. Of particular importance are the detailed instructions for use of the contents of the First Aid kits. These should be drawn up by an experienced doctor or pharmacist to correspond with the specific kit contents.

When putting together a First Aid kit for a trek or expedition it should be taken into consideration that the local population has a reasonable expectation to medical treatment too. For this reason the quantities of painkillers/antipyretics, heartburn remedies, bandages and dressings must be adjusted to take account of the number of contacts anticipated (specimen First Aid kit, see Annex, Page 289).

Listed below are a few ideas for more ambitious treks:

- **Clothing:** travel light (you can always wash it…), sports underwear and lightweight fleece pullover or sweater/shirt, anorak
- **Sun/Heat:** can become tremendous despite the altitude. A small umbrella can help. A good sun cream (e.g. Daylong®, Spirig) is essential: it should have an all-day action and not trigger allergies. A hat with a wide brim and a thin scarf or shawl will also be useful. And don't forget to pack two good pairs of sunglasses and an effective lip salve.
- **Bathing shoes** (surf shoes) made from Neoprene are helpful when it comes to crossing rivers – they provide significantly better grip in cold, fast-flowing water than, for example, Tevas or sandals.
- **Baggage weight:** if weight is a problem because of the flight, remember that you can buy pretty well everything that you need in all the larger trekking centres (Kathmandu, Manali, Leh…) – plus it will be even cheaper… toothpaste, shower gel, soap, detergent for washing clothes. Down jackets, mattresses, fleece clothing and other materials are very easy to come by and are often cheap – in addition you can, once the trek is over, donate them to the porters or the cook and do these undemanding and honest people a much-appreciated favour…
- **Sleeping bag:** your decision of a down or synthetic bag will depend on the trek/expedition. Down is warmer and is easier to fold up small, but does not tolerate damp as readily as synthetic fibres. An internal sleeping bag made from silk or cotton is to be recommended. A cat collar in the internal sleeping bag will do a good job of keeping out uninvited guests such as fleas, bedbugs and lice…
- In the majority of hotels and lodges the beds are so hard that even the smallest twinge of arthritis of the hip will mean that you sleep badly due to the pain – it is essential to take along a small, short, inflatable **mat** (e.g. small Thermarest®).
- When it comes to hygiene, lightweight bath towels made from synthetic material have proved a good investment.
- And don't forget to take along a few **wet wipes** which you can burn after use.

- We recommend that you choose high-sided **trekking shoes,** although many trekkers do go for trainers. The risk of spraining an ankle in rough terrain is considerable. In addition, sudden changes in the weather are a frequent occurrence.
- **Snacks:** the value of taking with you a few packs of nuts, almonds, chocolate or other food that you can snack on while walking along is undisputed. If you are really thirsty and there is no water available you can also tuck into snow at the same time; a small piece of chocolate and a mouthful of snow will provide liquid without drying out the roof of the mouth.

A special group of equipment is the electronic items. In this medical volume we can only give one or two brief details of this:

- A **satellite telephone** can be a vital factor when it comes to summoning help quickly. Information on which system (Iridium or Thuraya) works best in the relevant area can be obtained from the trekking organisation for the relevant country. These items of equipment are also available to hire.
- Whether a **GPS device** is likely to be of any use depends on whether one is trekking in a charted or uncharted region. In certain crisis areas (Baltoro–Pakistan) it is often forbidden to carry a GPS device.
- In certain heavily frequented trekking regions it is possible to charge up one's own battery-operated equipment (camera, mobile, MP3-Player etc.) in the lodges, for a small fee.
- One (unfortunately quite expensive) system for charging up all the equipment you can imagine (including computers) is the "Sunbag L" from Off-Grid, something which has proved invaluable on a long trek.

⇨ Certain countries do not permit the import of radio equipment (Oman 2008).

16.3 During the Trip

When on trips to tropical latitudes, a few simple rules can help to get the trek or the start of an expedition underway without diarrhea (and hence a weakening of one's general condition).

- **"Boil it, cook it, peel it or forget it"** still applies today: Avoid anything that you can't cook or peel! Drink only boiled water or drinks in bottles that you open immediately prior to consumption.

In addition: beer must only be made with pure water otherwise it goes cloudy. Beer is quite safe anywhere if the bottle has been kept closed.

⇨ The fastest way to clear up an attack of **diarrhoea on the trip** is to treat it with an antibiotic (Chinolon, e.g. Ciprofloxacin®, except in South East Asia where Azithromycin is the drug of choice), if necessary with the addition of small doses of loperamide (Imodium® or similar).

Usually a single dose will suffice. Starvation is now an out-of-date approach, the patient may eat whatever he fancies. Coffee (and also cola-based drinks) is, however, contraindicated due to the caffeine, which increases dehydration. It is important to ensure sufficient intake of fluids (e.g. tea with some sugar for better absorption) and electrolytes (e.g. soup, savory snacks).

The precise doses and the duration of antibiotic usage need to be explained by a doctor before the trip because details change frequently. Loperamide (Imodium® and others) can also help by ensuring that the patient does not lose too much water; at the start of an attack of diarrhea, assuming there is no fever, the patient can also take 1–2 Carbolevure® capsules; often the combination of charcoal and yeast will have the effect of stopping the diarrhea within 24 hours.

- **Long-haul flights** can have an adverse effect on the circulation in the legs and, in extreme cases, may even lead to a blockage of a large vein in the leg **(thrombosis*).** Anyone who suffers from slightly swollen legs when spending lengthy periods on their feet at home will benefit from donning a pair of lightweight support stockings for the flight. In addition it is advisable to drink as much as possible and walk about where this is feasible and/or move the feet and legs about as frequently as you can.
- In certain (emergency) cases the REGA can also provide specific details of hospitals and doctors locally (Tel. 0041 333 333 333), (see Section 9.1, Page 95).
- Many German embassies (e.g. in Delhi) employ a regional doctor who is up to date with regional ailments and who may be able to help with more serious health problems **(www.auswaertiges-amt.de).**

16.4 One or two Frequent Medical Problems on Treks and Expeditions

Blisters on the feet: there are innumerable tricks and tips for avoiding blisters on the feet. It Is definitely advantageous not to wear one's trekking shoes for the first time on the evening before embarking on the trek–we recommend that, wherever possible, you wear the shoes for some days (or in the evening…) at home, unless proper "running-in" is possible. Anywhere known to be susceptible can be covered with thin, elastic, self-adhesive dressings (Fixomull® stretch, for example), at the same time taking care to ensure that the dressings selected are large enough to avoid any risk of their rolling up as you walk. Another alternative is a "second skin" such as, for example, Spenco®. Prior to lengthy tours and treks it is advantageous not to wash the feet too frequently–especially not with warm water. Thin stockings under normal socks have proved a good idea while walking, as they form a sliding layer between the skin and the socks. We also think that people should go bare foot as often as possible, both at home and out of doors.

Treatment: Once a blister has formed you should on no account cut away the skin covering it. The blister can be drained by inserting a hypodermic needle or a scalpel blade to pierce the roof of the blister at several points. You can do the same thing with a sewing needle sterilized over a candle flame–the fine layer of soot that often continues to adhere does not matter. The blister is exposed to the fresh air for as long

* Under certain circumstances it makes sense to use a prophylactic such as Fraxiparin® or Fragmin® or similar medications (for prevention of thrombosis): for this the expedition doctor should be consulted.

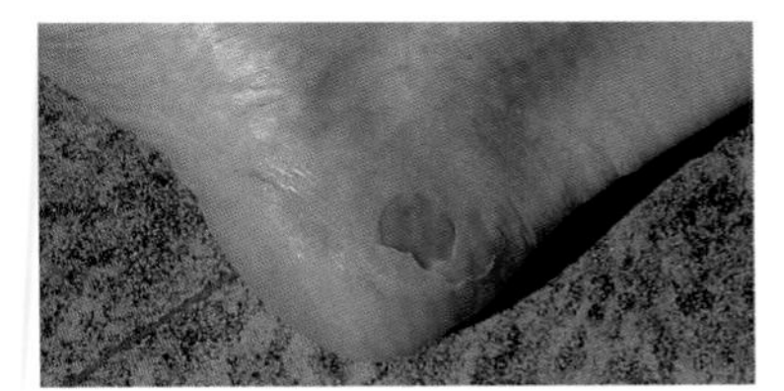

as possible and the dry skin on the blister left in place. Open, fresh blisters are very painful and can have a major adverse effect on progress.

Figure 16.3: *Unpleasant Companion on a Trek: A Foot Blister (U. Wiget).*

A simple and effective treatment in the field:

> After disinfecting the wound a piece of a (clean!) plastic bag (not the printed side) is placed directly on the wound and tied firmly or glued in place. Every 12 hours the non-adhesive dressing needs to be removed, the yellowish layer on the wound wiped away using a gauze or a clean cloth and the wound, once it has again been disinfected, should be left exposed to the air for as long as possible.*

Whenever a new dressing is required (nighttime, resumption of walking ...), the same procedure can be repeated until the wound has formed a scab.
A somewhat more expensive variant is a **hydrocolloid plaster,** which assume the function of a second skin (Compeed® and similar). They encourage the body's own healing mechanism, thereby accelerating the healing of the skin. By protecting the nerve ends they rapidly sooth the pain.

Hemorrhoids: are a tiresome complication of walking with a rucksack, where the abdominal muscles have to work harder than usual to compensate for the shift in weight of the upper body. As a result the pressure in the abdominal cavity is raised over a prolonged period encouraging the formation of hemorrhoids. Lack of hygiene exacerbates the complaint.
Should a painful pile protrude we recommend not using any suppositories or creams because these frequently cause additional inflammation of the highly sensitive skin in this area. In our own experience the simplest and best treatment on trekking and expeditions is right in front of the patient's nose, so to speak: ice-cold water and/or ice or snow. Cool the painful spot for as long as you can tolerate it and do it several

* This method originated from Dr. Dave Allan, a surgeon in Bangor/Wales. The author is also an enthusiastic advocate of this method and has never observed a single infection in 20 years. Due to the biofilm, plastic can indeed be a carrier of bacteria and it would therefore seem sensible to check the wound regularly and disinfect it. If need be you can "top up" the blister with betadine once you have popped it to encourage the floor of the wound to scab over but note that it is painful!

times a day. Non-stinging wet wipes (for babies) do an excellent job. You can utilize all these measures if the hemorrhoids bleed. In addition, one should be careful not to get constipated. If this happens, you should consume as much dietary fiber as possible (available in vegetables, rye flour [Tsampa] etc.) and maybe use a herbal remedy for constipation to help. In addition, an anti-inflammatory such as Brufen® 400 or 600 mg 2–3 times a day may help the pain to die down quickly.

High altitude cough: This very tiresome dry cough can crop up on lengthy expeditions or treks. Even doctors find that treating it is at best difficult or at worst impossible. It is a dry cough which is not unduly productive, without fever or any other physical indications. It tends to disturb patients predominantly during the night and unfortunately does not particularly respond to any medication. The best remedy has been shown to be frequent inhalations of hot steam (with Nasobol®), something which is possible at a high level camp. Although supplements are not necessary, herbal tea may also be taken.

Cracks in the skin (rhagades): Porters especially, who go bare foot, but also participants in treks and expeditions can develop very painful, deep cracks in the skin of the feet and/or fingers. Salves and other skin preparations have no effect on healing the skin during the trek. A tried-and-tested remedy here is to use a skin adhesive (for example, Histoacryl®). Cut open the vial of adhesive and carefully apply one drop directly into the cracks in the skin. The adhesive spreads immediately, closing off the base of the crack so that it is waterproof and thus enabling the crack to heal from the inside out because no water or dirt can now penetrate it. Occasionally it may be necessary to repeat the application after a few days.

Under no circumstances allow the adhesive to get into the eyes. Be very careful when cutting open and applying – it is best to wear spectacles during the procedure.

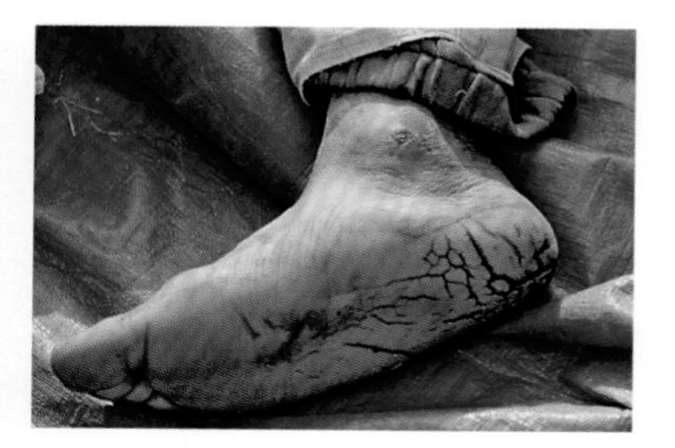

Treating pain: Wherever pain is present the most important factors are immobilization and protection from the cold. This also applies to pain not due to accidents.

Figure 16.4: *Deep and painful skin cracking on a Pakistani porter (U. Wiget).*

When treating severe pain, the only drugs that should be used are those that the helper or the patient are familiar with. In most cases, Paracetamol (Dafalgan®, Tylenol® etc.) will work, on its own or in combination with an anti-inflammatory medication such as Ibuprufen (Brufen® etc.). However, it is essential to ensure compliance with the instruction leaflet. **Spasmodic pains** such as renal colic or menstrual pains can be helped by anti-inflammatories as described above. Stronger remedies have more marked side effects, such as, for example, vomiting in the case of Tramal®. However, there are a whole range of popular remedies stretching back to antiquity that demonstrate some effect and which can be used anywhere without risk (see Table 15.1).

Sore throat, cough	Breathe in (inhale) steam (tea …) frequently
Stomach ache	Dip a large cloth in hot water, unwind and place as hot as possible on the skin of the abdomen and cover with a blanket; change at very frequent intervals (or use a hot drinking flask …)
Back ache	Improvised cummerbund, pull until taut (long johns, scarf, bandage if there is one available)
Headache	Cold, moist compresses on forehead and neck
Fever	Cold, moist leg compresses – cover with thick socks
Eyes	Wet teabags on (closed) eyes
Earache	Nose drops (in the nose!)
Sprain	Local cooling with snow or ice (over a bandage or socks)
Muscle pain	Same treatment as sprain, at least for the first two days

Table 15.1: *Simple medical treatment remedies.*

17. Mountaineering in Extreme Altitudes

T. Merz, M. Maggiorini

It is not the mountain we conquer but ourselves.
Sir Edmund Hillary

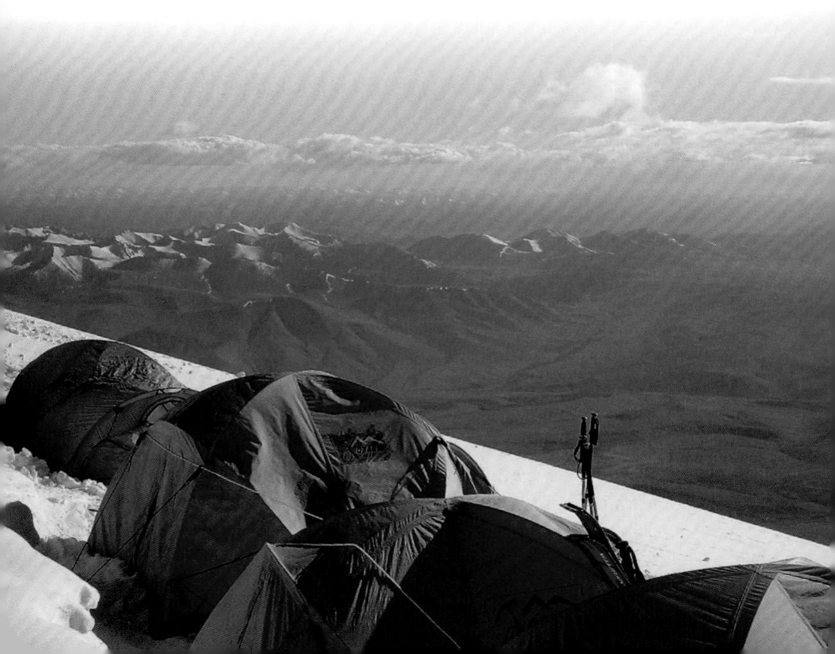

17.1 Physical and Physiological Principles

Air pressure is defined as the force per unit area that is exerted on a surface. The weight of the column of air above this surface ("force") determines the air pressure and allows the mercury thermometer at sea level to climb to 760 mmHg (experiment carried out by Torricelli). Factors such as air temperature and relative humidity affect the weight of the column of air above the point of measurement. The air pressure is greatest at sea level and decreases with increasing altitude as the height–and therefore the weight–of the column of air decreases. The density of the atmosphere and thus the height of the column of air is not uniform throughout: as a result of the Earth's rotation and higher air temperatures, a denser atmosphere exists above the Equator and this reduces towards the Poles. This effect is quite noticeable when mountaineering in Polar regions. There are various units of measurement for quantifying air pressure; it can be stated at sea level as 101.32 kilopascals (kPa), or 1013.25 millibars (mbar), 760 mmHg or 760 Torr.
The proportion of oxygen in the air is 21 %, regardless of the air pressure. The proportion of oxygen contributing to the air pressure is termed the partial pressure of oxygen and is equivalent at sea level to 159.6 mmHg (or 21 % of 760 mmHg) and, at 5000 m, with an air pressure of 40.6 mmHg, to only 85 mmHg (21 % of 406 mmHg).

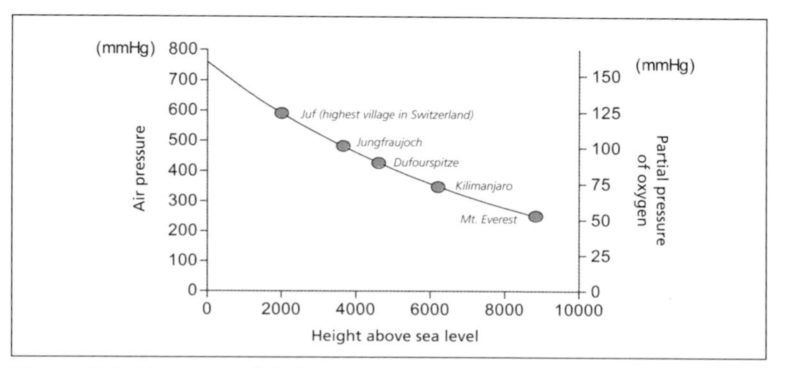

Figure 17.1: *Air pressure (left diagram axis) and partial pressure of oxygen (right diagram axis) depending on height above sea level.*
At 5500 m above sea level the air pressure and the partial pressure of oxygen correspond to roughly half and, at 8848 m above sea level, approximately one third of the pressure at sea level (assuming 0 % atmospheric humidity).

Only the partial pressure of oxygen in the air we inhale is of any significance as far as human metabolism is concerned; this can be increased by raising either the overall air pressure (hyperbaric chamber) or the proportion of oxygen (by adding oxygen from an oxygen cylinder).

At sea level and at heights of up to approximately 1500 m above sea level, the blood flowing through the lung is almost 100 % saturated with oxygen, i.e. each red blood cell/corpuscle (oxygen-carrier containing hemoglobin molecules) is filled with oxygen. Due to the fall in the partial pressure of oxygen at high levels, the diffusion of oxygen from the alveolus into the blood is limited. As a result, the blood can no longer be completely saturated with oxygen and many oxygen carriers leave the lung without having been loaded up with oxygen. This leads to a lower saturation of the arterial blood with oxygen, in particular during physical exertion (Figure 17.2).

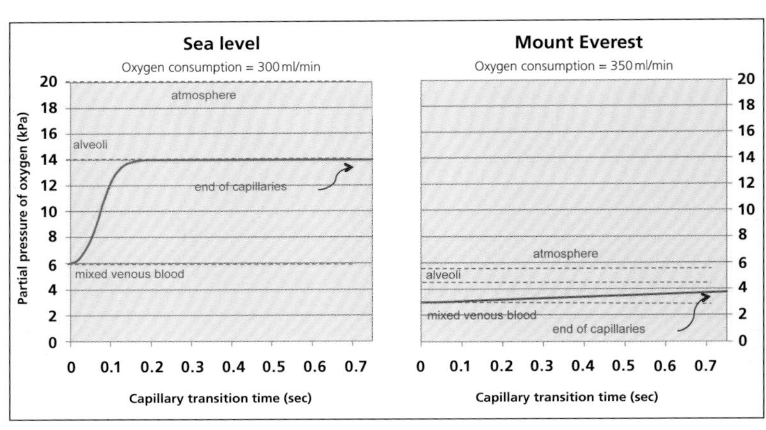

Figure 17.2: *Calculated change in partial pressure of oxygen during passage through the pulmonary capillaries.*
At sea level the partial pressure of oxygen in the blood rises very quickly and aligns itself with that of the air in the pulmonary capillaries. On the summit of Mount Everest the partial pressure of oxygen in the atmosphere and in the pulmonary capillaries decreases considerably, the gradient between the mixed venous blood and the alveoli becomes smaller and the blood is no longer able to enrich itself completely with oxygen. These changes are responsible for the limited oxygen diffusion at high altitude (diffusion limitation). Adapted from J.B. West and P.D. Wagner, Resp. Physiol 1980, 42:1 – 16.

Oxygen is of vital significance for the human organism because the provision of energy in the cells of the body is essentially based on the oxidation (burning up) of sugar, fat or protein. The lower quantity of oxygen available at high altitude leads to a reduction in the oxidative capacity of the muscle cells and hence to a reduction in performance capability.

Even at a height of 3000 m, maximum physical capability is still only about 85 % of **performance capability** at sea level. At 6000 m the mountaineer will still achieve around 60 % of his performance at sea level, but this falls to 20 % at the summit of Mt. Everest.

Figure 17.3 illustrates the relationship between altitude and oxygen saturation using the example of an expedition mountaineer on the ascent of Shisha Pangma (8046 m).

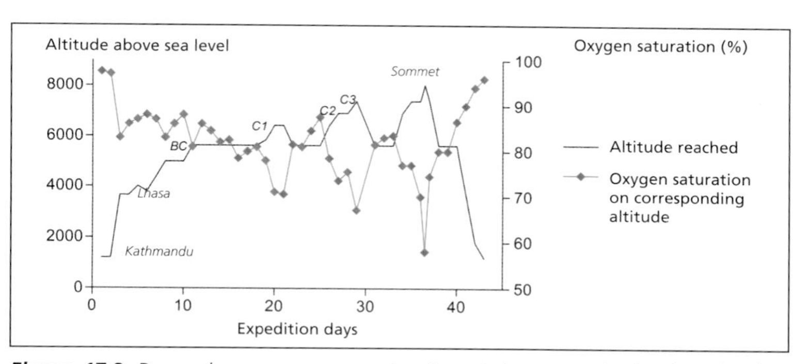

Figure 17.3: *Dependency on oxygen saturation at the respective level attained. This diagram shows the oxygen saturation of a mountaineer during an expedition to Shisha Pangma (8046 m), Tibet, taken on a daily basis using a pulse oximeter. The expedition route was via Kathmandu (1200 m) to Lhasa (3650 m) and from there on to base camp (BC, 5650 m). For the ascent of the mountain 3 high altitude camps were set up (C1, 6430 m; C2, 6920 m; C3, 7400 m). The arterial oxygen saturation varies between 98 % at lower altitudes (Kathmandu) and 58 % (at the summit of the mountain).*

17.2 Acclimatization

The human body's response to a reduction of oxygen in the blood is to bring into play adaptive mechanisms to ensure survival and help to reduce the performance losses at high altitude. The full complement of these adaptive processes is known as (altitude) acclimatization. The process of acclimatization is diverse and complex, beginning within a matter of hours of reaching a new altitude and lasts for up to 14 days. Acclimatization partially improves performance capabilities but cannot completely reinstate this due to the limited oxygen diffusion in the lung.

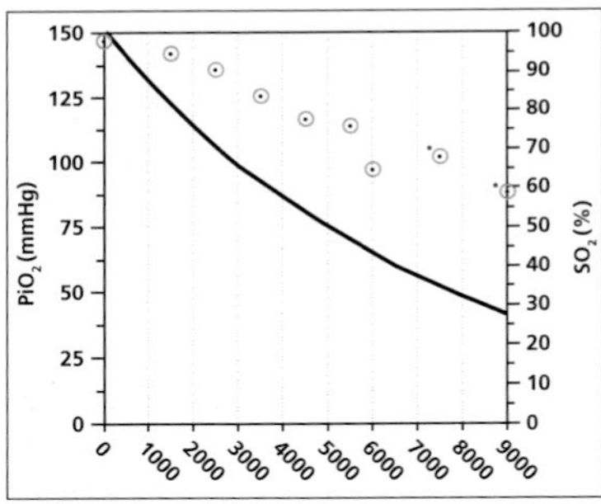

Figure 17.4: *Changes in oxygen saturation (%) in relation to partial pressure of oxygen at high altitude. The increasing difference between the partial pressure of oxygen (PiO_2) and oxygen saturation (SO_2) as altitude increases Is the result of hyperventilation (* = simulated height).*

Hyperventilation: The most important adaptation mechanism is the increase in breathing rate and depth known as hyperventilation. This accelerated breathing, which starts within minutes of reaching a new altitude, is triggered by chemoreceptors which react to the reduced partial pressure of oxygen in the arterial blood. Deepening of the respiration leads to improved ventilation of the lung and to increased amounts of carbon dioxide gas being expelled from the alveoli. Overall, these processes increase the oxygen content in the alveoli so that more oxygen can be transferred into the bloodstream (Figure 17.4).

Changes in the cardiovascular system: The decline of oxygen saturation in the blood leads, by stimulating the autonomic nervous system, to increases in the heart rate (pulse) and cardiac output (number of liters of blood that are transported by the heart in one minute). This physiological reaction serves to make more blood cells, laden with oxygen, available in the organs and muscles starved of oxygen. The increase in heart rate and cardiac output is directly proportional to the decline in oxygen saturation in the blood.

 Those mountaineers who suffer from a lack of oxygen have a higher **pulse.**

It is worth noting that the maximum heart rate achieved under exertion decreases with altitude. Whether this is in part responsible for restricted performance capability at high altitude has not yet been clarified.

Changes in pulmonary circulation: The low partial pressure of oxygen in the inhaled air leads, via a physiological reflex, to a narrowing and at the same time an increase in resistance of the pulmonary blood vessels (Euler-Liljestrand Reflex). Since the volume of blood flowing through the lung at any given minute stays the same, the heart is required to expend greater force (= pressure) in order to overcome the increased resistance. This increased pressure can be measured by way of raised blood pressure in the pulmonary arteries. As a result of the higher pressure in the pulmonary circulation, vessels in areas of the lung not previously supplied with blood are opened up whilst at the same time this reflex limits the flow of blood to non-ventilated sections of the lung.

Changes in acid base equilibrium: The acid content of the body (pH) is regulated precisely and within narrow tolerances by the human organism. Both too little acid (alkalosis) as well as too much acid (acidosis) will have a significant effect on biochemical processes and need to be corrected as quickly as possible. The hyperventilation caused by a lack of oxygen and described in the previous section will lead to increased exhalation of carbon dioxide gas and thus to a pronounced loss of acid from the body. The resulting alkalosis will be corrected by the body within hours/days through the discharge of increased quantities of alkalotic urine (altitude diuresis).

Increase in red blood cells (Polycythemia): A further effect of the reduction in oxygen content in the blood is the increased production of red blood cells. Although this does not increase oxygen saturation (it remains that only a certain proportion of the oxygen carriers are laden with oxygen), with the increase in the total number of oxygen carriers, the quantity of oxygen transported is also increased. However, this process of hematopoiesis (blood formation) takes days or even weeks to come about and is therefore of no significance as far as short term acclimatization is concerned. Longer periods of time spent at high altitude (e.g. during expeditions to the Himalayas lasting many weeks) will nevertheless lead to a considerable increase in the number of red blood cells (polycythemia) and, in combination with increased loss of fluids, also to an increased risk of the formation of blood clots (thromboses, embolisms).

Acclimatization Tactics

The human body needs a certain amount of time to acclimatize to a stay at high altitude. The faster the ascent and the greater the difference in altitude, the greater the risk that the acclimatization processes may not be sufficient to protect the body from the consequences of a lack of oxygen. In addition to exhaustion and increased susceptibility to injury, the primary consequence of neglecting acclimatization is the occurrence of altitude sickness. In order to avoid altitude sickness it is of paramount importance, especially at altitudes in excess of 3000 m above sea level, to undergo planned acclimatization. It should be noted that the onset of altitude sickness does not occur until several hours after arrival at a higher altitude. This means that the rules described in the following do not apply for daylong stays at high altitude (e.g. ski sports with overnight in the valley) but for periods of time amounting to more than 24 hours spent at high altitude.

Speed of Ascent: Above a height of 2500 m above sea level ascent should be no more than 600 m per day. This refers to the height at which the night is to be spent **(sleeping height),** whilst over the course of the day it is quite acceptable for ascents to higher altitudes to take place (e.g. in order to ascend a peak). Once an altitude gain of 1200 m has been attained, consideration should be given to an additional rest day. Once a height of more than 5000 m has been reached, several acclimatization days are recommended before tackling heights greater than 6000 m. It cannot be over-emphasised that acclimatization is the most important course of action when it comes to preventing altitude sickness!

Physical exertion: Significant physical exertion increases the risk of altitude sickness and should be avoided. A slow, steady walking tempo should be selected and any unnecessary pronounced effort should be avoid. Lack of sleep, lack of liquid or illness (colds, gastrointestinal problems) likewise increase the risk of altitude sickness.

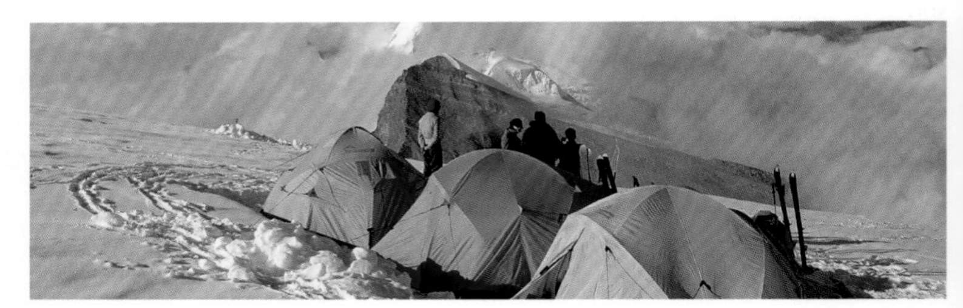

Figure 17.5: *Bedding down at 6400 m. Last high camp on the way to the summit of Putha Hiunchuli (Dolpo/Nepal) (A. Brunello).*

Acclimatisation Rules

- As of 3000 m above sea level do not increase sleeping height by more than 600 metres per day.
- Consider additional rest day after 1200 altimeters.
- During ascents over 6000 m, several acclimatisation days on an altitude of around 5000 m are strongly recommended.
- Avoid unnecessary and intensive activities.

17.3 Altitude Sickness

The cause of all forms of altitude sickness is, at the end of the day, the low partial pressure of oxygen and the resulting reduction of the oxygen content in the arterial blood. Failure to heed the acclimatization rules will inevitably lead to the development of altitude sickness. Altitude sickness can affect the lung and/or the brain:

- High Altitude Pulmonary Edema (HAPE)
- Acute Mountain Sickness (AMS)
- High Altitude Cerebral Edema (HACE) (final stage of Acute Mountain Sickness)

AMS and HACE are manifestations of varying severity of what is probably the same pathological process. Initially less serious symptoms of illness occur from which, however, the dreaded HACE may eventually develop, the outcome of which may be fatal. HAPE has a different pathophysiological mechanism and can occur either alone or in combination with AMS and HACE.

Acute Mountain Sickness (AMS) and High Altitude Cerebral Edema (HACE)
Pathophysiological mechanism: The brain is very sensitive to any decline in the supply of oxygen. Lack of oxygen will lead to unconsciousness in a few seconds and, within a matter of a few minutes, to permanent damage or even death.

Lack of oxygen and cerebral blood flow: in order to maintain the supply of oxygen despite a low oxygen content in the blood, the cerebral blood flow is increased by distension of the brain arteries (cerebral arteries) (vasodilatation) which leads to an increase in the cerebral blood volume. The hyperventilation due to a lack of oxygen (deepening and accelerating of respiration, see Acclimatisation, Page 210) with exhalation of carbon dioxide and alkalosis leads to the narrowing **(vasoconstriction)** of the blood vessels of the brain and counteracts vasodilatation due to a lack of oxygen. The cerebral blood flow is thus the result of a balance between vasodilatation due to lack of oxygen and vasoconstriction due to alkalosis (loss of acid). However, vasodilatation predominates so that the brain, despite a lack of oxygen, is adequately supplied with oxygen.

The increase in the blood supply to the cerebral blood vessels leads to an increase in the porosity of the vessel wall (leakage) and thus to the **exit of fluid** from the blood vessels into the tissue of the brain, at which point this increases in volume (cerebral edema). In its advanced state, the porosity of the blood vessels may be interfered with to such an extent that, in addition to the loss of liquid and proteins, small hemorrhages may also take place. In addition, the lack of oxygen in the tissues of the brain leads to a disturbance in the metabolism of the brain cells leading to **swelling** of the cell bodies and to a further increase in brain volume. The changes to the cerebral blood vessel walls and the disturbance to the metabolism of the brain cells are the cause of the classic symptoms of AMS and its final stage HACE.

⇨ Since there is, within the bony part of the skull, only very little reserve space for the brain to expand, any increased swelling will soon lead to a rise in pressure in the interior of the cranium which will further adversely affect brain function.

In extreme circumstances, the pressure inside the cranium may exceed the arterial blood pressure, which will interrupt the supply of blood to the brain resulting in brain death.

Identification of Symptoms: As a rule the signs develop 6 to 12 hours after arrival at high altitude. The transition from AMS to HACE is smooth and is characterized by the maximum possible increase in the symptoms described in the following.

- **Headache** is the main symptom of AMS and may develop from light pressure right through to the crushing feeling that one's head is "about to explode." Typically, the headaches occur at night or in the morning.
- Increasing loss of appetite develops as well as nausea up to the point of (uncontrollable) **vomiting.**
- There may be a degree of exhaustion and fatigue which is often played down by the patient and ascribed to other causes; in serious cases this increases to **lethargy** (sleepiness, listlessness) culminating in complete inability to act.
- Difficulties in falling asleep, or complete **insomnia.**
- **Dizziness** and balance disturbance are further signs of AMS.
- Often a rise in body temperature will ensue after a period of time.

Increasing brain swelling finally leads to clearly perceptible functional disturbances of the brain which define the HACE complex of symptoms. These include:

- Disturbances to gait and eventual **inability to walk**
- Increasing **confusion**
- Euphoria (exhilaration) and agitation (excitement), and finally **unconsciousness**

A simple test to diagnose an impediment to gait is **walking in a straight line.** In this the patient is asked to walk along a straight line, heel to toe; any balance disorder will be revealed in the form of stumbling or being unable to stay on the line.

Table 17.1 summarizes the most important symptoms and findings relating to AMS and HACE arranged in order of severity.

Severity		Symptoms	Findings
Acute Mountain Sickness (AMS)	Slight	Slight headaches, little appetite, slight nausea, disturbances to sleep	
	Moderate	Headaches, lack of appetite, nausea, sleeplessness, feeling of dizziness	
	Serious	Intense headaches (do not respond to headache tablets), vomiting, severe dizziness, listlessness, weakness	Temp >37.4 °C
High Altitude Cerebral Edema (HACE)		Violent headaches, constant vomiting, severe dizziness, drowsiness	Temp >37.4 °C, confusion, disturbances to gait, inability to walk, unconsciousness

Table 17.1: *Symptoms and findings–AMS and HACE.*

Prevention:

Careful acclimatisation is the most important course of action when it comes to the prevention of AMS and HACE.

Over ambition or lack of time often lead to any thoughts of acclimatization being thrown to the wind. This leads at best to unpleasant symptoms of illness which have the potential to significantly spoil one's pleasure on reaching the summit; or at worst to life-threatening situations. It cannot be over-emphasised that the preventive medication described in the following can **never** be a replacement for meticulous acclimatization!

If a slow adaptation to the altitude is not possible (e.g. in cases of direct flights to higher regions), one possibility is to start taking acetazolamide (Diamox®) in doses of 125 mg every 12 hours on the evening prior to the ascent, stimulating the excretion of bicarbonate in the urine and at the same time encouraging acclimatisation.

Increasing the elimination of bicarbonate generates a metabolic acidosis (over-acidification as a result of increasing the hydrogen ion concentration in the blood) which stimulates respiration (hyperventilation) and thus to an increase in the oxygen saturation in the blood. Many other medications, in particular those from the alternative medicine sector, claim to prevent altitude sickness. However, their effect has not been proven in clinical studies.

For projects on high mountains or repeated occurrences of pronounced altitude-related illness, the advice of a doctor with experience in altitude medicine should be sought. The Swiss Association for Mountain Medicine (SGGM) can put you in touch with appropriate contacts on request **(www.sggm.ch).**

Treatment: Whereas the milder form of AMS often occurs and, although it may be tiresome, is relatively harmless, a serious attack of AMS and, in particular, HACE represents an emergency situation and all possible therapeutic measures must be initiated without delay. Descent is always the best therapy, not only because of the higher air pressure at valley level but also due to the availability of what are, in most cases, better medical supplies. The therapy for AMS and HACE is based on three different action mechanisms:

- The increase in **partial pressure of oxygen** in the air we breathe and hence the supply of oxygen leads to a reduction in the increased supply of blood to the brain and to regression of the swelling of the brain.
- This can be achieved by increasing the pressure of the surrounding air (descent, mobile hyperbaric chamber) or by increasing the oxygen content in the inhaled air (bottled oxygen).
- **Corticosteroids** such as Dexamethasone (Decadron®, 4 mg 4 x daily) lead by way of what are still, to a major extent, unexplained mechanisms, to the stabilisation of the vascular wall of the cerebral vessels and thus to a reduction in the amount of fluid escaping into the tissue of the brain.
- Dexamethasone can, in an emergency, (if the patient is vomiting or is unconscious) also be given as an intravenous or intramuscular injection (dose: 8 mg into vein/muscle.; 2 ampules). Dextramethasone also has a strong anti-emetic effect and is slightly euphorigenic in its action. Taking Dexamethasone longer term is not to be recommended due to its less desirable effects (increase in blood pressure, blood sugar and susceptibility to Infection).

- **Acetazolamide** (Diamox®, 250 mg 2 x per day) has the effect of counteracting the impaired respiration that develops as a result of the fall in carbon dioxide in the blood, bringing about deeper and more effective breathing and preventing the pauses in breathing typical of high altitude. The alkalosis due to height is corrected faster and acclimatisation accelerated. Acetazolamide is suitable for therapeutic treatment of the tiresome slight to medium-grade AMS (persistent headache, nausea, fatigue and sleeplessness) whilst Dexamethasone is for treatment of serious AMS and HACE.

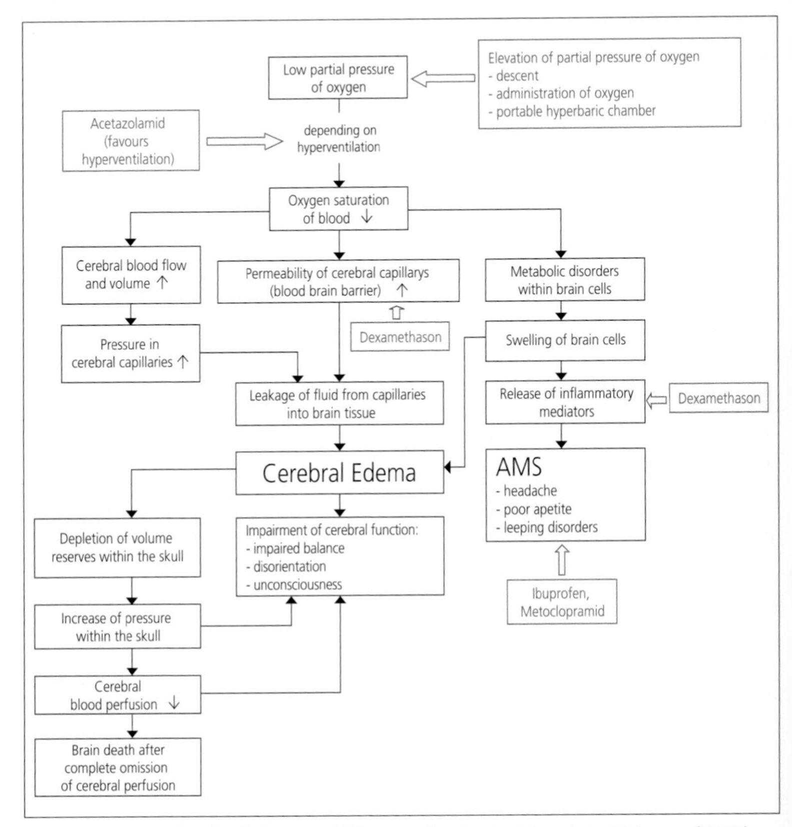

Figure 17.6: *Pathophysiology and Therapy for Acute Mountain Sickness (AMS) and High Altitude Pulmonary Edema (HAPE).*

In addition to the above therapy for AMS and HACE, unpleasant accompanying phenomena also often need to treated. These include in particular pain killers (analgesics e.g. Ibuprofen [Brufen®], 500 mg 3–4x daily) for headaches and medicines for nausea and sickness (anti-emetics, e.g. Metoclopramide [Paspertin®] 10 mg 3–4x daily). It is no good using medications such as Sildenafil (Viagra®) or Nifedipin (Adalat®) in the prevention and therapy of AMS and HACE as they have no effect!

Figure 17.6, Page 218 shows an overview of the pathophysiologic interrelationships and the therapeutic possibilities in AMS and HACE.

Table 17.2 summarizes the most important therapeutic measures in the case of AMS and HACE.

Degree of Severity		Therapy	Action
Acute Mountain Sickness (AMS)	Slight	No specific therapy required	No unnecessary exertion, consider a rest day
	Moderate	Acetazolamide Analgesics and anti-emetics as required	No unnecessary exertion, avoid ascending further
	Serious	Dexamethasone Analgesics as required Oxygen 2–4 L/min.	Descend without delay (min. 1000 m) If not possible, hyperbaric chamber
High Altitude Cerebral Edema (HACE)		Dexamethasone Analgesics as required Oxygen 2–4 L/min.	Immediate descent/ evacuation (min. 1000 m) If not possible, hyperbaric chamber

Table 17.2

Serious AMS and HACE are life-threatening situations! A patient with HACE can die within a few hours. Therapy and evacuation to lower altitudes are a maximum priority and must take place as quickly as possible.

Serious AMS and HACE –> descent–oxygen–Dexamethasone*

---

* According to priority

High Altitude Pulmonary Edema (HAPE)

Persons predisposed to HAPE display an excessive rise in vascular resistance (hypoxic vasoconstriction) in the pulmonary circulation at high altitude, which leads to high blood pressure in the pulmonary circulation (pulmonary hypertension). In addition, the increase in resistance appears not to be uniform, i.e. certain sections of the lung demonstrate increased hypoxic vasoconstriction, whereas other sections of the lung show less reaction. Since the increase in resistance predominately takes place in the arteries of the lung, this can lead to the exposure of lung capillaries to the full rise in blood pressure in sections of the lung without vasoconstriction (Figures 17.7 A and B).

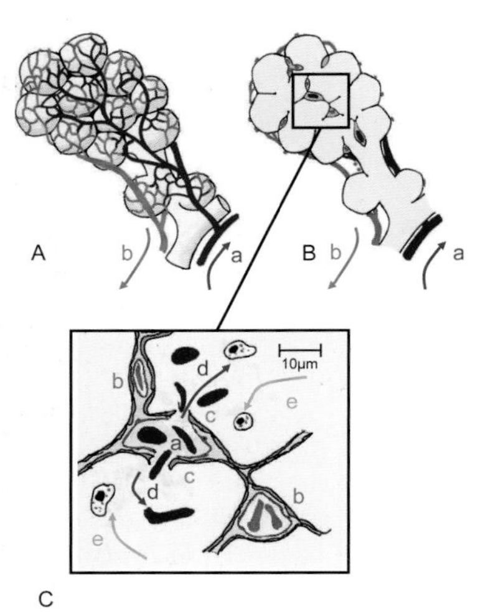

Figure 17.7: *Pathophysiology of High Altitude Pulmonary Edema (HAPE) A (plan view) and B (cross section) show the smallest airways (bronchioles) with branching into alveoli. It is in the alveoli that the interchange of oxygen and carbon dioxide between the blood and the air takes place. The alveoli are surrounded by a dense network of blood vessels: a) the arteries of the lung convey blood with a low oxygen content from the body's circulatory system to the alveoli; b) Veins in the lung transport the blood, enriched with oxygen, from the alveoli back into the body's circulatory system. The decline in partial pressure of the oxygen at high altitude leads to a rise in blood pressure in the arteries of the lung. C shows a detail view of the cross section through the alveoli of the lung with the embedded blood vessels. The occurrence of HAPE is caused by a rise in the blood pressure in the arteries of the lung. This leads to mechanical injuries to the very thin membrane (a few thousandths of a mm thick) between the blood vessels and the air-filled alveolar space (c), which means that fluids and blood cells are able to cross over into the alveolar space (d). The inflammatory reaction thus triggered with an accumulation of inflammatory cells and release of inflammatory mediators has the potential to further damage the alveolar wall (e).*

As a result of high pressure on the vessel wall, direct and shear forces develop which damage the membrane between the blood vessels of the lung and the alveolar space which is only a few thousandths of a millimeter thick. Very small injuries occur which enable the escape of protein-rich liquid and blood cells. The alveolar space, which is by now filled with liquid, is no longer available for the exchange of gases and the function of the lung is adversely affected. The blood and protein components in the alveolar space subsequently generate inflammatory reactions which further damage the alveolar membrane and encourage a further escape of liquid from the lung capillaries (see Figure 17.7 C, Page 220). These processes lead to a further reduction in the partial pressure of oxygen in the blood which, in turn, leads to a further increase in pressure in the arteries of the lung and to further damage to the alveolar walls.

It is important to recognize that the symptoms of HAPE are largely determined by the extent of the loss of lung function and the resulting lack of oxygen.

- The first symptom is often a sudden and unexplained **drop in performance.**
- First in the sequence is **difficulty in breathing** under exertion and later also at rest (orthopnea = increased difficulty in breathing when lying flat with improvement on sitting up).
- The patient starts coughing and often has a feeling of constriction in the chest; he will try to counteract the lack of oxygen by breathing rapidly.
- Despite this, the lips and finger nails may become tinged blue because of the lack of oxygen in the arterial blood **(cyanosis).**
- In the advanced stage, fluid collecting in the lung leads to coughing up **blood-stained froth.**
- Often, after a period of time, as with AMS and HACE, a rise in **body temperature** results.

Table 17.3 summarizes the most important symptoms and findings related to HAPE.

Degree of Severity	Symptoms	Findings
Incipient HAPE	Sudden drop in performance (Main symptom!)	
↓	Weakness, fatigue	High heart rate
	Feeling of constriction in the chest	Blue discolouration of lips and finger nails, peripheral oxygen saturation significantly lower than is usual for the altitude or compared to the day before at the same altitude.
	Difficulty in breathing under exertion	Very rapid breathing during low level exertion, decline in performance!
Serious HAPE	Dry cough	
	Difficulty when breathing and orthopnoea at rest	Difficulty breathing when lying down, very rapid respiration (> 25 breaths/minute)
	Coughing with frothy, blood-stained sputum	Audible, loose rattling when breathing
		Fever

Table 17.3: *Symptoms and Findings.*

Prevention: Careful acclimatization is the most important step toward preventing HAPE. This particularly applies to persons who have had HAPE symptoms previously on exposure to altitude.

⇨ The risk of a new attack of HAPE in the event of too rapid an ascent to above 3000 m is more than 50 % in persons who have already had one attack.

Where such persons are concerned, prevention with drugs following a consultation with a doctor trained in altitude medicine is recommended.
The Swiss Society for Mountain Medicine SGGM can on request (www.sggm.ch) put you in touch with the appropriate contacts.
The concept of prevention with drugs in the case of HAPE is based on stopping an excessive rise in blood pressure in the circulation of the lung.

Drugs aimed at prevention: Nifedipin (Adalat® CR 30–60) or Tadalafil (Cialis® 20 mg), one tablet daily starting 24 hours after ascent. Both medications can intensify the headaches associated with AMS. Recently it has been shown that it is possible, by taking a high dose of Dexamethasone (2 x 8 mg/day) as a prophylactic, to prevent HAPE. For longer stays at high altitude we would strongly discourage the use of a prophylactic incorporating Dexamethasone due to its undesirable side-effects.

Treatment: An attack of HAPE can rapidly develop into life-threatening lung failure. In addition, an attack of HAPE is associated with a very serious deficiency of oxygen which considerably increases the risk of other manifestations of altitude sickness (AMS/HACE).

⇨ If an attack of HAPE is suspected therapy must be commenced immediately and plans made for a descent.

- **Nifedipin** (Adalat CC®; 20 mg 3 times a day) reduces high blood pressure; it also works on the circulation in the lung and thus helps to improve the symptoms. A preparation which works more selectively on the circulation in the lung is Sildenafil (Viagra®), the recommended dose is 3 x 25 mg.
- Where moderate to severe AMS and HACE present concomitantly the therapy should be supplemented with **Dexamethasone** (Decadron®, 4 mg 4 times a day).
- If available, **oxygen** should be given at the rate of 4–6 litres per minute with the aim of raising oxygen saturation to above 88 %.
- An attempt should be made to ensure **immediate descent** by a minimum of 1000 metres of altitude.

If at all possible, the patient should be carried because physical exertion will increase the pressure in the blood vessels in the lung.

- If delays in transport occur the patient should be placed in a portable **hyperbaric chamber.**

⇨ Monitoring the patient is more difficult in the hyperbaric chamber. The patient must not be left alone; oxygen saturation, pulse and their state of consciousness must be checked regularly.

The portable hyperbaric chamber is, however, **never** a replacement for descent as the symptoms recur immediately on leaving the chamber.

HAPE represents a threat to life! Therapy and evacuation to lower levels have maximum priority and must take place as quickly as possible.
HAPE –> descent–oxygen–Nifedipin or Sildenafil–Dexamethasone (–> where applicable hyperbaric chamber) *

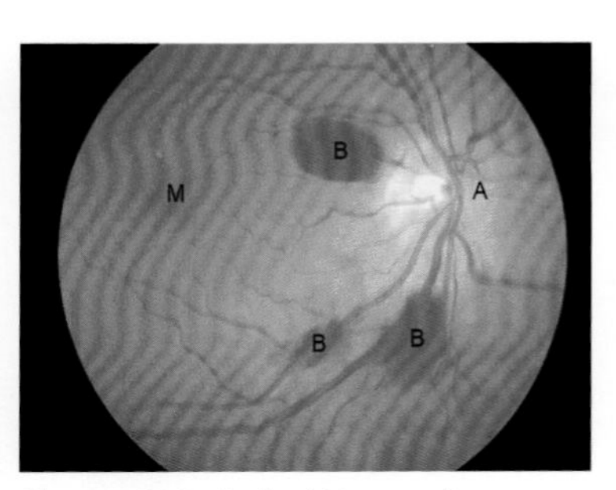

Figure 17.8: *Retinal Haemorrhages. This illustration shows the retina of a mountaineer on the ascent of Muztagh Ata (7545 m above sea level). The photograph was taken using a special camera on a medical research expedition.*
A: Head of the optic nerve; B: A number of retinal hemorrhages; M: Macula (Site of central vision) (M. Bosch).

Retinal Hemorrhages (High Altitude Retinal Hemorrhage [HARH])

The retina is subject to similar regulatory mechanisms as the rest of the circulatory system Lack of oxygen at high altitude leads to an increased supply of blood to the vessels of the retina. This increase in the supply of blood, which may be combined with damage to the vessel walls due to the lack of oxygen, often leads to small hemorrhages in the retina. As long as the hemorrhage is confined to the periphery of the retina it mostly goes unnoticed or leads to only minor disruption at the periphery of the field of vision. However, if the hemorrhage affects the macula (site of central vision) this will lead to the development of damaging **blind spots** (scotomas) (see Figure 17.8).

Prevention and Treatment: It is not known whether sufficient acclimatization reduces the risk regarding HARH, hemorrhages occur in more than 50 % of all mountaineers at heights of more than 5000 m, regardless of acclimatization. There is no therapy; the hemorrhages will disappear of their own accord within a matter of weeks.

* In accordance with priorities

4 golden rules of high altitude mountaineering:

- In the absence of evidence to the contrary, at altitude all health complaints and symptoms are assumed to have been caused by altitude sickness in one form or another.
- In the event of symptoms of any altitude sickness, improve acclimatisation.
- If you are ill, your condition worsens, your headaches do not go away and/or you find yourself vomiting regularly, or your performance capability starts to fall off rapidly, descend immediately.
- A patient suffering from any form of altitude sickness must never be left alone or left to descend alone.

18. The Cold

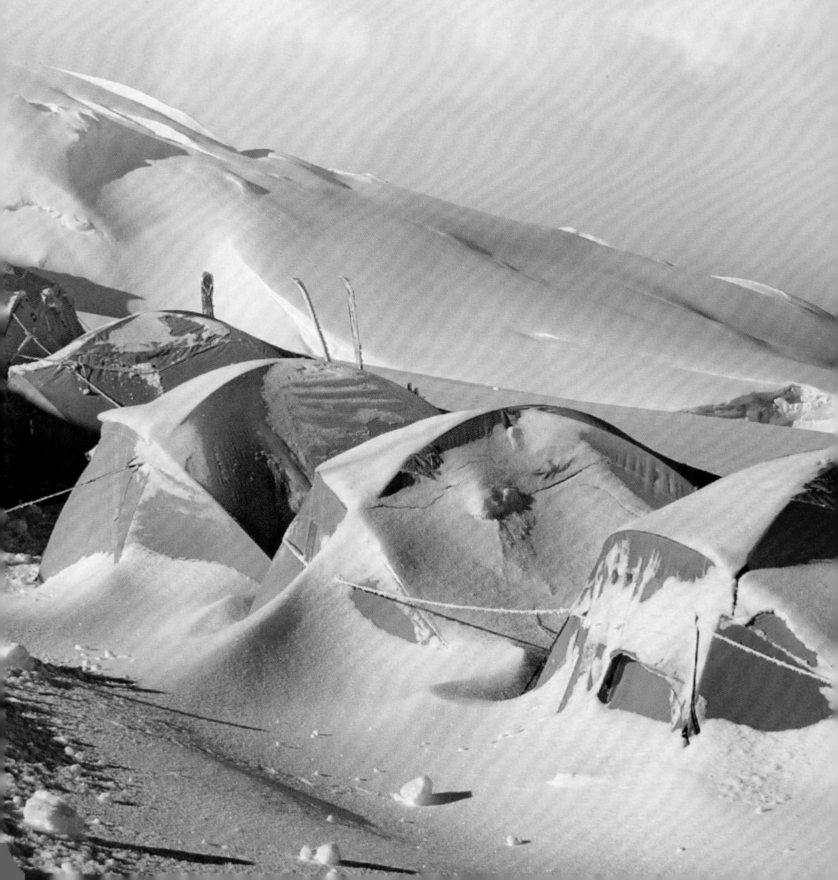

18.1 Localized Cold Injury

Prevention

All mountaineers must be aware of the risk of cold injury to themselves and other team members. Prevention is better than cure! Mountaineers who have previously suffered frostbite should take extra care. When exposed to temperatures around zero degrees Celsius or below, it is essential to wear warm clothes, to protect extremities from the cold and wind and to remove wet clothing. It is also important to maintain an adequate intake of food and drink. Energy requirements are higher in cold temperatures and warm fluids should be encouraged. Drugs which affect the nervous system, including alcohol should be avoided. There is evidence that caffeine affects peripheral circulation and therefore it is probably wise to limit its consumption.

⇨ Hypothermia tends to precede frostbite. Patients presenting with frostbite are usually found to be suffering with hypothermia as well. Such patients must be moved immediately to a safe place and warmed up. Only once there is no chance of refreezing should the frostbite be treated. Professional help is required!

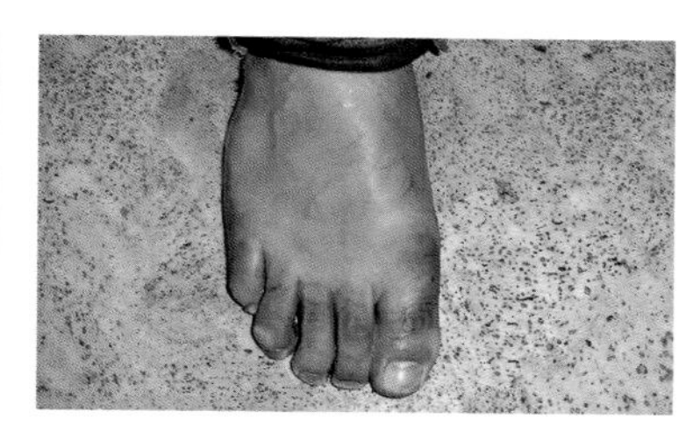

Figure 18.1.1: *Deep (4°) Frostbite affecting a mountaineer already suffering from hypothermia who was forced to set up a bivouac in the Swiss Alps at the end of December (B. Durrer), (see Case Study 18.2, Page 237).*

Definition

In minus temperatures, accompanied by wind, but also in temperatures above zero degrees, frostbite can develop predominantly in the area of exposed parts of the body such as the **hands, feet, nose and ears.** Ice crystals forming in the tissues due to the cold can subsequently directly damage the individual cell by causing the cell membrane to rupture. At the same time changes in the flow characteristics of the blood may develop with thickening of the blood, damage to the cell wall and *thromboses* (blood clots). As regards frost injury, a local inflammatory reaction invariably occurs. Once it is dead, tissue is irrevocably lost; the loss of fingers, toes, tip of the nose etc. may be the outcome.

Recognizing frostbite

Various degrees of frostbite may be identified. Classification into superficial (skin) and deep (muscles, tendons, nerves, bones) frostbite has proved a workable approach.

Frostbite can be recognized by whitish-tinged, dead areas of the skin, together with blistering, livid-black discolored, hard tissue. Frostbitten tissue may initially not be very painful or even painless. It is only after thawing that the pain tends to increase significantly, especially in the case of tissue that has not yet suffered definite damage.

⇨ If pain occurs after thawing, this is a good sign that the damage to the tissue is only superficial and that definite damage has not occurred to the nerves lying just under the skin.

Superficial Frostbite	1°	Whitish marbled skin	Spontaneous healing after thawing
	2°	Blistering, contents clear	Change in sense of touch possible
Deep Frostbite	3°	Blistering, contents bloody, reddening of the surrounding skin, muscles, tendons etc. involved	Permanent damage. Extent can only be definitively assessed after a few days
	4°	Cell death (necrosis)	Loss of tissue Amputation in due course

Table 18.1.1: *Frostbite: degrees of severity.*

Risks

The damage is caused by freezing of the tissue. Rewarming enables the displacement of liquid and electrolytes, and allows metabolic processes to resume. In this phase the tissue is extremely susceptible to any repeated exposure to cold. If a new attack of frostbite now occurs, massive damage to tissue may occur.

⇨ A frozen body part must only be warmed up again if all chance of re-freezing is excluded!

Once the tissues have thawed, there will still be a threat from general hazards such as thromboses, but the factor that gives rise to the most concern is **infection.** Demarcation of the necrotic tissue is normally present; the relevant body part will become completely devoid of feeling and blacken. This condition is called **dry gangrene.** Amputation is, as a rule, only carried out once demarcation is complete, that is, after a period spanning weeks or even months.

However, should an infection (so-called **moist gangrene)** occur, an operation will need to be carried out sooner than would otherwise have been the case. Amputation should never be carried out in the first few days.

Any cold injury should be treated in the same way as a **wound,** i.e. pack to ensure sterility and if need be, administer antibiotics and have the damage assessed by a specialist at home. Do not undergo any amputations abroad.

Treatment

Treatment can be divided into three distinct phases: The **preclinical phase,** which is the treatment given whilst on expedition, a **warm-up phase** and a **post-warming up phase** or thawing.

The warm-up phase and the post-warming up phase will wherever possible, be conducted in a hospital. On expeditions there may be specific instances where this may also have to take place in the field.

The following principles apply to the individual phases:

Preclinical Phase: The most important thing to remember is that the earlier an attack of frostbite is noticed the better. On visible parts of the body the following indicate an incipient frost injury:

- White discolouration of the skin
- Loss of sensation
- Pain prior to loss of feeling (feet)

If there is any doubt, the feet should be examined and warmed up again. In a wilderness environment this is only permissible if there is still no sign of general hypothermia, if any further cooling of the victim can be avoided and if there is no likelihood either of any further localized damage – otherwise there is no option but to turn back immediately! If the initial stages of frost injury are noticed (in particular on the feet) and rewarming is successful, it may even be possible to continue with the trip.

Successful re-warming is defined as full reinstatement of the blood supply to the foot within 10 minutes and complete reversal of dysaesthesia.

- If re-warming or prevention of further cooling is not possible in the wilderness environment – turn back!
- Protect against any additional mechanical injury; this means, for example, do not rub snow on the affected area and do not allow the patient to walk about on their frozen feet.
- Thaw only if any risk of further freezing can be excluded.
- Immobilisation, evacuation (in the event of frost injury to the feet, do not allow the patient to walk independently).
- In extreme situations, there is a possibility that a frost injury may only be noticed at a late stage or that direct treatment is not possible in those particular circumstances. Here, descending with a frozen foot may be preferable if it would result in a better outcome for the patient with faster treatment and better pain control.

It is not absolutely necessary to undertake an assessment of the extremities whilst still on the mountain. If cold injury (in particular to a foot) has already occurred and the decision to turn back has been made, the patient does not need to be undressed, and shoes should not be removed, especially if the patient is still going to have to descend further on his own. Protection against further cooling is of paramount importance. Hypothermia represents a threat to life; a frost injury by itself is not initially.

Warm-up Phase: Warming up must only take place in a **protected environment**. Place the affected extremity in hot water (approx. 40–42°C), add a few drops of a disinfectant solution containing iodine, and ideally leave in the solution for a few minutes over and above the thawing time so as to be sure that deeper-lying structures are also thawed.

Bathing should, however, not last for more than 30–45 minutes; otherwise the layer of skin will be completely soaked through, thus encouraging the penetration of germs and therefore infections.

- Do not massage extremities or the nose, ears etc.
- Give the patient something to drink in order to ensure that there is plenty of liquid in the body and in the bloodstream.
- **Combating pain** (strong drugs frequently necessary, see following page). In this situation the administration of acetylsalicylic acid (Aspirin® 75 mg PO, up to a max. of 300 mg PO) is indicated, circulation within the frozen body part can be improved by inhibiting the blood platelets.

Post-thawing Phase: this therapy is aimed at:

- Relieving pain
- Curbing the inflammatory reaction
- Preventing infections
- Optimising the supply of blood to the tissues

To reduce pain and inflammation, the combination of non-steriodal anti-inflammatories (NSAIDs, eg Ibuprofen 400 mg every 8 hours) in combination with Paracetamol (1 g every 6 hours) is a good option. For severe pain, a weak opiate such as Codeine or Tramadol can also be administered if required (Prescription only medicines). The affected extremity must be kept in the raised position.
If infection is suspected or a high risk of infection exists, preventive treatment with an antibiotic in tablet form should be considered (e.g. Co-Amoxiclav 2 x 1 g or 3 x 625 mg daily by mouth) unless a doctor can be consulted within an appropriate period of time. Further measures for preventing infection include:

- Changing of bandages/dressing and wound inspection daily
- Blister removal – NB be sparing and ensure cleanliness
- Sterile dressing
- Tetanus top-up (booster) or immunisation

Optimization of the circulation can be achieved by means of an adequate supply of liquid. Aspirin may help as discussed above. The importance of completely avoiding smoking during recovery from any frost injury should be emphasized to the patient.

In the event of excessive pain and/or new occurrences of discomfort, swelling or redness of the skin of the affected body part, consult a doctor. as there is a significant risk of **compartment syndrome** (post frost injury).

This is a serious condition where the volume of muscle increases due to disturbance of the circulation and a corresponding inflammatory reaction. As the muscle is trapped in a connective tissue tube, high pressure develops within it potentially causing irreversible damage. This also causes compression of nerves and blood vessels within the muscle, causing further serious complications. This is very painful and an emergency operation may be necessary.

Frost injuries must be shown to an experienced doctor. Any amputations should be deferred for as long as possible. Any such operation will only make sense in the event of a life-threatening infection (this also includes overseas). Frost injuries should be photographed every day and documented.

18.2 Hypothermia

The effect of cold can lead to generalized hypothermia (cooling of the entire body) and local cold injuries (cooling of peripheries). Either they may occur in isolation or in combination, although one is likely to hasten the onset of the other.

What happens in the cold?

Metabolic processes important to life are only possible within particular temperature limits (24–42 °C). Warmth is produced as a result of metabolic processes and by working the muscles. Loss of heat is possible as a result of convection (loss of the warm blanket of air that envelops the body when it is windy), conduction (in water, on cold ground), radiation and evaporation.
The following factors can lead to hypothermia and localized frost injury:

Nature

- Temperature: Damage caused by cold can also occur at temperatures above 0 °C.
- The wind is constantly blowing the warmed blanket of air away from the body. Wind chill: as the speed of the wind increases the effect of cold on the body is augmented, thus accelerating the rate of cooling.
- Wet conditions can speed up the rate of cooling many times over.

Human being

- Clothing: multi-layer, loose layers of clothing do a better job of insulating.
- Exhaustion, being in poor physical condition with regards to diet and training. This may result in inadequate thermoregulation. Someone who is physically fit will be able to actively produce heat for longer.
- Immobility due to injuries, illnesses, alcohol intoxication: active heat production through movement is no longer possible.
- Alcohol, vasodilating drugs: vasodilating means that more heat is given off more quickly.
- Nicotine: as a result of narrowing of the blood vessels there is a greater risk of localized injuries from the cold.
- Age: Children and older people are at a greater risk of hypothermia.

Wet and **windy conditions** simultaneously will cause more rapid cooling in an injured person.

Practical recommendations for preventing injuries as a result of cold

- Protection from the wind: even low strength winds will encourage faster cooling.
- Protection against wet: wet clothes cause faster cooling.
- Several loose, thin layers of clothing do a better job of insulating than just one thick one.
- Movement exercises will keep you warm. In the event of exposure to danger, you should monitor each other and keep each other alert.
- Avoid alcoholic drinks or vasodilating drugs. Avoid smoking.
- Maintain adequate warm fluid intake.
- Massage any at-risk parts of the body, working in the direction of the heart, and ensure active movement. Tissues that are already frostbitten should not be massaged as this may worsen the damage.

Generalized Hypothermia

The body's response to the effects of cold is first of all to increase heat production by shivering, increased respiration and circulation and to try and maintain its normal temperature. As soon as this regulatory mechanism is no longer adequate, the core temperature of the body starts to fall. When this happens, the blood supply to the skin is reduced and correspondingly the latter cools more quickly. This leads to a centralization of the circulation i.e. the body tries to maintain the temperature in the core of the body (head and trunk) for as long as possible.
In a situation where serious general hypothermia is present, the respiration and circulation activities of the body are slowed down and may stop altogether (suspended animation). At the same time, however, cooling protects the vital organs from a lack of oxygen. For this reason, persons apparently lifeless and suffering from hypothermia can be resuscitated successfully in special clinics even after several hours of cardiovascular arrest. The lowest core temperature recorded to date in an individual with hypothermia who was subsequently successfully resuscitated was 13.7 °C.

Definition

If the core temperature of the body falls below 35 °C, then we refer to it as generalized hypothermia. In mountainous terrain, generalized hypothermia may develop as a result of exhaustion or obstruction, falling into cold water, as a result of an accident involving a crevasse or in an avalanche.

The degree of severity of generalized hypothermia (Hypothermia, HT) is categorized by reference to the state of consciousness, shivering and cardiovascular function (existing, nonexistent). Recently, additional measurement of the core body temperature at the location of the emergency has enabled a more precise allocation to be made by the rescue services.

Category	Sign(s)	Temperature °C
HT I	Clear consciousness with shivering	35–32
HT II	Cloudy consciousness, without shivering	32–28
HT III	Unconscious, slow pulse and respiration	28–24
HT IV	Suspended animation (cessation of cardiovascular activity, no pupil reaction)	24–13.7?
HT V	Death	<13.7?

Table 18.2.1: *HT = Hypothermia (generalized sub-cooling). Where apparently lifeless persons are concerned, the core temperature is measured in the esophagus (Source: B. Durrer et al. 1998)*[1]

⇨ **Think!**

An apparently "lifeless" person may be in stage IV of an HT. This is the reason why a medical layperson must never diagnose death at the site of an emergency. The rescue personnel must always exclude serious HT before diagnosing death, especially in the wilderness and when the ambient temperature is low. The layperson will do well to remember the following:

Someone suffering from hypothermia is not dead until they are warm and dead.

First Aid

With all patients suffering from hypothermia in the wilderness, it is absolutely essential that they should be protected from further cooling, especially if it is wet and windy.

Measures aimed at protection from further cooling:

- Move the patient to a location that is warm and protected from the wind.
- Wrap up in insulating blanket to protect against cold, dampness and wind plus appropriate improvisations as necessary (duvet jacket, bivouac bag, warm clothing, hot water bottles etc.).
- Where possible change wet clothing for dry warm clothing.
- Place chemical thermal bags on torso (not directly on the skin due to the risk of burning!)

Hypothermia Category I

- Hot, sugary drinks.
- Active movements are permitted in the interests of producing heat.
- Protect against further cooling, see above.
- If no existing injuries, evacuation to a hospital is not necessary.

Hypothermia Category II

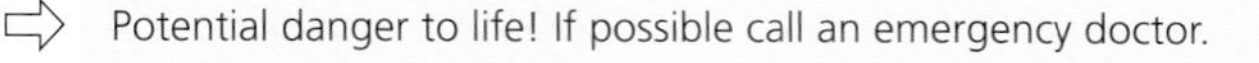

Potential danger to life! If possible call an emergency doctor.

- The patient must not be encouraged to indulge in active movement because this could bring about a so-called *"post-rescue death"* (cardiac arrest as a result of increased mixing of warm core blood with cold blood from the skin). Abrupt movements during and after rescue are to be avoided.
- Evacuate lying down with strict monitoring and readiness to perform resuscitation. Administer oxygen if possible.

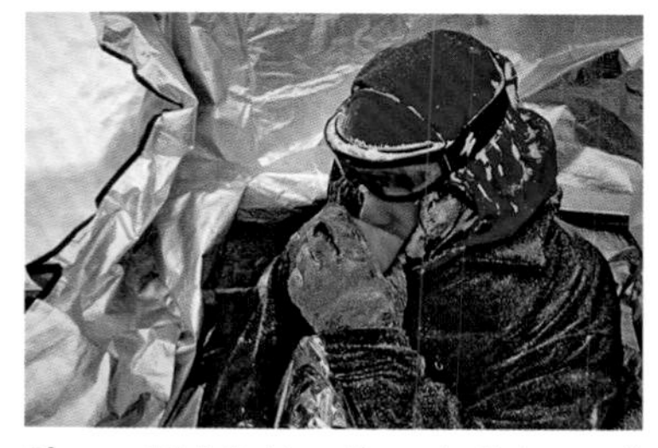

Figure 18.2.1: *Hypothermia Category II First Aid on Lauitor, Bernese Oberland (B. Durrer).*

- Protect against further cooling. As long as the person suffering from hypothermia can swallow properly, here too hot drinks alongside other measures to protect against further cooling are indicated.

Hypothermia Category III

> Direct threat to life! The risk of a so-called "post-rescue death" is higher than in the case of HT II.

- Protect from further cooling
- Place patient in stable position on his side with strict monitoring (see Section 9.4, Page 127)
- Be prepared to perform resuscitation measures.
- Evacuation to a specialist hospital (active warming facilities: e.g. heart/lung machine)

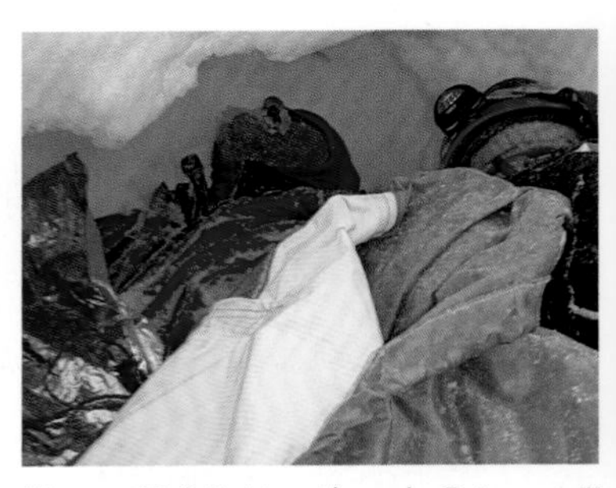

Figure 18.2.2: *Hypothermia Category III unconscious and suffering from hypothermia at 4000 m (B. Durrer).*

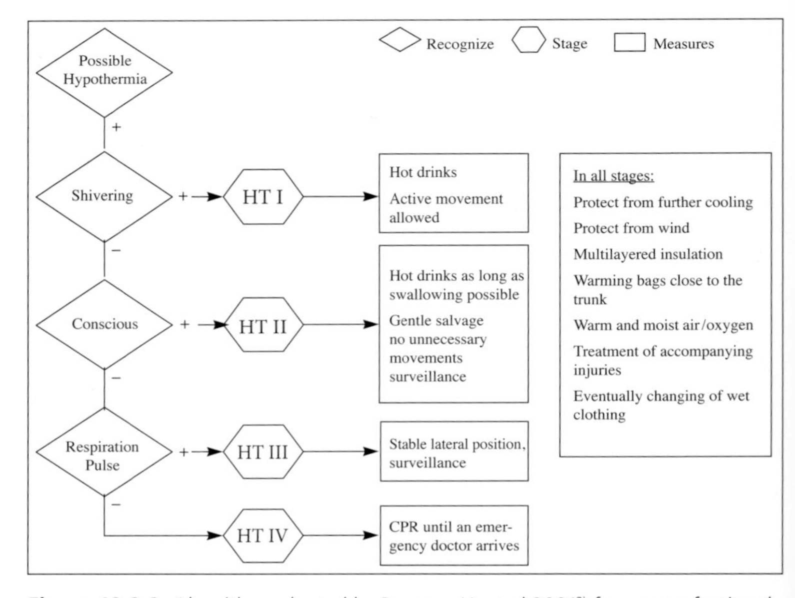

Figure 18.2.3: *Algorithm adapted by Brugger H. et al 2001[2)] for nonprofessional rescuers.*

Hypothermia Category IV

- Resuscitation measures as detailed in Section 9.2, Page 102.
- Protect from further cooling.
- Evacuation to a specialist hospital (active warming facilities: e.g. heart/lung machine).

In the case of patients with HT II and III, there is the threat during implementation of all such measures and during the evacuation process of acute cardiovascular arrest as a result of a so-called "post-rescue death."

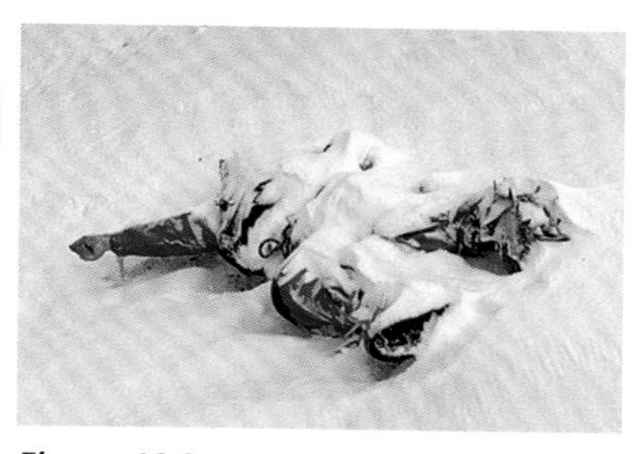

Figure 18.2.4: *Hypothermia Category IV (B. Durrer).*

Case Study

Two brothers plan a ski trip from the Jungfraujoch via the Lauitor as far as the Hollandia Hut at the end of December. While descending on a rope at nightfall XX falls into a crevasse. XY, not familiar with the technique of improvised crevasse rescue, pushes his ski into the ground and fixes it in position. XY gets no answer from the crevasse, so he panics and returns to the Lauitor at night on foot with the idea of using his mobile phone to raise the alarm. Here he finds himself overtaken by a snowstorm with wind speeds of up to 150 km/h with no bivouac equipment. The combined terrestrial/air rescue service, encountering poor visibility and storm force winds, takes 23 hours to arrive. XY is still only just responsive with no shivering (HT II) and has localized frostbite on his hands and feet. XX had been able to climb out of the crevasse using the fixed rope and managed to reach the Hollandia Hut in the snowstorm without hypothermia or localized frostbite after spending three nights in snow holes.

Literature:

1) Durrer B, Brugger H, Syme D (1998). The Medical On Site Treatment of Hypothermia. Recommendation REC M 0014 of the Commission for Mountain Emergency Medicine (ICAR).
2) Brugger H, Durrer B, Adler-Kastner L. On-site triage of avalanche victims with asystole by the emergency doctor. Resuscitation 31;11–6 (1996).

19. Eyes and Skin under Alpine Conditions

D. Barthelmes, R. Meyrat

Only mad dogs and Englishmen go out in the midday sun
Noel Coward, 1928

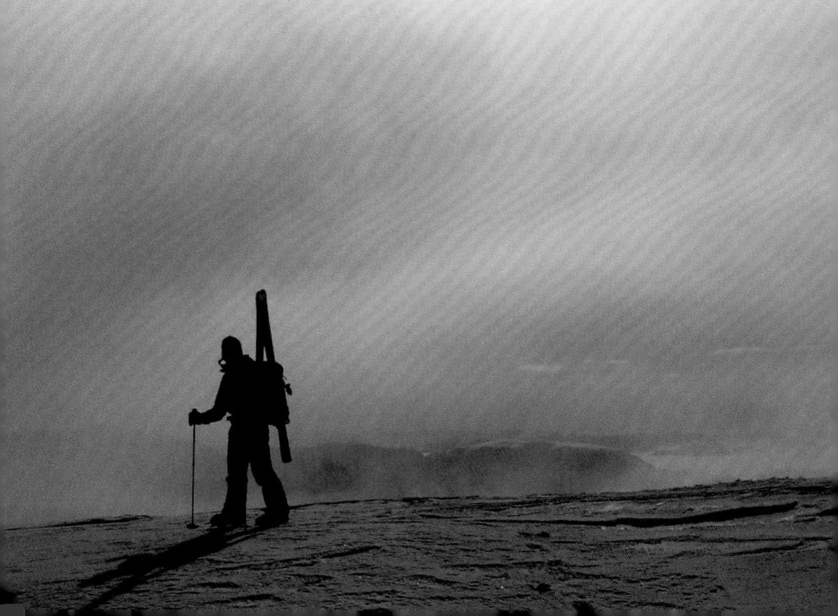

19.1 The Eye

In the same way as the rest of the body, the eye is exposed to particular stresses in the mountain environment and these may lead to changes in relation to function, i.e. visual impairment. As a rule, on trekking expeditions or multiple day trips, specialist personnel and equipment are not available to diagnose and treat eye conditions. Therefore, the following chapter will explain a few significant problems faced by mountaineers, while also suggesting some possible solutions.

Changes at Altitude

At high altitudes the amount of moisture in the air is subject to extreme variations. At the same time this fluctuates between very low and very high values, depending on the temperature, the wind and other factors. Increased sweating and increased rate and work of respiration can lead to physical dehydration. In the case of the eye, this primarily affects the conjunctiva and, to a lesser extent, tear secretion. These changes culminate in the development of so-called **"dry eye."**
The **retina,** located at the back of the eye, is very well supplied with blood vessels and receives adequate oxygen, even under extreme conditions at high altitude. The cornea of the eye, which does not contain any blood vessels, is supplied with oxygen mainly from the air. This is especially important for wearers of contact lenses as all contact lenses reduce the supply of oxygen to the surface of the eye and thus may contribute toward the development of infections related to lack of oxygen by damaging the surface of the eye.

UV Exposure

UV radiation can have a damaging effect on the eye across the entire range of the spectrum. Depending on the altitude, in mist and cloud up to 50 % of UV rays impact the Earth's surface. UVB/C rays impact predominantly on the cornea and conjunctiva of the eye, UVA and B waves penetrate as far as the lens of the eye and visible light as far as the retina.

The younger the person, the greater the absorption of the radiation in the front section of the eye.

A common, acute form of damage to the unprotected eye caused by UV radiation, especially in the high mountains or by the sea, is **"snow blindness,"** which occurs as a result of swelling and inflammation of the cornea, linked with diffuse inflammation of the conjunctiva (Photokeratitis actinia corneal).

The symptoms become apparent gradually after several hours (e.g. overnight) and take the form of pains in the eyes on both sides, tears, reddening of the conjunctiva and blepharospasm. In the majority of cases the symptoms die down after 48–72 hours. It is essential to remove contact lenses. Localized numbing drops (not too much, maximum six times per day, since these impede healing!) and the application of cool packs can have a soothing effect.
Chronic damage accumulating over a number of years will affect the conjunctiva and the iris in the form of chronic inflammation. Any opacity will be accelerated in the area of the lens and this, together with inflammation of the cornea, will contribute to premature cataracts.

Protecting the Eyes

Even on cloudy days it is advisable to wear sunglasses with adequate sun protection. The incidence of rays from the side and from below, especially on snow, needs be taken into account.

The sunglasses should have CE certification and ensure 100 % protection up to a wave length of 400 nm. In the high mountains attention should also be paid to an adequate blue light filter. The "Blueblockers," as they are known, provide 100 % protection, however, it is important to understand that the color perception is distorted.
Incorporating a polarization effect in the lenses will give protection against unpleasant glare, especially any such reflected from snow, ice or aquatic surfaces.

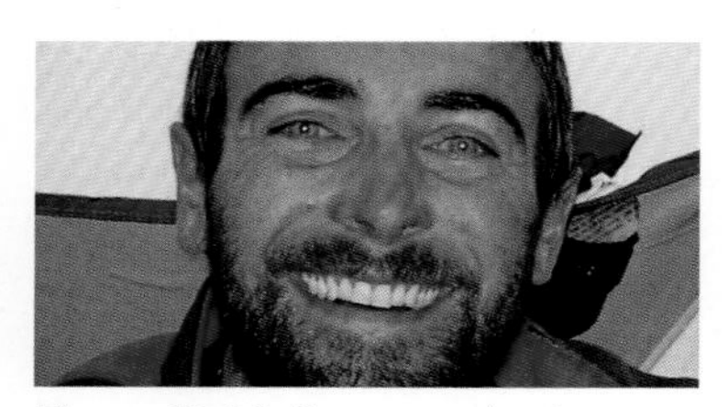

Figure 19.1.1: *Pronounced redness affecting dry eyes on a young mountaineer who has just ascended the Cerro Aconcagua (6962 m, Mendoza, Argentina) (F. Brunello).*

Dehydration-related Problems

Early signs are cumulative blinking and increased tear production, especially when it is windy. As the symptoms become more apparent, burning and reddening of the conjunctiva may be added to this. Often there is also a definite sensation of a foreign body ("as if there is something in the eye"). There is seldom any adverse effect on the visual acuity.

In an extreme case, the surface of the cornea may be so badly damaged due to dehydration that visual impairment and very severe pain may be experienced.

A check will need to be carried out in case a foreign body or contact lenses are present; if necessary rinse the eye with water (boiled water on trekking expeditions).

Treatment:

- Moisturising eyedrops: Lacrycon®, Oculac®, min. 6–8 times a day
- Moisturising gels: Viscotears®, Vismed® Gel, 3–4 times a day
- Vitamin A or Bepanthen eye ointment (esp. at night)

Water on its own is not to be recommended because it washes out the fats that the surface of the eye needs and, in so doing, makes the symptoms even worse. It may be an idea to wear fully enclosed spectacles so as to limit the evaporation on the surface of the eye.

Problems associated with Contact Lenses

Soft contact lenses often exacerbate the moisturizing situation in relation to the cornea because they absorb water from the surface of the eye and, together with a reduction in the blinking stimulus, lead to increased evaporation. This effect is very noticeable, even at sea level.

If the cause of the problem is not a foreign body, treatment will consist of dispensing with contact lenses/wearing glasses if possible plus eye drops/ointment as for "dry eye."

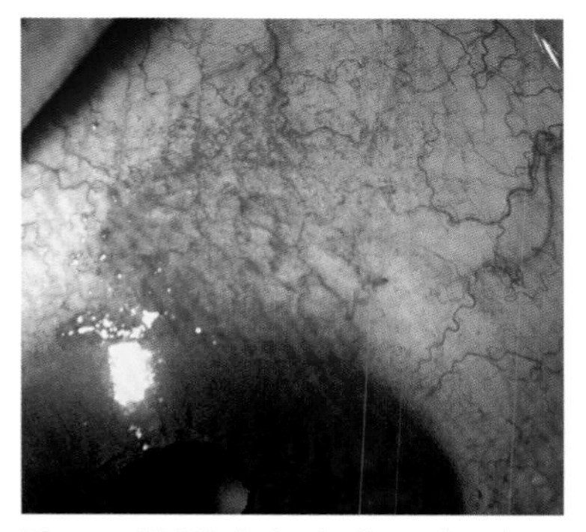

Figure 19.1.2: *Dehydration-related damage to cornea and conjunctiva (keratoconjunctivitis sicca).*

Contact Lens-associated Keratitis (= bacterial inflammation of the cornea as a result of wearing contact lenses)
Mostly very severe pain, reddening of the eye to a major extent, excess tear production and extreme sensitivity to light, so much so that significant effort is required to open the eye.

⇨ Major suffering as far as the patient is concerned!

There may be a significant reduction in the sharpness of vision. As a rule it is not contact lens hygiene that is the problem, rather it is the dehydration of the surface of the eye together with the reduction in the supply of oxygen which renders the surface of the eye susceptible to infection. There may possibly be hygiene-related problems in addition to this.
These problems occur only in wearers of contact lenses and frequently develop within 12–24 hours, taking the form of intense, increasing pains. The lens will need to be removed and the cornea observed; it is probable that there will be a small whitish spot seen in the cornea. If so, it is possible to be relatively certain of the diagnosis.

Treatment: Take a break from contact lenses.

⇨ Taking a break from contact lenses = **not wearing lenses!** Continuing to wear the lenses can have a highly adverse effect on progress.

As a rule, where infections of this kind are involved, intensive therapy with antibiotic eye drops will be necessary as follows:

- Floxal® drops: 48 hours every 30 minutes for as long as possible (including at night)
- Floxal® eye ointment (to cover the time when the drops are not being administered)
- After 48 hours 5–6 times 1 drop for 7 days and Floxal® eye ointment at night
- Alternative: Vigamox® 4–5 times a day for 7 days

⇨ In cases involving **fungal** infections or infections with other unusual germs (from water) the therapy may be ineffective. Even under normal conditions and with good medical care (e.g. in hospital), it is still possible for these infections to progress rapidly and lead to blindness or even to **loss of the eye.**

Continue to avoid contact lenses for at least two months and visit an ophthalmologist as soon as possible.

Problems following Operations on the Cornea

(Transplant, LASIK = Treatment with a laser to correct either long or short sight.)

Since a cornea transplant and a LASIK both involve the destruction of the delicate nerves of the cornea, the sensitivity of the cornea is reduced. Very often patients will suffer from a **dry eye** and will, as a rule, already be using moisturizing eye drops. These dry eye symptoms may increase at high altitude. For recognition and treatment see "Dry Eye."

Cornea and Lack of Oxygen: The cornea is made up of a number of layers. The task of the inner layer, the endothelium, is to keep the water content of the cornea at a constant level by pumping water out of the cornea. This helps to ensure the transparency of the cornea. The endothelium is very sensitive in its reaction to the lack of oxygen. If the supply is inadequate, its function will be reduced, water will collect in the cornea and the tissue will swell. As a result, the transparency will be reduced and visual acuity may, under certain conditions, deteriorate significantly to the point all that is possible is the ability to distinguish light from darkness. Normally this process is painless. As soon as the supply of oxygen reverts to normal, the cornea will clear and as a rule the patient will once again be able to see as well as before.

In other situations too, e.g. following a corneal transplant (complete transplant), in elderly patients and with conditions affecting the endothelium and where a patient has undergone previous operations on the eye, a reduction in the function of the endothelium may occur so that water may collect. If a reduction in function of this nature is already present, it is possible that the deficiency in the supply of oxygen at high altitude will lead to a much more rapid loss of visual acuity.
This clinical picture is characterized by a clear loss of vision, no reddening of the eye and, as a rule, an absence of pain.

Treatment: Administer oxygen, if available, descend, if necessary and where available, administer 5 % NaCl drops to reduce swelling and drain the cornea.

If Acetazolamide (Diamox) is being taken, it should be stopped because it will have a further adverse effect on the function of the endothelium and may even trigger the problems mentioned.

Special Problems following LASIK–Flap Repositioning

Sudden blurring of vision, pain, pronounced sensitivity to light. A LASIK involves making a small incision in the surface of the cornea (like a lid = flap). After treatment with the laser, the flap is folded back on to the site of the operation and held in position. The incision does not heal completely; even years later it will still be possible to lift the flap and, for example, embark on a new course of laser treatment. In the event of an accident or extreme dryness, displacement of the flap may come about which will cause the symptoms described at the beginning.

Treatment: Visit the ophthalmologist to have the flap repositioned. Make sure that the eye is very well moistened (frequent applications of moisturizing eye drops or vitamin A eye ointment, see Page 241) and, if possible, keep closed, in order to avoid any further damage. If need be, wear an eye patch or bandage.

Sudden Loss of Vision

Sudden, painless loss of vision can occur within the space of a few minutes or hours and is mostly unilateral.

From outside the eye looks completely normal.

The precise cause can in most cases only be established by the ophthalmologist within the framework of a complete examination which will not generally be possible under expedition or trekking conditions. Frequently the causes will be found at the rear of the eye, where they may be identified (e.g.) in the form of blood vessel obliteration or even a detached retina, although this is a very rare occurrence. There is no emergency therapy in expedition conditions. It is essential to consult an ophthalmologist quickly.

Painful Loss of Sight (Glaucoma)

As a rule, a worsening of vision develops quickly in association with pain. Often glaucoma occurs following an injury to the eye. Signs include reddening of the conjunctiva, tears, sensitivity to light and an increase in the internal pressure of the eye. This can be felt with a finger exerting slight pressure on the closed eyelid. The affected eye will feel "rock hard" in comparison to the opposite side.

Treatment: Descend and consult an ophthalmologist. Emergency medication:

- Diamox® 2 × 500 mg orally per day
- Subsequently up to 4 × 250 mg per day (including once the pain problem has improved)
- Pain medication (e.g. Ibuprofen)

Inflammation

Conjunctivitis

This is a very frequent ailment which, in the great majority of cases, is triggered by **viruses.** With viral infections, the eye is reddened, the patient complains of similar problems as with dry eye (see above). In the morning, yellowish crusts can sometimes be found on the eye. Visual acuity is normal, very seldom is there any pain. In a few cases infection with **bacteria** may also develop. In such cases the eye will also be reddened and there will be copious amounts of whitish-yellowish discharge. The eye will be painful, visual acuity may be very poor, especially if the cornea is also affected. The conjunctiva are reddened and often slightly swollen.
The presence of a foreign body must be excluded. Has there been an injury? Does the patient wear contact lenses? Has there been any contact with people who have an infection?

Treatment:

- Moisturising drops (Lacrycon®, Oculac®) once an hour (as long as visual acuity is good and there is no pain).
- Antibiotic eye drops (Floxal® one drop per day and eye ointment at night, Neosporin® or Vigamox® 3–4 times a day).

⇨ If there is any suspicion of a bacterial infection (pains, pus, poor visual acuity), an ophthalmologist should be consulted as quickly as possible.

Hand hygiene is important so as to ensure that other people/the other eye are not infected. Take a rest from contact lenses!

Visual Acuity and Ocular Pressure

In the normal eye visual acuity undergoes only minimal change at high altitude; in fact, a slight transient improvement tends to occur.
At high altitude ocular pressure is relatively stable; there may be slight fluctuations but these are of no consequence from a clinical point of view.

Recommendations for an Expedition

Wearers of contact lenses: In principle, it is quite possible for contact lenses to be worn on a high altitude expedition.

Lens cases, along with lenses, must be kept warm at night, e.g. in a sleeping bag (risk of freezing!).

Recommendations as far as hygiene is concerned are the same as at sea level (hand hygiene, keep cases clean, use cleaning fluids in accordance with the instructions). Since problems as described above (and which should also not be underestimated) may occur, wearers of contact lenses should take one normal pair of glasses and one pair with dark lenses – with ground ophthalmic lenses or a pair that can be worn over normal spectacles – along with them on the expedition. In addition, it is advisable to pack some spare lenses.

Medication: Because, when making preparations for an expedition or a trek, there is a multitude of things to remember and it is impossible to cover all eventualities, the following recommendations should be regarded as a compromise between what is possible and what is feasible.

- For those who have no problems with their eyes and who do not wear contact lenses, moisturising eye drops (Lacrycon®, Oculac®) or at least an antibiotic (e.g. Neosporin®) should suffice.
- For **contact lens wearers,** it is without doubt sensible to take along moisturising eye drops as well as antibiotic eye drops (see Appendix, Page 288) for use in an emergency together with a pair of sunglasses (with standard and prescription lenses) as well as replacement lenses.
- Persons who are in regular contact with an ophthalmic specialist due to **eye problems** should consult their specialist prior to embarking on any planned expedition or lengthy tour in the mountains.

Any eye problem may make an interruption to the trip or even repatriation necessary!

In addition to boiled water, in an emergency tea, mineral water or NaCl 0.9 % may also be used for flushing the eye. Under no circumstances should milk or similar substances be used.

Literature:

1) Bloch, K. E., A.J. Turk, et al. (2009). "Effect of ascent protocol on acute mountain sickness and success at Muztagh Ata, 7546 m." High Alt Med Biol 10(1): 25–32.
2) Bosch, M. M., D. Barthelmes, et al. (2009). "New Insights into Corneal Thickness Changes in Healthy Mountaineers during a Very High Altitude Climb to Mt Muztagh Ata." Arch Ophthalmol.
3) Bosch, M. M., D. Barthelmes, et al. (2008). "High incidence of optic disc swelling at very high altitudes." Arch Ophthalmol 126(5): 644–50.
4) Bosch, M. M., D. Barthelmes, et al. (2009). "Intraocular Pressure During a Very High Altitude Climb." Invest Ophthalmol Vis Sci.
5) Bosch, M. M., T.M. Merz, et al. (2009). "New insights into ocular blood flow at very high altitudes." J Appl Physiol 106(2): 454–60.

19.2 The Skin

The Sun and Ultra-Violet Radiation

Every second, within the gigantic fireball we know as the Sun, 564 million tonnes of hydrogen are converted at around 20 million °C into 560 million tonnes of helium through the thermonuclear processes. The loss of mass (amounting to 4 million tonnes per second) is released in the form of radiation energy, of which fortunately only a small fragment reaches the Earth's surface.
This radiation features a range of highly diverse wavelengths. The longer waves – "Infrared" – we perceive as heat. The shorter wavelengths we perceive in the form of what is, to the human eye, visible light, that is, light in the narrower sense. The "light" with the shortest wave and the highest energy is "ultraviolet" (UV). The problem here is that UV rays are not visible to the human eye, neither can they be felt.

Sun Exposure and Climatic Influences

The UV spectrum can be divided up as follows:

- **UVA** proportion (320–400 nm long wave): causes a direct but unstable browning/tanning of the skin.

- **UVB** range (285–320 nm short term): in the top layers of the skin leads to cell stimulation, inflammation ("sunburn") and indirect but stable browning/ tanning.

These biophysical effects on the skin are complex and diverse. Since the 1980s there has been an average estimated increase in UVB radiation (which triggers sunburn and skin cancer) of 10 +/- 5 % per decade, reaching its peak in the winter and early spring months (measured at a height of 3570 m on the Jungfraujoch). Whereas the ozone values in the high layers of the stratosphere fluctuate depending on the season and bring about an increase in UVB solar radiation depending on the time of day, the high ozone concentrations in the lower layers of the atmosphere (troposphere), together with air pollution in low-lying regions, may increase, thus leading to a variable decline in UV global radiation. Further influences determine the biological/ pathological effectiveness of UV rays on the skin:

- **Geographical latitude:** In southern latitudes UV radiation increases by 10–15 % per thousand kilometres (need clarification – is this per thousand km south of the equator?).
- **Height above sea level:** As altitude increases, the intensity of UV rays also increases by 10–15 % per 1000 m, with a slightly greater increase in the UVB range. The reason for this is the reducing filtration effect of atmospheric layers (see Table 19.2.1).
- **Time of day and season** depending on the angle of the sun: a 10 % increase/decrease in UV radiation can be reckoned with for every hour before and after the sun attains its highest position in the sky. As the sun's altitude increases over the course of the year, a monthly increase of 15 % in mid-latitudes from March to June can be discerned with a similar decrease between July and October.
- **Meteorological conditions** play a particularly important role as far as the change in UV exposure is concerned. The reflection of the rays on snow, for example, can increase exposure to UV by more than 50 %, particularly when areas of intensive radiation protrude some kilometres into the environment (Albedo: Reflection of ground radiation).

	UVA	UVB
Sea level	100 %	100 %
Height of 1000 m	117 %	120 %
Height of 2000 m	127 %	135 %
Height of 3000 m	134 %	150 %

Table 19.2.1: *Intensity of ultra-violet intensity of radiation in relation to sea level.*

When skiing, the sun, the cold, the wind and the dryness of the air all have an effect on the skin. Rainfall and snowfall moisten the skin of the face and reduce resistance to radiation. Clouds and mist can, despite the cold, allow more than 80 % of UV rays to permeate.

Damage to the skin may also take place due to the combined effect of wind and dehydration as a result of not noticing a fall in temperature. For example, a skin temperature of -20 °C may be caused by a wind strength of 18 km/h and an absolute temperature of -10 °C.

Skin Damage resulting from UV Radiation

Throughout our lives our skin is exposed to sunlight and hence to UV radiation, in descending order, from our heads, the backs of our hands, the dorsal sides of our forearms, legs right down to the torso. Here it is important to distinguish between physiological skin aging phenomena (pigmentation, slackening and wrinkling) on the one hand and on the other hand, premature pathological **aging** as a result of increased UV damage to the cells caused by cumulative damage over years and decades.

"The skin is very unforgiving."

UVB has a very much greater involvement in this than UVA, which, due to its greater depth of penetration, leads to a loss of elasticity as well as to shrinkage and wrinkling. UVA on the other hand works primarily on the rapidly regenerating cells of the epidermis, as the top layer of skin is called, and can cause immunodeficiency and degenerative processes. These commence as early as the point where UVB reaches 2/3rds of the threshold erythema dose (MED) (corresponding to the length of time it takes for any reddening to become visible), that is, before any sunburn occurs.

Sunlight level in MED%	Acute Consequences	Subsequent Consequences
Higher than the threshold erythema dose (MED)	Sunburn	Immuno-suppression. Risk of melanoma and epitheliomas
Between 66 and 99 % of MED	Momentary irreparable damage to cell with no visible effect	Chronic sun damage, acceleration of the aging process, actinitic keratoses. Skin carcinomas, Hautkarzinome
Less than 66 % of MED	None	None

Table 19.2.2: *Threshold erythema dose (MED) of UVB corresponding to period of time up to when reddening becomes visible and direct long-term consequences.*

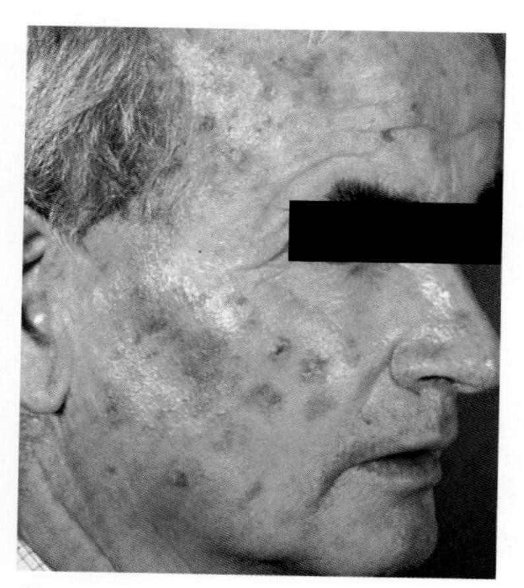

Figure 19.2.1: *Preliminary stage of a skin tumor (precancerous) (R. Meyrat).*

As already mentioned, the facial area is the most likely location for skin damage, subject to **Pigmentation Type,*** lifelong UV exposure, the effect of nicotine on the skin and genetic factors.

As a result of the process of continuous regeneration–growth–death the cells of the epidermis are exposed to a particularly pronounced risk of degeneration which, at best, will progress over a period of years without being visible. In addition, with increasing age, the systems which regulate the repair of genetic information tend to become exhausted. As a result the damage becomes visible and preliminary stages of skin tumors (precancerous or actinitic keratoses) and malignant cell changes (basal cell carcinomas and squamous cell carcinomas) develop.

* 1975 by the American dermatologist Thomas Fitzpatrick. The most important factor as far as determination of skin type is concerned is the colour of the skin in daylight when not irradiated, nevertheless the observation of browning/tanning behaviour and a tendency to sunburn are relatively reliable indicators (depending on the quantity of melanin produced by each individual). The Groups (I-IV) may be divided up on the basis of very light skin-type (I) to dark negroid skin-type (IV).

All three forms tend to become increasingly evident after the age of 40 on exposed parts of the body.

Precancerous lesions (very frequent!) usually develop in groups as opposed to single manifestations. Their appearance is initially a pale pink color with superficial scaling and slight thickening.

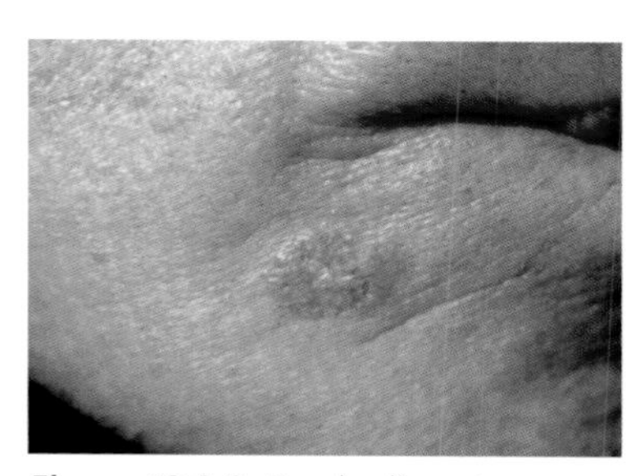

Figure 19.2.2: *Basal cell carcinoma (R. Meyrat).*

Basal cell carcinomas (very frequent!) are single lesions with a range of different aspects, mostly consisting of a scirrhous mole formation, skin pigmented through to pink, with a smooth or tuberous surface, surrounded by a rim as it increases in size over a period of months or years, with a tendency to bleed. These are the most frequent skin cancers, locally destructive, but do not tend to form metastases.

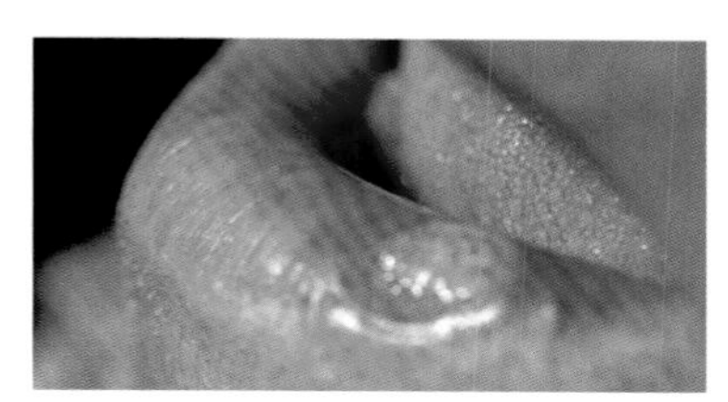

Figure 19.2.3: *Damage to the lower lip caused by squamous cell carcinomas. The lower lips are more exposed to the effects of the sun than the upper lips. (R. Meyrat).*

Squamous cell carcinomas develop from the spinous cells of the epidermis, often on the basis of a pre-existing precancerous lesion, on photo-damaged skin in older people. The tumor manifests itself as keratinizing after the manner of a wart or as a crater-shaped ulcer in older people and may metastasize if it has penetrated deep.

Any localised inflammation, thickening of the skin, wound which fails to heal within a matter of a few months must be examined and treated by a doctor.

In the case of **Melanoma,** the "black skin cancer" which develops from the melanin-forming pigment cells of the epidermis, the circumstances are different. Its development is, with one or two exceptions, not so closely linked to direct exposure to UV as is the case with squamous and basal cell carcinomas. Melanoma is unpredictable: it may present as an irregular dark speck and grow slowly over a period of years or also grow at lightning speed adopting a nodular format, spread prematurely to other organs and lead to death within the space of weeks or months.

Melanomas may occur at any age once growth has stopped and can occur in any location in the body, even at sites that have not been subject to exposure.

The following may be regarded as the most significant **risk factors** for the malignant form of melanoma: pale, fair-skinned pigmentation type, accumulation of episodes of sunburn in childhood, an above-average number of irregular naevi (moles) over the entire body, family history of melanomas.

⇨ The melanoma is one of the few fatal tumours to affect humans that can be easily identified at an early stage when it is still curable and an operation performed to remove it.

An annual (self) examination of the skin of the entire body based on the A-B-C-D rules should focus on:

- **a**symmetry of the lesion
- irregular demarcation of the **b**orders
- **c**olour changing to patchy brown, dark to black
- **d**iameter with favourable prognosis at D </= 5mm

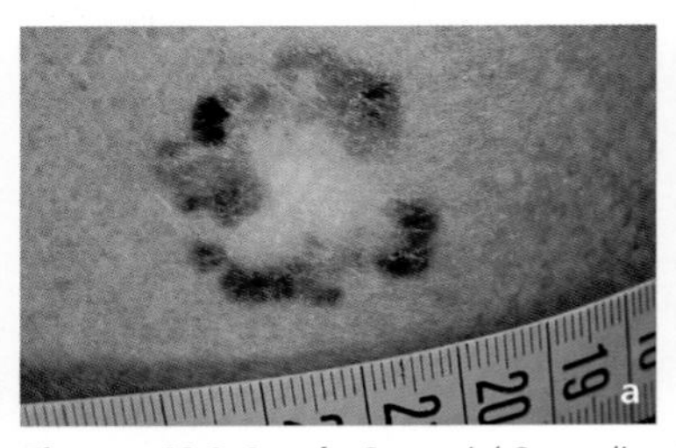

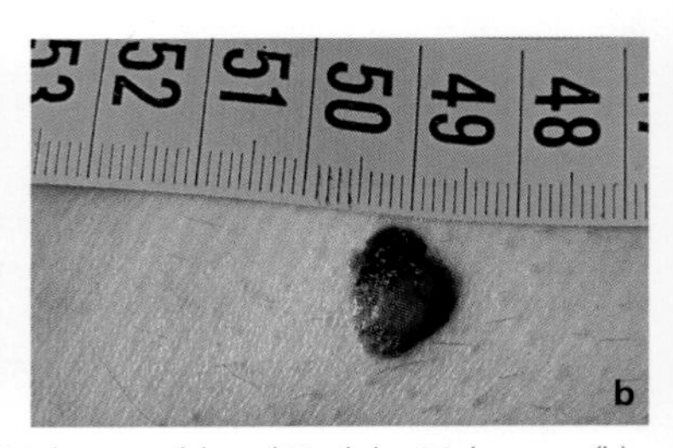

Figures 19.2.4, a–b: *Supercial Spreading Melanoma (a) and Nodular Melanoma (b), melanomas may present under a range of highly diverse aspects (R. Meyrat).*

Melanomas are not palpable, they do not itch, they are not inflamed. In the early stage they are flat and only very slightly raised. Injuring a mole does not lead to a risk of melanoma.
By far the greatest increase in the white-skinned population worldwide during the last 50 years has been recorded in relation to melanomas. Experts all over the world agree that the change in **leisure-time behavior** has paved the way for an increasing epidemic of skin cancer. At the top of the list is Australia (the black aborigines have no melanomas!), in Europe the highest rate of increase in melanomas has been identified in Switzerland.

Skin Adaptation and Protective Measures

Of the **skin's own ways of protecting itself,** the genetically predisposed tanning type or acquired pigmentation (tanning through melanin regeneration) represents the most effective response when it comes to counteracting UVA and UVB damage. Nevertheless, it is still far too little to prevent cell damage under the conditions of exposure which are standard today, especially with regards the face. Dry or mature skin with a thin or chronically damaged depleted stratum corneum increases sensitivity to UVB.; The same applies to cosmetic peeling procedures or external/internal vitamin A acid preparations, for example, as used in acne therapy. After moderate permanent sun exposure the skin forms a reactive thickening of the upper stratum corneum of the skin (so-called **"actinic keratosis"),** which is fully developed after approx. 3 weeks and represents an approximately fourfold increase in UV tolerance.

External Protective Measures: Alongside avoidance of unnecessary sun exposure (over the midday period from 11.00 to 15.00 hrs, and also not forgetting to cover up adequately) there is an immense diversity of effective sun protection preparations in both the UVA and the UVB range and these need to be used correctly. The choice of preparation is based on individual sensitivity and foreseeable skin exposure.

Sun filters: Chemical and physical filter substances exist, the first of which generate UV absorption biochemically in different band widths whilst the latter, in the shape of "biological" substances in an extremely finely dispersed form, create, by means of diffusion, reflection and absorption, a broad protection band in the UVA and UVB range with good skin tolerance, stability and an absence of reabsorption. Nowadays it is possible to circumvent the problems associated with these substances where fair skins are concerned and to largely eliminate them with new formulations.

Confusion reigns with regards to the **protection (SPF)** factors stated. USA standards are different to European ones, there are efforts underway within the EU to instigate a further 4 categories between "low" and "very high." Today, for example, a factor 10 means a 50 % reduction in UV, factor 20 one of 95 %, a factor 50 will give a 98 % reduction in UV.

Water-resistant preparations attach themselves to the stratum corneum; for winter conditions water-in-oil emulsions are better as these give additional protection against the cold.

Three areas of the face that are at special risk are **nose, margins of the ears and lips.** The latter develop hardly any pigment and do not incorporate a stratum corneum.

Crayons, with high protection factors and applied on several occasions over the course of the day, will provide additional protection against dehydration and cracking. Coloured lipsticks for women as well as make up pigments that can be applied to the face and giving good coverage likewise provide high-quality UV protection. Similar consistent applications of lip salve will also reduce the occurrence of cold sores contingent on UV (Herpes simplex solaris).

With regards to **exposure in mountainous terrain,** the consistent application of UV protection to the face to counteract any reddening (and hence damage) due to sun-exposure is necessary throughout one's life.

- For fair skins, long-term UV exposure and pre-existing skin damage caused by UV, preparations with maximum protective action in the UVA and UVB range should be selected (sunblocks, medical UV protection).
- All UV protection preparations should be rubbed into the dry, untreated skin/lips in the mornings one hour prior to exposure to the sun, with a repeat application as necessary over the midday period.
- Re-exposure to the sun for further tanning is not advisable. Self-tanning cosmetics are harmless to the skin, but remember that using them will not protect you against UV!

Lip Herpes (Herpes simplex solaris)

Following initial infection, herpes blisters tend to reappear on repeated occasions over a number of years, mostly localized in the lip/chin area. In addition to sunshine, they tend to be encouraged by stress, colds, lack of sleep, alcohol, menstruation and other things. In the acute weeping stage they can be passed on by direct contact. Spontaneous recovery takes 8–10 days, assuming no complications.

As soon as the symptoms occur (tingling, hypersensitivity and swelling of the affected area) localised intensive treatment may be initiated with the application of anti-viral substances every 1–2 hours, if possible prior to development of the blister stage.

Where serious relapses are known to be a risk, oral herpes medications are available which also need to be taken for several days as soon as the symptoms appear.

19.3 Emergencies: Sunstroke, Heatstroke, Sunburn

Sunstroke and Heatstroke

Hot weather, combined with excessive physical exertion, unsuitable clothing promoting a build up of heat (dark colors, helmets) and a lack of fluid intake may lead, in the absence of opportunities for cooling and transpiration, to health problems which may range from minor to very serious.

⇨ At particular risk are elderly people and children.

Both of the above mostly begin with dizziness, nausea and headaches. In the case of **sunstroke,** stimulation of the central nervous system occurs as a result of direct thermal radiation. Although the head may be bright red and hot, the rest of the skin feels cool to the touch, a general state of restlessness is accompanied by weakness and possibly vomiting and collapse.
Heatstroke, on the other hand, may occur even without any direct action on the part of the sun as a result of the effect of heat building over a long period, followed by a rise in body temperature to more than 40 °C, a fall in blood pressure, flickering before the eyes, confusion and unconsciousness. Treatment is as follows:

- Lay the patient down in a shady, cool place, open up clothing.
- Cover the warm parts of the body, in particular the head, with cloths soaked in cold water.
- Keep drinking fluids containing salt (one teaspoonful of cooking salt per litre of water/tea).
- Keep a close eye on the patient and start life-saving measures (see Section 9.2, Page 99) if necessary.

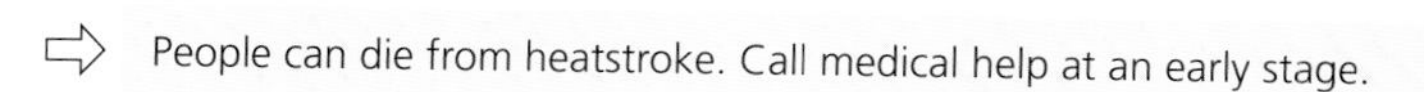
⇨ People can die from heatstroke. Call medical help at an early stage.

Sunburn

The sunburn that is prone to develop under alpine conditions occurs after a latent period of 2–4 hours after UV damage, predominantly in the area of the face/head, on the backs of the hands and the dorsal sides of the arms. Depending on the degree of severity, painful reddening linked with variable swelling of the tissue, possibly with pronounced swelling of the lids (making it impossible to open the eyes) may develop as well as grotesquely thickened lips. In cases of severe damage from the sun's rays, scattered small blisters or larger blisters filled with light-colored fluid may also develop on all reddened and inflamed and hot areas of the skin. The treatment is as follows:

- Avoid sun and exertion.
- In the acute stage, apply cold, wet cloths, snow etc. as quickly as possible for 1–5 minutes at a time in order to prevent any additional swelling or inflammation.
- Subsequently frequent regular applications of cooling creams, foam, lotions, if possible with a corticosteroid supplement at half-hourly/one hourly intervals.

Greasy salve products are contraindicated. Conduct a new assessment of the superficial area of the skin during a subacute phase after 12–24 hours. If blisters have formed, open up the lid section of the blister carefully and, without probing too deep, discharge the wound secretions without removing the lid section of the blister. Where the surfaces of the wound are weeping, treat as for burns using disinfectant or topical antibiotic medications (lotions, creams), loose net/gauze dressings. After 3–4 days, once the wound surface has dried out change to greasy topical preparations.

Severely sun-damaged skin is the equivalent of a burn and will require a period of 1–2 months to regenerate. Depending on the degree of severity, the site (especially the face, nose and ears) may remain super-sensitive in the extreme and UV-intolerant for a number of years.

20. Special Alpine Emergencies

B. Durrer

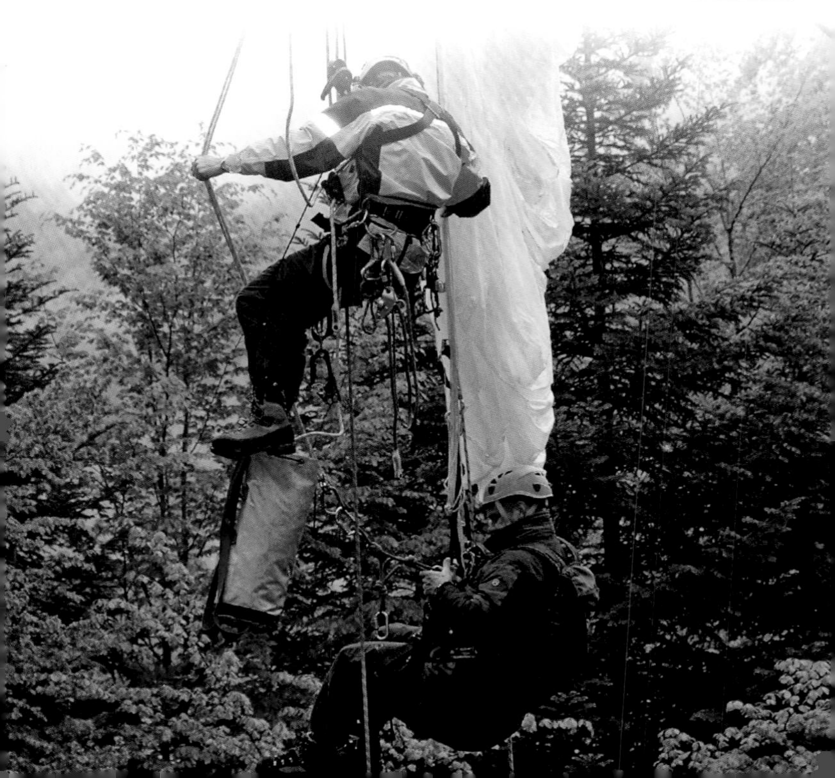

20.1 Accidents caused by Lightning Strike

Accidents caused by lightning strike tend to be rare occurrences in the Swiss Alps where they account for barely 1 % of all mountain emergencies. Although the majority of accidents due to lightning strike do not have a fatal outcome, around 1000 persons do nevertheless die from them worldwide. Many such accidents could be prevented if people find safe refuge in good time and take appropriate precautions.

Precautionary Measures

Thunderstorms with lightning occur predominately in high summer and frequently during the afternoons and evenings. Frontal storms often occur in advance of a cold front and are not dependent on the time of day. Those responsible for planning tours must therefore always keep an eye on the weather reports.

The following applies in high summer: make an early start on the tour so that you are not caught by lightning on exposed ridges and summits and are able to get back to your hut in good time.

Flashes of lightning may occur several kilometers before a storm front and–in the truest sense of the word–strike like a bolt from the blue. The beginning and the end of a thunderstorm are particularly dangerous periods.
To help avoid incidents, people in English-speaking countries apply the "30-30" rule:

Danger exists when you see a flash of lightning and cannot count up to 30 before hearing the thunder (lightning/thunder time). You should only leave the safe area once 30 minutes have elapsed since you saw the last flash of lightning or heard a clap of thunder.

In the mountains it is not always easy to get to a safe place in a reasonable time.
If there is a risk of lightning in the mountains, remember to avoid ridges and summits, and also proximity to individual trees, pylons or ski-lift masts.

The safest place when there is a risk of encountering lightning is in a hut, staying away from open doors or windows. Ground currents can be conducted within small, open shelters. Because of the vertical poles, tents are not protective against lightning strikes. Large caves and recesses are safer than small caves and couloirs. Flat glaciers are just as dangerous as open spaces. Near a vertical wall there is an equilateral **safety triangle,** made up of the height of the wall and the same distance on the ground. However, to avoid ground currents it is important to stay at least 1–2 meters away from the wall. (See below).

The safest body position to adopt is a squatting position with knees and feet together and maintaining as little contact with the ground as possible to avoid step voltages causing injury as a result of ground currents. Under no circumstances should you lie down. Your helmet will provide protection against any injuries as a result of rebounding and falling. The mountaineer should always stay belayed, especially when descending on a rope (Figures 20.1.1 a–b).

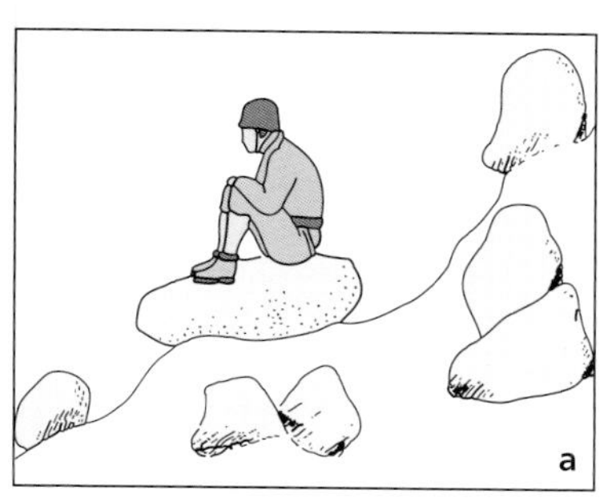

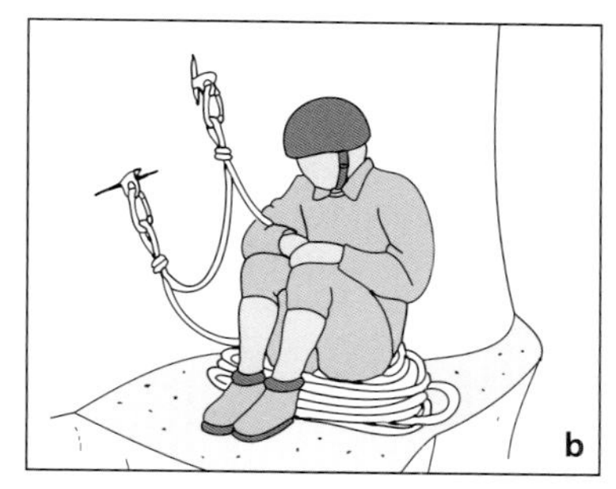

Figures 20.1.1 a–b

Metal will not attract a lightning strike but it is a good conductor of electricity. Any items protruding above the shoulder/head area will increase the risk of a direct lightning strike, e.g. skis, ski poles, ice axes and radio antennas. Metal equipment such as carabiners, nuts, crampons, ice axes and ski poles must not be kept anywhere near the body because, in the event of lightning strike, there will be an increased risk of burns.

⇨ Lightning currents can be transmitted via a wet rope. On a via ferrata you should get away from the rapidly conducting steel ropes and ladders as quickly as possible and set up a belay sling on the rock.

Should your hair stand on end due to static electricity or your skin start to creep, you should immediately get into the squatting position. Crackling noises or visible glowing (St. Elmo's Fire) also indicate an immediate threat of danger from lightning.
Mobile telephones and radio equipment must be stored deep down in your rucksack so as to protect them from discharging.

If an entire group is at risk of lightning strike, safe distances should be maintained between the group members where possible in order to minimize the risk of ground currents or current sparking.

Accident Mechanism

A lightning flash is a massive flow of current of very short duration. Injuries are caused by both the current and the heat generated.
Various mechanisms of injury exist:

- People rarely survive a direct strike on the body due to the very high energy impact.
- More often, injuries occur as a result of sparking currents from nearby tall objects (a tree, a mast or a person).
- A contact injury occurs as a result of contact with a conductive item (via ferrata, wet rope).
- In the event of a lightning strike to the earth, the current may disperse. If different body parts are in contact with the ground at the same time (e.g. straddled feet, hand on a belay device) injuries may occur as a result of step voltages.
- Accompanying mechanical injuries can occur after a fall due to the shock wave created by a lightning flash or as a result of muscle contractions caused by the electrical current.

The majority of people killed by lightning strike die from cardiac arrest. People rendered unconscious or with paralysis, temporary blindness and/or deafness have a good chance of survival.
Current entry and exit points are usually associated with deep-seated burns. However, most burns are superficial due to the extremely short duration of discharge. The typical feathery, red skin marks following a lightning strike (Lichtenberg's markings) are not burns but are caused by the effect of electricity.

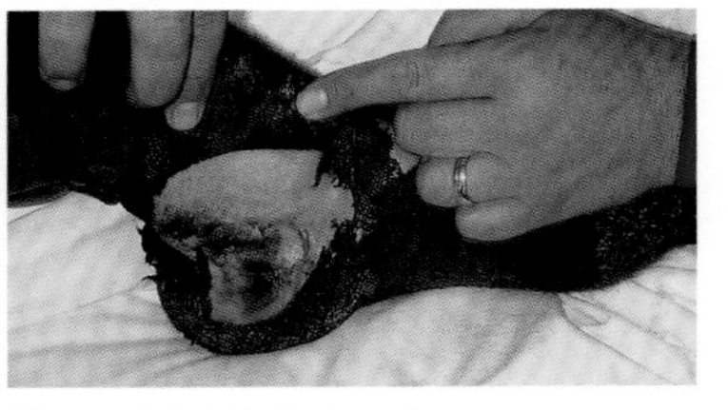

Figure 20.1.2: *Serious burns may occur at the entry and exit points of the strike (B. Durrer).*

First Aid following a Lightning Strike

First Aid following an accident involving a lightning strike primarily means help from colleagues because any organized (air) rescue facility will often only become available once the storm has passed. Initial action is based on the ABC of First Aid (see Section 9.2, Page 97).

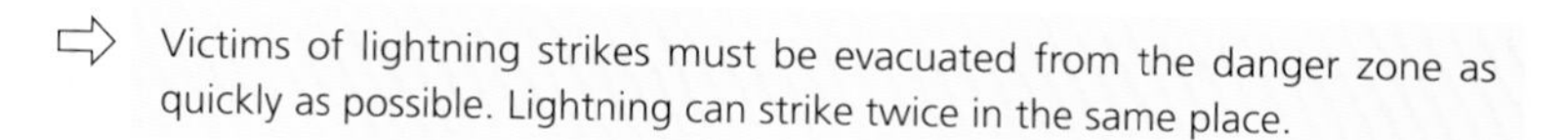

Victims of lightning strikes must be evacuated from the danger zone as quickly as possible. Lightning can strike twice in the same place.

Victims of cardiocirculatory/respiratory arrest have a good chance of survival and cardiopulmonary resuscitation should be initiated immediately as a priority. Where lightning strikes are concerned, dilated pupils which do not react to light are not a reliable indicator of brain damage. Injuries should be treated as detailed in Section 9.4, Page 125.

Where **burns** are involved, the following should be observed:

- Only remove those items of clothing that are not stuck to the wound.
- Cool the affected area for a minimum of 20 minutes with lukewarm water: this prevents the heat injury from extending any deeper and alleviates pain.
- Do not use water that is too cold or ice for cooling–this could increase the severity of the injury!
- If possible remove rings, belts, watches and shoes before swelling of the injured area makes it impossible.

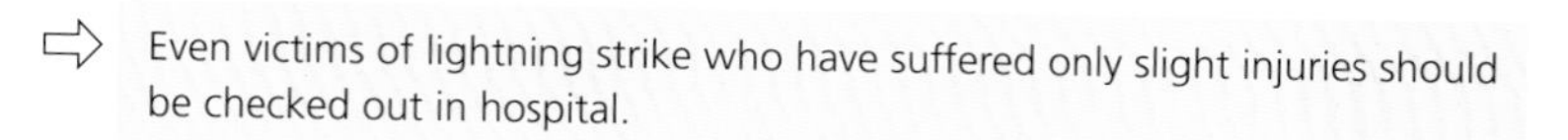

Even victims of lightning strike who have suffered only slight injuries should be checked out in hospital.

Literature:

Zafren Ken, Durrer Bruno, Herr Jean-Pierre, Brugger Hermann: Prevention and on-site treatment of lightning injuries in the mountains. Official guidelines of the International Commission for Mountain Emergency Medicine and the Medical Commission of the International Mountaineering and Climbing Federation (MedCom ICAR and MedCom UIAA).

20.2 Snakebite

Snakes are found throughout Switzerland. With regard to habitat, the two native venomous types of snake, **Vipera aspis** (the **Asp viper)** and the **European adder,** tend to favor sunny hillside locations in the Jura and the Alps. Mountaineers and hikers can therefore expect to encounter snakes from March through to the middle of October. It is difficult to distinguish venomous from harmless snakes from a safe distance. In addition, the color and markings of many snakes are highly variable. Therefore, people are advised to exercise caution in relation to any snake.

⇨ Snakes are shy creatures. They never attack people unless injured or provoked.

The majority of poisonings that occur as a result of snakebite run their course with only mild symptoms. As a rule, a period of monitoring in hospital will suffice when it comes to treating the symptoms. Only in exceptional circumstances may antivenin serum be required. Since 1960 there has only been one fatality. Similarly to insect bites/stings, it is primarily **allergic reactions** that present a threat to life.

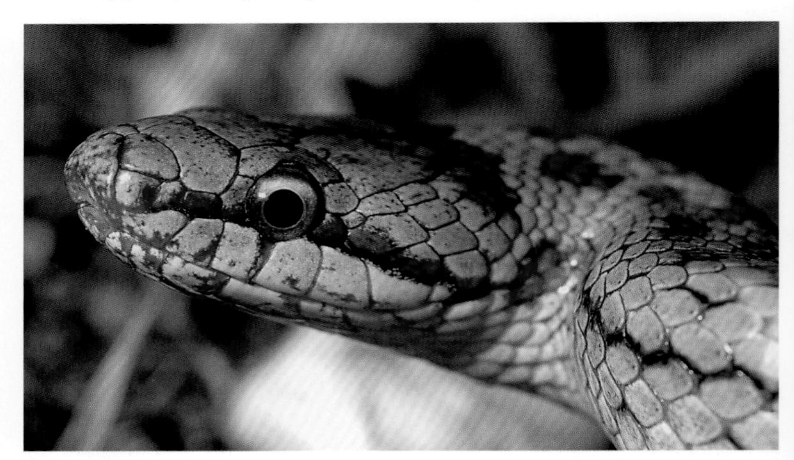

Figure 20.2.1 Smooth Snake: *The smooth snake can be identified by the typical markings on its head. It has a horseshoe-shaped mark on the top of its head and a line that runs from the nostril across the eye to the back of the head. Smooth snakes occur in almost the whole of Europe. The snake will defend itself vigorously if attacked, however, its bite is nonvenomous. Length up to 0.9m (Karch, Coordination Unit for the Protection of Amphibians and Reptiles in Switzerland).*

Prevention

Preventive measures include sturdy **footwear** and possibly a stick with which to penetrate dense shrub cover and undergrowth. Particular care should be taken when poking about in cracks and crannies in piles of logs, dry-stone walls, sawn planks and flagstones. Small children should not be allowed to play in unsupervised locations with dense overgrowth. At night a head torch is recommended. In snake-infested areas only sleep in a tent or on a camp bed.

- Swiss snakes with a length in excess of 90 cm are harmless. Vipera aspis (the Asp viper) and the adder are invariably shorter.
- Shouting and calling out will not help. Snakes are deaf to airborne sound.
- Snakes that lie still without moving are not necessarily dead but may be sleeping or relying on their camouflage. Pass by quietly, giving them a wide berth (at least 2 m).
- Snakes that approach a human being will certainly not have noticed him/her and will under no circumstances try to attack. Any movement will cause the animal to flee.

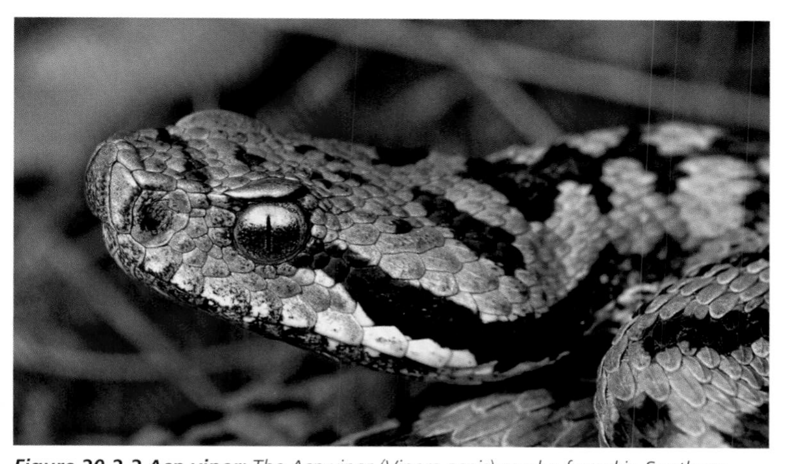

Figure 20.2.2 Asp viper: *The Asp viper (Vipera aspis) can be found in Southern Europe, in the Black Forest, in the Jura and in the Alps. It is similar to the Adder. The males have a zigzag band on their backs whereas the females sport more insignificant coloring. Asp vipers inhabit steep and sunny slopes. Their bite is venomous but not life-threatening (exception: allergic reaction). Length max. 0.85 m (Karch, Karch, Coordination Unit for the Protection of Amphibians and Reptiles in Switzerland).*

First Aid

Stay calm and keep the patient calm. In Switzerland, snake bites are rarely serious. The ensuing panic is often more dangerous than the bite which may only cause pain and swelling. Poisoning can take several hours to reach its peak and there will therefore be sufficient time to locate a medical facility.

⇨ A 24-hour period of monitoring in hospital is nevertheless indicated following any snake bite.

- Disinfect the area of the bite (as a rule two fine puncture marks next to each other).
- Remove rings, watch and bracelets (see Section 9.4, Page 153).
- Immobilise the affected limb (see Section 9.4, Page 125). Movement will only help to disperse the venom. A pressure bandage is not necessary with European snake bites. Administer pain killers as necessary.
- Transport to medical facility or hospital via car or rescue helicopter, keeping the patient as comfortable as possible. The casualty should not be allowed to exert himself.

⇨ A bite from a snake may trigger an **allergic reaction** in some individuals. Dizziness, unconsciousness as well as a rapid and weak pulse are signs of a dangerous allergic reaction (see Section 21.4, Page 286).

You are advised to refrain from:

- Applying tourniquets using belts or cords
- Incising, sucking or injecting the wound
- Snake anti-venom is rarely necessary and will only be administered by the doctor where there are serious complications.

Literature and Sources:

Leaflet, Coordination Unit for the Protection of Amphibians and Reptiles in Switzerland (karch) 3005 Bern: www.karch.ch.
TOX-Centre 145 (Tel. +41 44 251 51 51)
Schweiz Med Forum Nr. 32/33 13. August 2003. Die medizinisch bedeutsamen Giftschlangen der Schweiz Teil 1: Biologie, Verbreitung und Giftzusammensetzung (The medically significant venomous snakes of Switzerland Part 1: Biology, Distribution and Venom Composition) Jürg Meiera, Christophe Berneyb.

20.3 Harness Hang Syndrome (Suspension Trauma)

Long-term suspension, free on a rope is, for mountaineers, one example of a rare accident that may occur after a fall in rocky terrain or on ice or a fall into a crevasse. Suspension trauma may come about in technical caving and in new trending sports such as rope adventure parks, paragliding and hang-gliding or base jumping. In addition to any injuries sustained during a fall, suspension in a climbing harness is, on its own, quite capable of leading to serious circulatory problems, possibly culminating in cardiac arrest and death. Even in a combined chest/seat harness it will not be long before a free-hanging victim will find himself in a life-threatening situation.

Within a few minutes, **collapse of the circulatory system** with unconsciousness may well occur.

Restriction to breathing, disturbances to return blood flow and the increasing toxic metabolic waste products will ultimately generate an acute threat to life.

Mechanism

Hanging in free suspension in a climbing harness will cut off the blood flow to the legs and blood is prevented from flowing back from the lower to the upper part of the body (heart). This leads to pooling of blood in the legs and a reduction in the amount of blood in the active circulation.
In the event of unconsciousness after a fall or where injuries are involved, the victim will no longer be able to move the leg muscles in order to pump the blood from the legs upward. In such cases the phenomenon described above will occur much more quickly, hence provoking collapse of the circulation.

In an incapacitated victim, who also happens to be carrying a heavy rucksack, tilting into the head-down position may occur. This may significantly accelerate the occurrence of suspension trauma.

Sudden post-rescue death syndrome

Should insufficient care be exercised in laying the casualty down or the operation be carried out incorrectly (e.g. laying the patient flat too quickly) the increase in the return flow of blood enriched with harmful substances may lead to sudden heart failure.

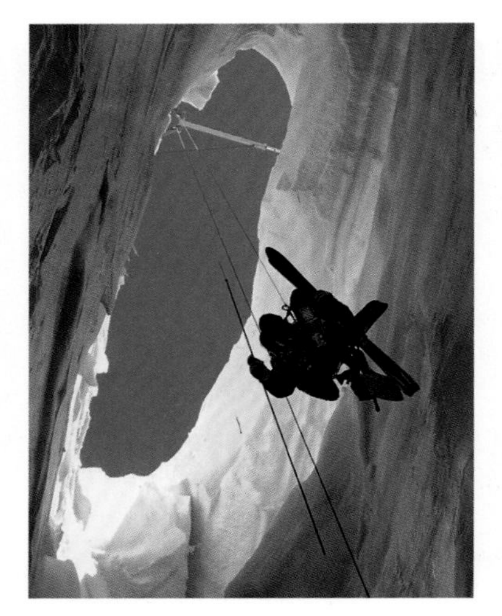

Figure 20.3.1: *Free suspension in a glacier crevasse (by kind permission of Rega Archive).*

Precautions:

- Use climbing harnesses that fit well and are properly adjusted (e.g. combined chest-/seat-belts on glaciers together with rucksack). A belt that proves painful in a suspension test will encourage the rapid onset of suspension trauma.
- Prepare and keep to hand, **foot slings** to relieve pressure with a Prusik or belay device.
- Participate actively in rescue courses so as to familiarise yourself with the improvised rescue techniques.

Rescue and First Aid

Where the person concerned is able to move, pressure on the feet should be relieved by means of a Prusik sling or belay device. Moving the legs activates the muscle pump which promotes the return flow of blood from the legs toward the heart. Elevation of the upper part of the body is recommended.
The rescue of unconscious victims should proceed quickly and carefully, wherever possible crouched in a seated position or seated with outstretched legs and with the upper part of the body erect.

⇨ Following rescue from a suspension trauma situation, the victim should not be laid flat or placed in the **recovery position** during the first **10–20 minutes** (risk of sudden post-rescue death syndrome!)

Only then should slow, careful repositioning of the patient take place, from an elevated upper body position into a position where he is lying on his side (see Section 9.4, Page 128).
These patients must be monitored closely and where required, it must be possible to initiate resuscitation promptly.

21. Other Acute Incidents in the Mountains

Various Authors

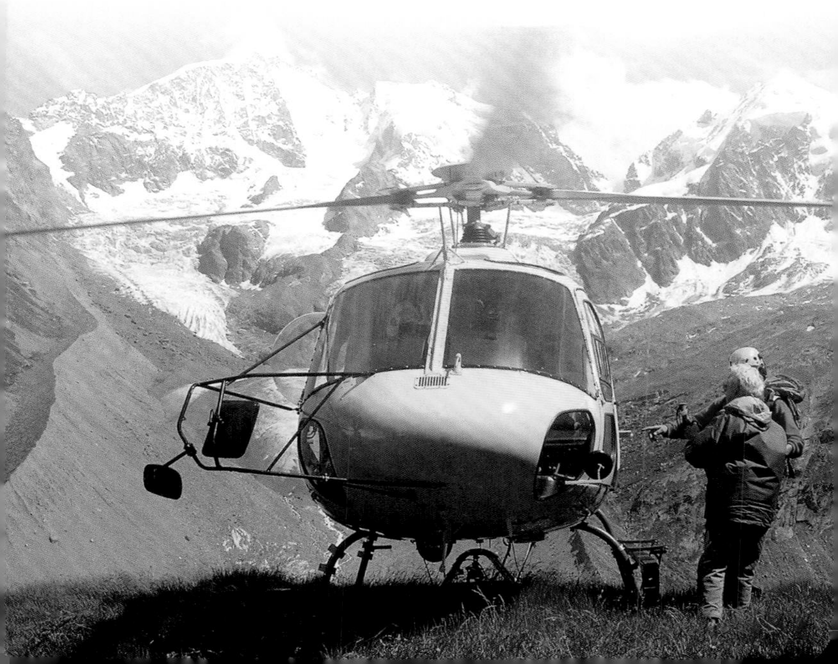

21.1 Acute Low Back Pain in Adults

Low back pain means pain in the lower back, extending from the lower ribs as far as the gluteal folds, with or without radiation into the legs. Muscle tension and reduced range of movement may also be observed in these areas. Acute low back pain means sudden onset pains which are of less than 12 weeks' duration and which may demonstrate variable intensities of pain. **Recurrent low back pain** describes constantly recurring episodes of low back pain with a symptom-free interval of at least 6 months. By contrast, in the case of **chronic low back pains,** the pain is uninterrupted and present for longer than 12 weeks.

⇨ 75–85% of the total population will suffer low back pain at least once during the course of their lives and sometimes on more than one occasion. Younger people are more often affected than older people.

Usually, it is possible to distinguish between **musculoskeletal back pain** (joints, bones and muscles) and back pain emanating from the **internal organs** (gastrointestinal tract, kidney and urinary tract and uterus together with ovaries). The latter are rare and occur in approx. 2 % of cases.

Musculoskeletal back pains (approx. 98 %) are classified into acute uncomplicated low back pain, **radicular** low back pain and complicated low back pain. Radicular low back pain signifies low back pain which radiates as far as the area below the knee or even as far as the area of the foot.

Acute uncomplicated low back pain (>80 %):
Synonyms: lumbalgia, lumbago, non-radicular low back pain. Criteria as follows:

- Age 20–50 years.
- Low back pain which radiates as far as the buttocks and/or thighs. Typically, the pain does not go below the knee area. Diffuse pain distribution over the affected areas.
- Movement-related pain: changing position may make things better or worse.
- Good general condition.

Radicular low back pain (approx. 5 %):
Synonym: Ischialgia, lumbar ischialgia. Criteria as follows:

- Unilateral leg pain worse than the back pain.
- Radiation into foot or toes.
- Numbness, tingling and "pins and needles."
- Positive *Lasègue's Test* (see Figure 21.1.1).
- *Loss of reflex,* paralysis or numbness in the area supplied by the nerve roots. Paraesthesia (impairment of sensation) frequently occurs in bands extending from the buttocks as far as the foot.
- Pain on coughing radiating as far as the feet.

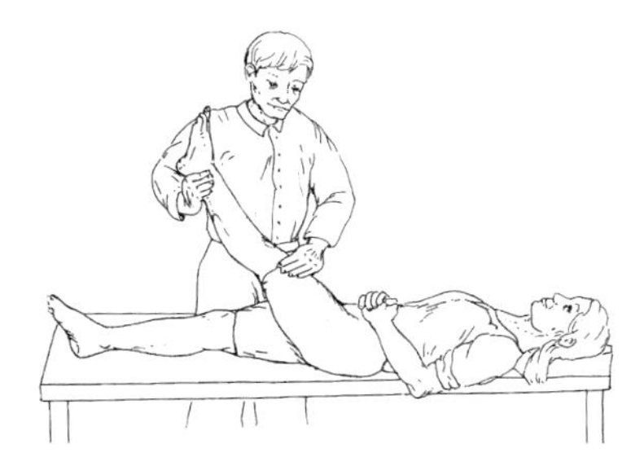

Figure 21.1.1: *Lasègue's Sign (named after the French physician Ernst Charles Lasègue's [1816–1883]) describes pain associated with stretching the sciatic nerve and/or the spinal nerve routes in the lumbar and sacral segments of the spinal cord. In this case, the patient is in the supine position.*

The physician slowly raises the affected leg, which should be relaxed. Should the pain increase below a lift angle of 45°, this is a clear sign that the nerve roots are the cause of the pain in the lumbar spine.

Complicated low back pain (= severe course):
1 % of all low back pain may be ascribed to ***fractures,*** infections, deformities, inflammatory rheumatic diseases or tumors. The clinical picture is very similar to that presented by uncomplicated low back pain. The more of the criteria listed below that are identified, the greater the likelihood that complicated low back pain is present.

Criteria as follows:

- Age between 20 and 50 years.
- Increasing pain, unrelated to movement, or persistence of symptoms despite treatment.
- Poor general condition, potentially known malignant disease, unexplained night sweats.
- Fever (e.g. with purulent structures–*abscess*–in the area of the back).
- Co-existing *trauma*, making a fracture likely.
- Drug abuse, advanced HIV infection, weak immune system.
- Cortisone therapy or known osteoporosis.
- Definite loss of neurological function such as paralyses and sensory disturbances.
- *Saddle anaesthesia, bladder* and *bowel disorders.*
- Indications of inflammatory rheumatic disease.

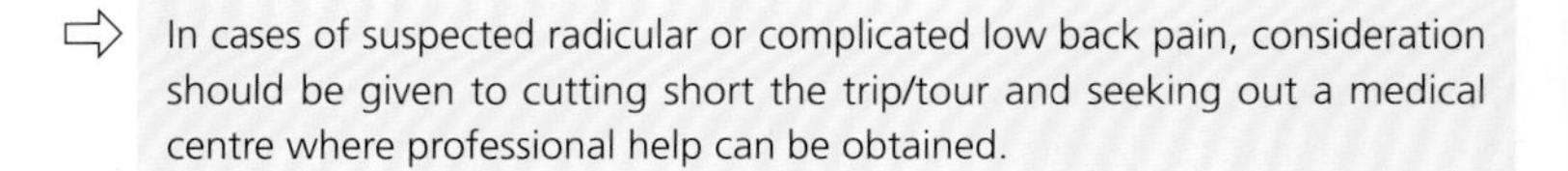

In cases of suspected radicular or complicated low back pain, consideration should be given to cutting short the trip/tour and seeking out a medical centre where professional help can be obtained.

Key questions:

- Are nerves affected (tingling, numbness, muscle weakness)?
- Is there an underlying dangerous disease?
- Are there factors (e.g. depression, dissatisfaction with tour group, worrying about the next project) that are likely to affect further progress?

Physical examination where low back pain is a factor:

- Pain points
- Muscle tension
- Bruising *(haematoma)*
- Skin lesions

In the event of pain radiating into one or both legs, including the lower leg and/or feet *(radicular pains)*, particular attention should be paid to the following:

Muscle strength	Calcaneal gait
	Tiptoe gait
	Standing on one leg with knee bent
Reflexes (side/side comparison*)	Achilles tendon reflex
	Patellar tendon reflex
Tactile sensation	Instep
	Lateral foot and sole of foot
	Medial foot
Nerve stretch pain	Lasègue's Sign
	Reverse Lasègue's Sign

Table 21.1.1

Indicators for further investigations (curtailment of trip/tour)

- Particularly severe pain.
- Therapy-resistant symptoms.
- Uncomplicated backpain after 4 weeks.
- Radicular low back pain after 1–2 weeks.
- Severe neurological disorders (*saddle anaesthesia*, disorders of the bowel/rectum or urination disorders, paralyses).
- Warning signs of inflammatory or malignant diseases or trauma (complicated low back pain).

Treatment:
Uncomplicated low back pain:

- Fastest possible resumption of usual daily routine.
- Gentle sporting activities.
- Exercise with normal body movements (no stinting here!).
- Supportive drug therapy (see Table 21.1.2).
- Possibly muscle-relaxant medication, pain point infiltrations, manual therapy.

* Reflexes tested by a physician or a person who has undergone medical training.

Radicular low back pain with paralyses and numbness:

- Fastest possible resumption of mobility with slow build-up of activity.
- Support therapy with drugs (see below, where applicable muscle-relaxing medication *muscle relaxants*).
- If tiptoe and/or calcaneal gait and/or standing on one leg with bent knee is not possible, then the trip should be cancelled immediately and a visit paid to a medical centre with appropriate qualified facilities.
- If tiptoe and/or calcaneal gait and/or standing on one leg with bent knee is still possible, the trip may be continued. However, the situation should be reassessed on a daily basis and a medical assessment should take place at the next opportunity.

Complicated low back pain:

- Drug-based pain support therapy.
- Immediate attendance at a medical centre for an assessment and therapy.

⇨ In 80–90% of cases, uncomplicated low back pains die down within 4–6 weeks. Should the pain be persistent or progressive, or in the event of neurological loss of function or complicated lumbago, a visit should be paid to a medical centre.

	Quantity	**Morning**	**Midday**	**Evening**	**Night**
Paracetamol	1 g	1	1	1	1
Diclofenac	50 mg	1	1	1	0
Pantoprazole	20 mg	1	0	0	0
Diazepam*	5 mg	1	0	1	0

Table 21.1.2: *Example of a medication scheme.*

* It may be possible to make use of a combined preparation (e.g. Paracetamol and Codeine). However, it is important to be aware of side effects, including a reduction in concentration. (See also Annexe "First Aid Kit," Page 294).

In the case of stomach problems, kidney disease, allergies or other diseases, a prior consultation with a specialist as regards the use of medications is to be recommended or the patient should discuss the subject with his GP before setting off on the trip.

Precautionary Measures: It is possible to prevent and combat back pain by adopting active measures. Correct training is important, in addition to education in posture and back hygiene. Any type of sport in which the muscles of the back and the abdomen are uniformly loaded to a sustained extent (cycling, jogging wearing the correct shoes, Nordic walking and swimming) is suitable. Rapid rotational movements of short duration are harmful to a back that is already under strain (tennis, gymnastics, golf, bodybuilding etc.). Here other types of balancing sports are recommended.

	Low back pain		
	Acute uncomplicated	Radicular	Complicated
Age between 20 and 50 yrs			
Age over 50 or under 20 yrs			
General condition: Good			
General condition: Poor			
Pains:			
Low back			
Buttocks			
Thighs			
Lower leg			
Foot			
Toes			
Position-related increase in pain			
Leg pain associated with coughing			
Diffused thigh pain			
Leg pain along nerve pathway			
Leg pain > low back pain			
Low back pain > leg pain			
Numbness extending to toe: nerve pathway			
Lasègue's Sign			
Reverse Lasègue's			
Missing or weakened reflexes			
Motor Skills:			
Calcaneal gait restricted/not functioning			
Tiptoe gait restricted/not functioning			
Standing on one leg with knee bent restricted/not functioning			

	Low back pain		
	Acute uncomplicated	Radicular	Complicated
Other Factors:			
Intense trauma			
Fever			
Inflammatory rheumatic disease			
Accumulation of pus along back			
Intravenous drugs consumption			
HIV/Aids			
Cortisone therapy			
Known tumour			
Night sweats			
Weight loss			
Increasing pain			
Bladder disorder			
Bowel disorder			
Saddle anaesthesia			
Haematoma			
Total No. of Points (total number of orange fields per column)			

Table 21.1.3: *Questionnaire relating to the Classification of Back Pain. The column with the highest number of colored fields selected provides an impression of the types of pain involved.*

Literature:

1) Spinal Disorders, Fundamentals of Diagnosis and Treatment (Norbert Boos, Max Aebi et al.), Springer Verlag, ISBN 978-3-540-40511-5.
2) Guidelines No. 3 Low Back Pain.
3) Gen. Med 2007; 83: 487–494; Chenot JF et al. Update of the DEGAM Guidelines.
4) Swiss Med. Forum 2001;9: 205–208: Diagnostics: Lumbar Back Pain.
5) Swiss Med Forum 2006; 6:542–548: Lumbar Pain and Ischialgia with no Loss of Function – The Importance of Physical Activity in Treatment.
6) Swiss Med Forum 2006; 6:928–929: Physical Activity in relation to Lumbar Pain and Lumbar Radiculopathy.

21.2 Dental Problems

It is an unfortunate fact that teeth are also well able to cloud our enjoyment of a beautiful day and pleasure in a successful climb to the summit.

Preventive measures will reduce the likelihood of having to undergo a painful experience and careful daily attention to dental care at home lays the foundation for this. Regular dental support will promote healthy conditions in the oral cavity and we can forget about the possibility of any sudden dental disorders. Nevertheless, accidents involving injuries to the teeth can still occur. Whether it is on a one-day trip or a tour lasting several days in the Alps, immediate treatment will be required if a fall results in damage to a tooth or teeth. In all other situations, pain killers can be used to afford relief pending the next possible visit to a dentist.

Accidents involving Dental Injuries

Splitting/crushing wounds to lips: Wounds should be cleaned, disinfected and covered. Any extensive splitting/crushing wound should be assessed in due course by a doctor who will deliver the appropriate care.

Easily movable tooth: Impact to a tooth can cause it to become movable. This may be associated with slight pain. Treat the tooth with care until normal mobility is restored. A checkup at the dentist's is to be recommended.

Broken tooth: A broken tooth that does not bleed after rinsing with water can, in an emergency, be left untreated for several days. Although a sharp edge may be a nuisance, the tooth is neither at acute risk nor will major pain occur. Once the tour is over the tooth should be treated by a professional.

A tooth bleeding from the fractured surface indicates that the blood vessel and nerve fibre have been damaged. Immediate dental treatment is essential. Without it the nerve will first become inflamed and then decay.

This process is painful during the first few days. The pain will then die down temporarily, before possible resumption of intense pain after an indeterminate period due to bacterial infection.

Displaced tooth: A tooth that has been displaced following a blow can be repositioned in the original location by applying gentle but consistent pressure with a finger. Afterwards handle with care and have it splinted by the dentist as quickly as possible.

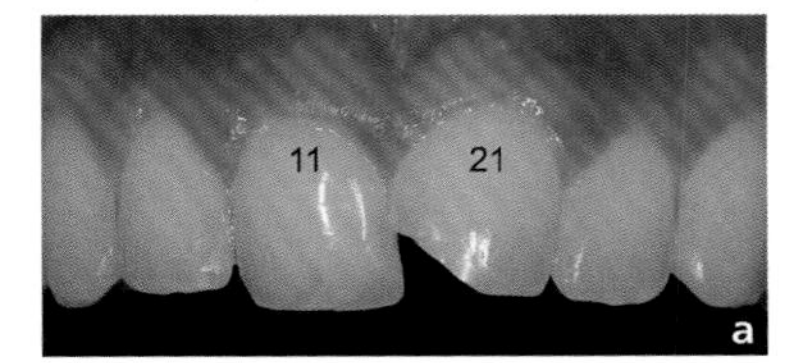

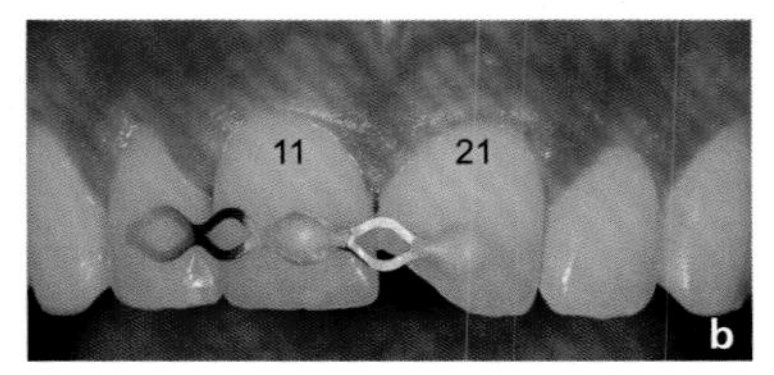

Figures 21.2.1 a–b: *a: Displaced tooth 11 and broken tooth 21 b: repositioned and splinted tooth 11.*

Tooth that has been dislodged but is still intact in the root area: the root of an intact tooth terminates in a slightly "rounded tip." Possible injuries include a sharp-edged surface fracture or a crack. With appropriate action, an intact tooth can heal again although this will require help from a dentist. When faced with an accident of this type, a decision will need to be made as to which is the priority–the tooth or the success of the expedition.

Should you decide **in favor of the expedition,** the healing process with the lowest risk is if the tooth is not reinserted. Subsequent treatment of the gap will become more complex.
If the decision is **in favor of the tooth** and if it is possible to get to a dentist, the tooth can be removed in the meantime. Ideal for this is the Dentosafe® "Tooth-Rescue-Box" (small box containing a cell nutrition liquid; cells can survive in this for up to 48 hours. Available in pharmacies or at some schools and swimming pools in Switzerland) (see Figure 21.2.2).

In the short term the tooth can be transported in a container or plastic bag with UHT milk (first choice), milk, physiological saline solution or water (last resort). NB: The root of the tooth should never be touched.
If none of these are available and if the dentist cannot be reached on the same day, and if the other mountaineers have the courage to do it, an intact tooth can be pushed back into the bone socket.

The tooth could still fall out again and be swallowed or inhaled. The surface of the root should not be touched. Any dirt on the surface may be rinsed off with water but not rubbed off.

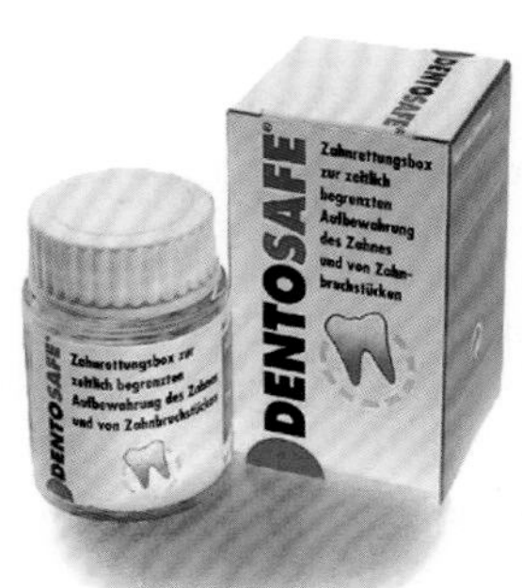

Figure 21.2.2:
Dentosafe® "Tooth-Rescue-Box."

Once the tooth has been reimplanted antibiotic therapy is indicated. A follow-up visit to the dentist is essential.

Diseases of the Oral Cavity

In the case of expeditions lasting several weeks in areas where there is no guarantee that dental care will be available, it is important to be aware of the following injuries and diseases.
Caries and periodontal disease affect the oral cavity and are caused by a lack of oral hygiene. Both are unobtrusive at the beginning but may develop into a painful swollen jaw.

Periodontitis is inflammation of the gums and bone. This happens when layers of plaque and bacteria accumulate along the gum line and between the teeth and are not removed.

Caries is demineralization of the tooth surface and decay on the inside of the tooth. Acid in the mouth, which we absorb by ingesting food or which may develop due to bacteria from sugar, attacks the surface of the tooth. As the surface of the tooth breaks down, the process of decay sets in underneath. In the advanced stage this may lead to painful nerve inflammation (see Figures 21.2.3 a–b).

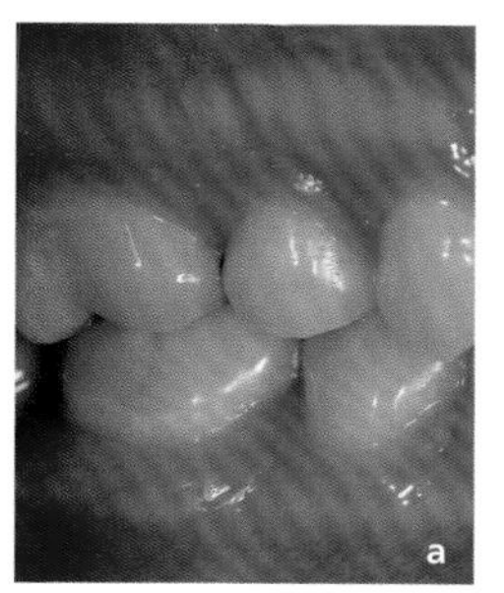

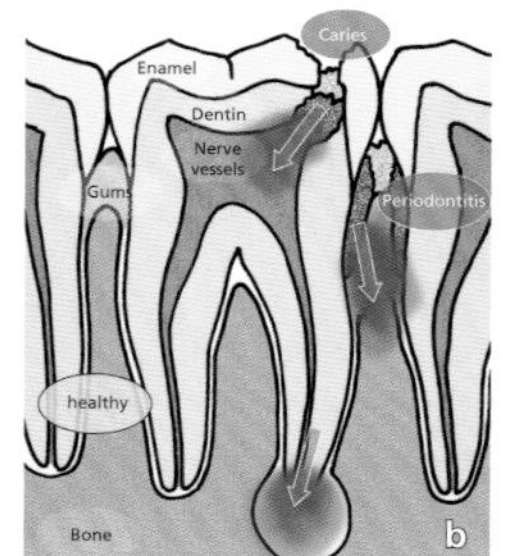

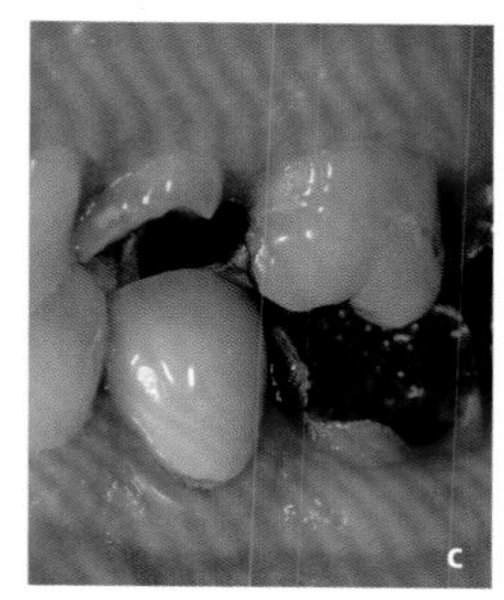

Figures 21.2.3 a–c: *a: Well-cared for and healthy set of teeth, c: neglected and decayed teeth.*

Preventive measures, such as good dental hygiene and regular visits to the dentist, are essential. If these have been neglected it is advisable, before a planned expedition, to make an appointment for another checkup.

Arrange for a dental check-up **before** an expedition! This should be arranged **several weeks** beforehand so that any treatment that may be required can be carried out properly and the healing process monitored.

It is advisable to embark on the trip with a healthy oral cavity and teeth. Starting on the expedition with periodontitis or an inflamed wound from a bad fall off a mountain bike are equivalent – everything may be fine but you may still find yourself having to call the trip off as a result of purulent abscesses. With a healthy oral cavity and normal diet you can be fairly sure that there will be no painful surprises in store for you on the journey, with the exception – of course – of any accidents.

Infections and Abscesses: Infection is indicated by a reddened and painful area of the mouth. This can turn into an abscess – an increasingly painful swelling filled with pus. You need to consult a dentist. If this is not possible the bacterial infection will need to be brought under temporary control using a broad-spectrum antibiotic e.g. Augmentin®.

Treatment:

- Augmentin®: 625 mg 3x a day for 6 days.
- Dalacin® C where there is a known allergy to penicillin.
- Pain killers as required (see Annexe "First Aid Kit," Page 289).

Antibiotic therapy will not guarantee a successful outcome unless the root cause is eliminated by a dentist. In addition, there is a danger that the inflammation may erupt again once a period of time has elapsed.

If the patient's **general condition** deteriorates and the swelling spreads to take in the area around the angle of the jaw and where the oral opening is reduced, there is a danger to life and urgent action is indicated. Contact a hospital before the inflammation spreads along the oesophagus into the cardiopulmonary region.

Oral hygiene on the go

After breakfast and the midday meal food residue should be removed, i.e. the teeth should be cleaned or the oral cavity at least thoroughly rinsed with water. In the evening the teeth should be cleaned thoroughly using a toothpaste containing fluoride; a soft toothbrush is ideal for this. The spaces between the teeth should also be cleaned conscientiously with dental floss, tooth picks or brushes. As there is hardly any flow of saliva during the night, cleaning in the evening is particularly important. After this you should restrict yourself to sugar-free drinks only. If oral hygiene is only neglected in the short term and not repeatedly there will be hardly any consequences to worry about. However, if this happens over a lengthy period of time or repeatedly there is increased risk of developing periodontitis or caries. Eating habits also have a major influence on the health of the oral cavity. Saliva has the ability to neutralize the acid; this takes about half an hour. We can make the saliva's work easier by rinsing the mouth with water after eating or drinking. However, launching a new attack on the teeth, even after just half an hour, in the shape of sticky Powerbars or acidic sports drinks will soon lead to caries. On the odd days when maximum performance is required, food and drink rich in carbohydrates may be ingested without any consequences. However, on rest days, it is a good idea to take a rest from this habit too.

21.3 Poisoning by Plants and Fungi

Poisonous Plants

There are a number of native plants in Switzerland that are poisonous or highly poisonous. Ingesting even a small amount of a highly poisonous plant may have fatal consequences. The most frequent cause of poisoning is confusion between berries, leaves or roots, some types of which are poisonous and others that are not.

The **highly poisonous** wild plants occurring in Switzerland include the following:

- Monkshood (Aconitum napellus) (Figure 21.3.1)
- Deadly Nightshade (Atropa belladonna)
- Autumn Crocus (Colchicum autumnale) (Figure 21.3.2)
- Foxglove (Digitalis ambigua: grandiflora, Digitalis lutea: yellow, Digitalis purpurea: Common Foxglove)
- Yew (Taxus baccata)
- White hellebore (Veratrum album)

Poisonous wild Swiss plants include:

- Cuckoo Pint (Arum maculatum)
- Lily of the Valley (Convallaria majalis)
- Spindle Tree (Euonymus europaeus)
- Spurge (Euphorbia sp.)
- Euphorbia cyparissias (Cypress spurge)
- Euphorbia esula (Green Spurge, Leafy Spurge)
- The following species of Hellebore: Christmas Rose (Helleborus niger), Green Hellebore (Helleborus viridis) and Stinking Hellebore (Helleborus foetidus)

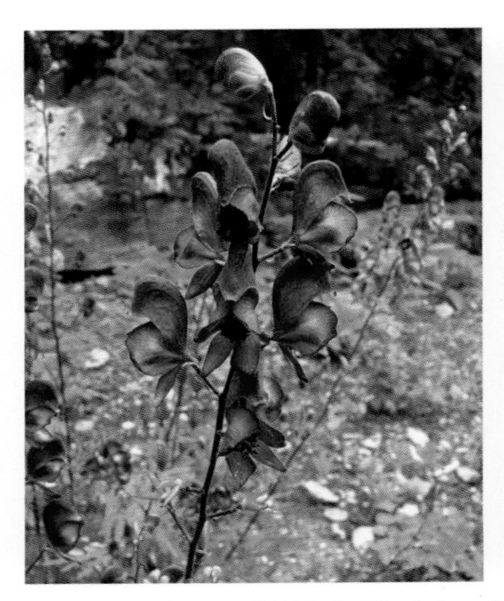
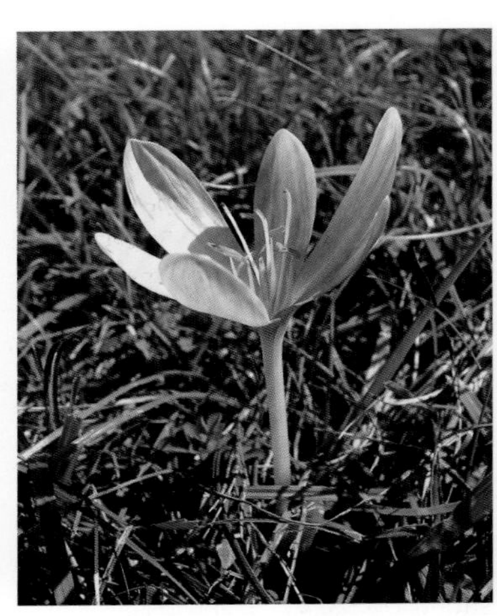

***Figures 21.3.1 and 21.3.2:** Monkshood (Aconitum napellus) and Autumn Crocus (Colchicum autumnal).*

The individual plants are listed below, together with hazardous quantities, the potential for confusion and the signs of poisoning:

> If a highly poisonous plant is ingested in a quantity known to be hazardous, a doctor or a hospital should be contacted without delay. Keep the plants and take them with you!

Signs of poisoning vary from mild symptoms (nausea, vomiting, dizziness) right through to life-threatening ABC problems (see Section 9.2, Page 97). If a highly poisonous plant is ingested in a dangerous quantity, the best course of action is to take liquid charcoal without delay but at the latest within 1–2 hours of ingestion (1 gram per kg body weight, subject to the patient being conscious). Then contact a doctor or the Toxicology Information Centre (Tel. 145).

Monkshood (Aconitum napellus)
Potential for confusion: Leaves may be confused with parsley leaves.
Hazardous quantity: Small amount of plant material.
Symptoms: Monkshood contains aconitine, one of the strongest plant toxins. Initial symptoms occur within 10–20 minutes and include initially burning and numbness in the mouth, which subsequently spreads to the limbs and entire body. Added to

this is a feeling of cold, nausea, vomiting, colicky diarrhea, severe muscle pains and possibly even convulsions. In severe cases of poisoning, cardiac dysrhythmia and a fall in blood pressure may occur.

Deadly Nightshade (Atropa belladonna)
Potential for confusion: Blackberries, blueberries.
Hazardous quantity: 1 berry or more.
Symptoms: Tropane alkaloids in belladonna cause dilation of the pupils with blurred vision, feeling hot, reddening of the skin, a dry mouth, hoarseness, difficulties in swallowing, vomiting, intestinal paralysis, difficulties with urination, palpitations, agitation, disturbance of gait and confusion. Hallucinations, convulsive seizures and coma may also occur.

Autumn Crocus (Colchicum autumnal)
Potential for confusion: Wild garlic leaves, although the leaves of wild garlic smell strongly of garlic, have a stalk and are shorter and wider.
Hazardous quantity: Small quantity of plant material.
Symptoms: The main alkaloid Colchicine causes the following 3-phase symptomatology: Phase 1: Following a latency period of 2–18 hours, severe gastrointestinal symptoms occur with nausea, (blood-tinged) vomiting, colic and (bloodstained) diarrhea. Phase 2: 24–72 hours after ingestion multi-organ failure may occur. Phase 3: recovery phase follows 7–10 days after ingestion.

Foxglove, Grandiflora-, Yellow, Purple (Common Foxglove)
(Digitalis ambigua, Digitialis lutea, Digitialis purpura)
Hazardous quantity: Small quantity of plant material.
Symptoms: The cardiac glycosides can lead to cardiac dysrhythmia and cardiac arrest. In addition gastrointestinal upset may occur as a result of saponins causing localized irritation.

Yew (Taxus baccate)
Potential for confusion: Needles can be confused with pine needles.
Hazardous quantity: The red aril is nontoxic but biting through seeds or needles may cause symptoms.
Symptoms: Yew toxins, the taxines, are quickly absorbed from the gastrointestinal tract and may lead to gastrointestinal disturbances including vomiting, abdominal pains and diarrhea within just 60 minutes of ingestion. After consuming a large quantity of needles or chewed seeds coma, convulsions, dilated pupils, cardiac dysrhythmia with slowing of the pulse, respiratory paralysis and cardiac arrest may occur.

Cuckoo Pint (Arum maculatum)
Potential for confusion: Wild garlic leaves.
Hazardous quantity: Small amounts of plant material though not life-threatening.
Symptoms: Cuckoo Pint contains oxalic acid and calcium oxalate crystals. These typically irritate the mucous membranes. The symptoms include burning, pain, reddening and the formation of blisters in the mouth and throat and sometimes swelling. In addition, nausea, vomiting, stomach, abdominal pains and (bloodstained) diarrhea may occur.

First Aid: In this case, contrary to other plant poisoning, charcoal should not be administered. Instead, give drinks or foods containing calcium (such as milk and ice-cream). The cooling action alleviates the pain and the calcium will act as a binding agent for the oxalic acid.

Lily of the Valley (Convallaria majalis)
Potential for confusion: Wild garlic leaves.
Hazardous quantity: Plant material in relatively large quantities.
Symptoms: As in the case of foxglove, the cardiac glycosides may lead to cardiac arrhythmia and cardiac arrest. However, more plant material is required here than in the case of the foxglove because the lily of the valley glycosides are less readily absorbed than the foxglove glycosides. In addition, gastrointestinal disturbances occur as a result of saponins acting as local irritants.

Spindle (Euonymus europaeus)
Hazardous quantity: More than 5 of the caps.
Symptoms: The various constituents of the euonymus cap (steroid glycosides, an alkaloid, a lectin and triterpene) cause severe irritation locally and trigger violent diarrhea with vomiting.

Cypress Spurge (Euphorbia cyparissias), Leafy Spurge (Euphorbia esula)
Hazardous quantity: A small amount of milky sap.
Symptoms: The milky sap contains a variety of constituents that, depending on location, may cause severe irritation or may even be corrosive. They are highly corrosive to the cornea and can cause serious injuries if the eyes are not immediately washed with water. On the skin, they cause inflammation and, if ingested, a gastrointestinal disorder.

Stinking Hellebore, Christmas Rose, Green Hellebore
(Hellebores foetidus, niger, viridis)
Hazardous quantity: Large quantities of plant material.
Symptoms: The toxins of the various species of Helleborus tend to be irritants whilst others may be cardiac glycosides, although these have only been identified in Helleborus foetidus and viridis. In larger amounts, the irritant substances trigger gastrointestinal symptoms in the form of nausea, vomiting and diarrhea. The cardiac glycosides cause palpitations, marked slowing of the heart rate and disturbances to cardiac rhythm.

Toxic Fungi

The majority of the fungi to be found in Switzerland are inedible; some are edible but a few are potentially capable of causing severe poisoning. A large group of fungi (mycorrhizal fungi) are found in association with deciduous and coniferous trees. Their incidence is therefore directly dependent on the location of these trees. The other major group (saprophytes) survives by exploiting dead wood and therefore tends to appear in a number of different locations. The root system of fungi often survives for many years in the soil or in host plants, hardly visible to the human eye. The season, temperature and humidity determine whether fruiting structures will appear.
Switzerland, with its diverse regions, contains habitats for a large variety of fungi. The northern side of the Alps differs from the southern side not only in relation to fauna and flora but also in terms of the incidence of fungi.

Probably the most toxic fungus in Switzerland is the **Green Death Cap** (Amanita phalloides) and its white cousins (Amanita virosa and Amanita verna). These lamellae fungi, reminiscent of mushrooms, contain Amanitins (see Figure 21.3.3).

Amanitins cause liver failure within the space of just a few days which, if left untreated, will lead to death.

Symptoms and treatment: Following consumption of these fungi, incessant vomiting and watery diarrhea ensues after a period of 6–8 hours. After a short period of apparent improvement rapid liver failure develops. Therapy consists of the early administration of charcoal and intravenous fluids. An antidote (available in hospitals) can slow down the absorption of the toxin in the liver.
Every year in Europe people die from Death Cap poisoning or have to undergo a liver transplant in order to save their lives.

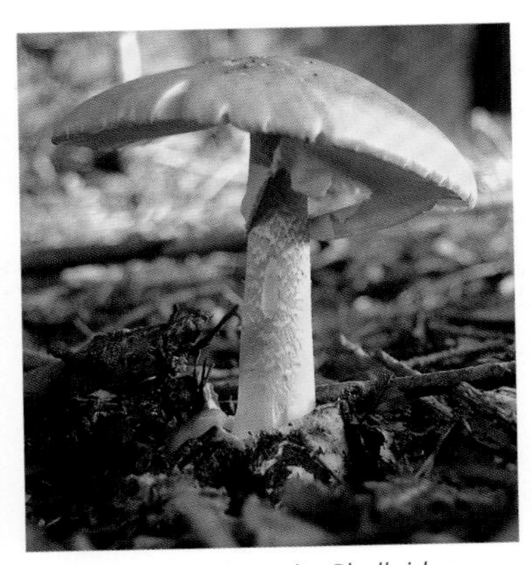

Figure 21.3.3: *Amanita Phalloides.*

Amanitins also occur in other fungal species, namely Lepiota sp. and Galerina sp., and ingestion of these may also lead to life-threatening poisoning. Similarly, ingestion of many other fungi, sometimes with unknown toxins, will also cause gastrointestinal symptoms (vomiting, nausea, diarrhea). In such cases the symptoms tend to emerge within 1–3 hours of ingestion. The most severe symptoms are seen following consumption of **livid entoloma** (Entoloma sinuatum), **sulfur tuft** (Hypholoma fasciculate) and **Satan's mushroom** (Boletus satanas). The latter is one of the few poisonous boletes. The symptoms usually die down over a period of 1–3 days with simple fluid replacement therapy and leave behind no permanent damage.

From time to time fungi are also ingested in order to promote intoxication. Due to their highly variable content of toxins their effect on the central nervous system is difficult to predict and can be extremely unpleasant for the individual concerned. On rare occasions children may be affected when they find and consume these fungi. The **Psilocybes** (Psilocybe sp.), and **Panaeolus** (Panaeolus sp.) varieties may contain the toxin Psilocybin. This generates euphoria, hallucinations, panic states and, in a worst-case scenario, convulsive fits. These symptoms will die down with tranquilizers under medical supervision within a period of 12 hours to a maximum of 3 days.

Toxic species e.g. Clitocybe dealbata (ivory funnel) and the majority of fungi in the genus Inocybe (Inocybe sp.) contain the active ingredient muscarine which also acts on the central nervous system. Within a short period of time (15–120 mins.) they cause sweating, slow pulse, constricted pupils, tears and salivation which may be combined with gastrointestinal upset. These symptoms can be treated in hospital with an antidote (*Atropine*). These fungi are often wrongly identified as edible mushrooms.

Fly agaric (Amanita muscaria) does not–as its name may suggest–contain muscarine but instead ibotenic acid and muscimol. These substances, which also occur in the Panther Cap (Amanita pantherina), cause an increase in pulse rate or even ventricular tachycardia, dry mucous membranes and a state of confusion within the space of 15–120 minutes. Dilated pupils are often a feature. On occasions hallucinations may occur and, in serious cases, coma, which in some circumstances may persist for longer than 24 hours. The white veil residues on the cap of the Fly agaric (which can be easily washed away in a downpour) often leads to the Fly agaric being confused with the extremely tasty Caesar's Mushroom (Amanita caesarea).

Emergency action where mushroom poisoning is suspected:

- Charcoal administration (charcoal suspension; 1 g/kg body weight) if possible and/or.
- Immediate transfer to the nearest hospital.
- Take any remains of the meal, peelings or waste along for examination.
- The consumption of unknown fungi not subject to statutory controls is to be discouraged as a matter of principle.
- Round-the-clock information in the event of suspected fungal poisoning may be obtained from the Swiss Toxicology Information Centre Tel. 145.

Risk of Confusion with Edible Mushrooms

Reliable information with regards to edible mushrooms growing in the wild can be obtained from official fungi control offices. Specimens other than the popular porcino ("penny bun") mushroom (Boletus edulis) have been known to lead to violent gastrointestinal upsets.
The False Chanterelle (Hygrophoropsis aurantiaca) and the Jack O'Lantern (Omphalotus olearis) are deserving of particular mention due to their potential confusion with the Chanterelle (Cantharellus cibarius): both have gills but no ridges. The False Chanterelle is often consumed without any symptoms, whilst violent gastrointestinal symptoms may occur after tucking into a plate of Jack O'Lanterns.
With all gill mushrooms it is essential to be aware of the risk of Death Cap poisoning. For this reason, the consumption of gill mushrooms that have not undergone the appropriate checks should be strongly discouraged.

Accidents often happen when fungi have not been assessed by specialists at recognised fungal control centres prior to consumption. Information on official fungal control centres can be found by visiting **www.vapko.ch** or may be obtained from any local council office.

21.4 Allergic Reactions

An allergic reaction is an abnormal, extreme reaction to otherwise readily tolerable substances. The most important allergy-inducing substances (allergens) are absorbed via the respiratory tract: pollen, mites, hair, mold. However, these may also include medications (penicillin, pain killers), food (nuts, kiwi fruit, strawberries), insect venom (bee and wasp stings) and materials (latex).

Symptoms: Reddening and itching, urticaria. Swelling of the airways can cause life-threatening airway obstruction and a generalized reaction can cause circulatory collapse.

Treatment: For laymen, treatment is restricted to removing the allergy and to the administration of First Aid in accordance with the ABC rules. Where symptoms are mild (no immediate effect) antihistamines may be administered. Serious reactions are treated with cortisone (if available) and where necessary adrenaline (people who suffer severe allergic reactions often carry suitable medications with them).

A severe allergic reaction incorporating respiratory or circulatory problems is a life-threatening emergency.

21.5 Panic Attacks, Hyperventilation

Panic attacks manifest themselves in the form of sudden attacks of anxiety with accompanying physical symptoms. Under situations of physical and/or emotional stress, those affected by panic attacks may experience palpitations, dizziness or excessive sweating. They interpret these symptoms as life-threatening and react with panic, which in turn intensifies the symptoms. **Hyperventilation** can be a feature of panic attacks or psychological stress. Often those affected are young women. The picture may look very dramatic but is not dangerous given the appropriate action. Hyperventilation is a rapid, superficial form of respiration where more carbon dioxide than necessary is exhaled. Due to a fall in acid levels in the blood, this leads to a relative shortage of calcium and the typical symptoms similar to tetanus.
Symptoms: These may vary widely: cardiovascular problems, hyperventilation and shortness of breath, breaking out in sweats, dizziness and fear of death. One of the classic features associated with hyperventilation is tingling feelings in the hands and around the mouth culminating in spasm of the hands ("paws").
Treatment: Responding to a panic attack in a patient may take the form of calming words and/or finding a quiet place if possible. Panic attacks on a mountain tour[1] may require a change of plan in the short term.

Where a fear of heights is the problem, make sure that hands and feet have a firm hold and allow sufferers to sit. A short belay rope can work wonders at a psychological level.

A hyperventilation crisis can be controlled with advice on how to breathe and breathing the air that one has just exhaled back into a plastic bag (so increasing the level of carbon dioxide in the blood). Where recurrent panic attacks are a problem professional help should be sought.[2]

No tranquillisers on a mountain tour! (Risk of falling as a result of disordered perception.)

Literature and Links:

1) The Alps 6/2008, When Heavenly Heights turn into hell, Martin Roos Scientific and Alpine Journalist, Munich/Valencia.
2) Anxiety and Panic Helpline, Hotline 0848 801 109, www.aphs.ch.

22. Appendix

Various authors

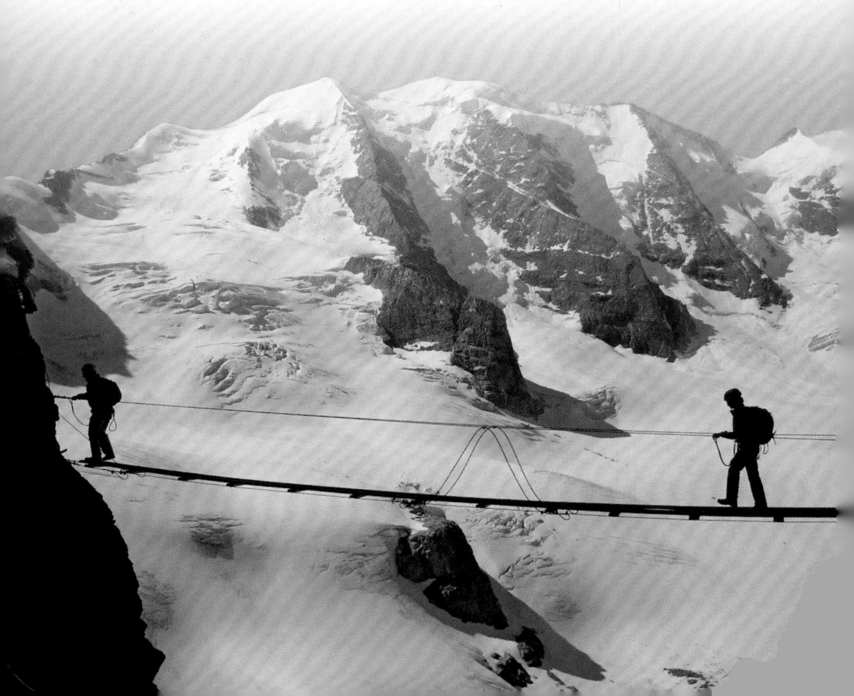

22.1 First Aid Kit

Mountaineering means moving about in terrain where medical help is not generally available. This makes it all the more important to carry a suitable first aid kit with you. This should not be too bulky, plus it should be clear exactly how the individual items of medication are to be used. Basically, you should only take with you what you can actually use. A basic stock of bandaging and dressings material is also essential; sometimes it is possible to improvise here using items of clothing.

⇨ Only take with you what you are going to be able to use.

For **one-day excursions** walking in the Alps it is advisable to take at least 2 different pain killers, Tegaderm wound cover, 1 SAM® splint, 1 elastic bandage (4 or 6 cm) as well as Leukotape. For **longer tours and trekking expeditions** Module 1 points the way forward. Based on this, it is possible to get together a relatively small First Aid kit (e.g. painkillers/antipyretics, travel sickness medication, heartburn, insomnia, diarrhea, vomiting). Module 2 incorporates a supplement for mountaineering guides or persons who are already familiar the use of the medications. In Module 3 we have listed the medications required for treatment of the various types of **altitude sickness** (as per Chapter 17, Page 206) which may befall people on trekking tours and/or expeditions at higher altitudes.

The following list of items of equipment is intended to serve as a guide. It has been put together on the basis of experience collected by a number of doctors. Nevertheless, it is worth arranging a prior medical consultation or obtaining advice from the pharmacist so as not to overlook any contraindications that may be present. Any side effects will be discussed only superficially in overview, details can be gleaned from the packaging slip. Each individual is responsible for taking his own medications with him (e.g. insulin and blood sugar monitors for diabetic mountaineers: ampuls in impact-resistant containers and duly protected from the effects of cold). The quantity is dependent on the number of participants and personal requirements and is not definitive (see recommended literature).

Little is known about the shelf life/effectiveness of medications under **extreme conditions** (altitude[1], cold and heat[2]). Once ampoules have been frozen and/or the content is no longer crystal clear and its colour has changed, they should no longer be used. Capsules and suppositories are as fragile as glass in their frozen state and at higher temperatures will potentially lose their efficacy. Numerous substances (including Nifedipine, Nitroglycerin) are UV-sensitive: don't leave lying around in the sun if you can help it!

Literature:

1) Küpper T, Efficacy of Medications. Yearbook of the Austrian Society for Alpine and High-Altitude Medicine, Innsbruck 2008.
2) Küpper T, Milledge J, Basnyat B, Hillebrandt D, Schöffl V: Consensus statement of the UIAA Medical Commission Vol 10: The effect of Extremes Temperatures on drugs. With note on side effects and use of some other drugs in the mountains. Bern/Switzerland, 2008.
3) ICAR Recommendation REC M 0004 of the Commission for Mountain Emergency Medicine of 1996 Contents of a Mountain Refuge's Pharmacy ICAR Recommendation REC M 0005 of the Commission for Mountain Emergency Medicine of 1998.
4) A Modular First Aid Kid for Alpinists, Mountain Guides and Alpinist Physicians.
5) Thomas Hochholzer: Trekking and High Mountain Climbing – A Medical Companion, Lochner Verlag.
6) A.J. Pollard & D.R. Murdoch: The High Altitude Medicine Handbook (Second Edition).
7) J-P. Richalet & J-P. Herry: Alpinism and Mountain Sports-related Medicine, Masson Verlag.

General:

As req. = As required, drg = dragée, h = hr/s, no info. = no information, BW = body weight, Cps = capsule(s), min. = minimum, p/o = oral, by mouth, sac = sachet, syr = syrup, sl = sublingual, supp = suppository, tbl = tablet, drp = drop, x = times, sl = sublingual, Kurotex, 2nd skin, sun cream, oral rehydrating solution.

22.1.1 Modul 1: For mountaineers (tours of several days'duration/trekking trips at low altitudes)

Symptom	Ingredient(s)	Examples*	Dose/Application
Allergic reactions, hay fever	Cetirizin	Zyrtec®	10 mg 1 x 1 tbl daily p/o
Diseases affecting the airways (common cold)	Cineol, Levomenthol, Oil of Rosemary, Oil of Thyme	Nasobol®	Tbls to dissolve and inhale 2–3 tbls (3–4 x daily) p/o
Conjunctivitis, snow blindness	Acidum fusidicum	Fucithalmic® liquid gel (a number of variants)	1 drop every 12 hrs local application
Disinfectant	Iodine, Octenidine hydrochloride	Betadine® Octanisept®	Apply generously to wound undiluted
Diarrhoea	Loperamide Live yeast Activated carbon Intestinal flora	Imodium® Carbolevure® (see Index) Bioflorina® (see Index)	Imodium: 1–2 cps (2291 mg), then 1 cps after each attack (max. 8 cps daily) p/o
Sore throat	Lysozyme, Bacitracin	Lysopaine®	4–8 tbls daily p/o
Infections: Throat/ nose/pharynx, middle ear, oral cavity, skin soft tissue, lungs	Amoxycillin Clavulanic acid	Augmentin®**	625 mg every 8 hrs for 7–10 days p/o
Infections of the intestine and the urogenital tract	Ciprofloxacinum	Ciproxin®**	500 mg 2 x a day for min. 3 days p/o
Minor burns, sunburn, insect repellent and stings/bites	Dimethindine maleate Proplyene glycol Silver sulfadiazine	Fenistil® Flammazine®	Gel, ointment, foam-based salve for local application
Minor sprains, bruising	Arnica Globuli	Similasan®	3–6 x daily p/o
Disturbed sleep	Zolpidem	Stilnox® Zolpidem Mepha®	10 mg 1 x daily (tbl) p/o
Pain, esp. locomotive system	Ibuprofen	Brufen®	400–600 mg up to 4 x daily (tbl) p/o

* Several possibilities

** Worth considering for tours lasting several days. Discuss application and alternatives with a doctor prior to the trip (e.g. penicillin allergy).

Symptom	Ingredient(s)	Examples*	Dose/Application
Pain, fever, cold symptoms	Paracetamol Mixed preparation	Dafalgan® Neocitran®	0.5–1 g max 4x daily 3 pouches or efferves-cent tablets daily
Rhinitis, for reducing swelling in the nasal mucosa	Dimethindine	Vibrocil®	3–4 drops 3–4x daily nasal
Heartburn, acid regurgitation, stomach pains	Omeprazole	Nexium® Omeprazole Mepha® Oprazol Spirig®	40 mg 1x daily (tbl) p/o
Dry, crusted or injured nasal mucosa	Dexpanthenol	Bepanthen®	local application
Nausea, vomiting, bloating, heartburn	Domperidone	Motilium lingual®	10 mg up to 3x daily before food (tbl) sublingual

22.1.2 Modul 2: Supplement for Mountaineering Guides or Persons familiar with the Use of the Medications

Symptom	Ingredient(s)	Examples*	Dose/Application
Abdominal cramps, renal colic	Scopolamine	Buscopan®	10 mg 1–3x daily (tbl) p/o
Serious allergic reaction	Dexamethasone	Decadron® Dexamethasone®	4–8 mg p/o until doctor arrives
Very severe pain	Tramadol	Tramal®	50–100 mg up to 4x daily p/o
Constipation	Bisacodyl	Dulcolax®	1–2 drg p/o

**

22.1.3 Modul 3: Trekking and Expeditions at High Altitude

Symptom	Ingredient(s)	Examples*	Dose
Acute mountain sickness	Ibuprofen	Brufen®	400–600 mg up to 4x daily p/o
Acute mountain sickness	Acetazolamide	Diamox®	125 mg 1–2 tbls 2x daily p/o
Pulmonary edema	Nifedipine	Adalat CC ®	20 mg 3x daily p/o
Severe acute mountain sickness	Dexamethasone	Decadron ® Dexamethasone®	4 mg 4x daily, initially 8 mg p/o

⇨ At high altitude there will also be fever, dry cough and mucosa, sore throat and eye problems to be reckoned with. For the appropriate treatment see Module 1.

* Several possibilities

** For the most important side-effects and observations, see Index of Medications.

22.1.4 Checklist for Children's First Aid Kit

Symptom	Treatment/Medication*	Dose **
Allergy	Cetirizine®, in cases of severe allergy Dexamethasone®	From 6 years of age: Cetirizine: 1 tbl daily, (10 mg) for 4 wks p/o
Diarrhoea	Rehydration p/o antibiotics if necessary, Imodium® as applicable	Loperamide for children from 6 yrs of age, start with 1 tabl. Max. 3 tbls daily p/o
Purulent ophthalmia	See Module 1	
Vomiting	Itinerol® Supp	1 supp. daily (age-dependent dosage, supp.)
Fever	Dafalgan® or Brufen®	Discuss application and dosage with doctor prior to embarking on trip
Sore throat	Lozenges (various possibibilities)	
Urinary tract infection	Bactrim® tbl, Syr.	Discuss application and dosage with doctor prior to embarking on trip
Cough	In certain circumstances Augmentin® tbl, drops, sachet, syrup	Discuss application and dosage with doctor prior to embarking on trip!
Pain	Paracetamol* tbl, drp, supp., Brufen® tbl, granulate	Paracetamol: approx. 15 mg/kg BW in 4 daily doses, Brufen: 20 mg/kg BW administered on several occasions, supp. or p/o
Snow blindness	Close eyes and bandage Black tea bags, Brufen®	Brufen®: 20 mg/kg BW administered on several occasions p/o
Rhinitis	Nose drops (Vibrocil®)	1–2 drops 3–4 x daily nasal
Sunburn	See Module 1	
Burns	Cool, Flammazin® as applicable, clean cover	Local application
Nappy rash	Zinc ointment, Miconazol	Local application
Wound	Tissue adhesive, Fucidin gauze if applicable, Augmentin® tbl, syr. (in cases of infection)	Discuss application and dosage with doctor prior to embarking on trip
Altitude sickness	**IN GENERAL DESCENT IS CALLED FOR !!!**	
AMS	Paracetamol***, Brufen®, Itinerol® supp, where applicable Dexamethasone®	Dexamethasone: 0.4 mg/kg BW every 12 hrs p/o
HAPE	Adalat CC®	Children > 12 yrs: as for adults
HACE	Dexamethasone®	0.4 mg/kg BW every 12 hrs p/o

* Trade name

** Make sure that, where children are concerned, all medications are dispensed strictly in accordance with body weight.

*** A number of preparations on the market (e.g. Dafalgan®, Tylenol®).

21.1.5 Other Items for the First Aid Kit

Triangular cloths	Bandages, fixations, immobilisations
Alcohol swab	Disinfecting skin
Elastic bandages (4 or 6 cm)	2nd layer dressing, loose or compression dressing
Clinical thermometer	Esp. when travelling with children
Fixomull® Stretch	Adhesive strapping for anchoring full surface wound cover, in particular on joints, mobile and contoured parts of the body
Gloves	Personal protection
Cooling, heating	Cooling spray, auto-heating packs for hands and feet
Metal tweezers (Brucelle)	Splinter removal
Plasters – different types and sizes	Conventional, blister pads (www.spenco.com, www.compeed.com)
Rescue materials, various	Rescue foil, mirrors, candle, light source, plastic bags, scissors, emergency information sheet, pencil, whistle (children)
Scissors or scalpel blade	Opening up blisters, small operations
Splint (e.g. SAM® Splint)	Fixations
Self-adhesive field bandages	2nd dressing layer (no patch needed) loose or compression bandage
Special material	Histoacryl® (see Medi List), hydrocolloid dressings
Syringes	For administering medication (intravenously or by mouth – children!)
Sterile needle	For opening up blisters, removing splinters, injections, drawing up medications
Steristrip	Wound care for use with clean wounds and very flexible edges (cuts)
Tape 2 cm	Support bandage for joints

22.1.6 Medications Index

Preparation	Active Ingredient	Form/Price	Dose*	Action/Indication	Notes
Adalat® CR 20–30CR Bayer	Nifedipin	20 x 28 mg tablets CHF 17.30	Precautionary: 1 tbl 24 hrs prior to ascent Treatment: 20 mg 3 x daily	High Altitude Pulmonary Edema (prevention and treatment) high blood pressure, Angina Pectoris	Potential exacerbation of headaches contingent on altitude. Medication to lower blood pressure!
Arnica Montana Similasan	Arnica, among others	Globules No info	3–6 x daily 7 Globules	Slight sprains, bruising	Increased tendency to bleeding
Aspirin® Bayer	Acetylsalicylic acid		100 mg daily p/o max. 300 mg (frostbite) 500 mg (heart attack)	Local frostbite, heart attack	Risk to sensitive stomach mucosa, esp. at high altitude (gastric ulcer). Platelet inhibition for approx. 7 days; pronounced tendency to bleed
Augmentin® GlaxoSmithKline	Amoxycillin + Clavulanic acid	10 x 625 mg foil-wrapped tablets CHF 40.30	625 mg every 8 hrs for 7–10 days	Antibiotics to counter infections of the throat/nose/pharynx/lungs, inflammation of the middle ear, infections of the soft tissue underlying the skin, dental infections	Diarrhoea may occur as a side effect. Avoid in the event of allergy to penicillin, be alert to side effects. Discuss application with doctor prior to embarking on trip
Bactrim Forte® Roche	Trimethoprim (TM) and Sulfa-methoxaz-ole (SMZ)	10 tablets CHF 10.00 100 ml Syrup CHF 7.65	1 tbl 2 x daily	Infections of the gastrointes-tinal and urogenital tract	Medication of choice for children, available in retail outlets in syrup form, NB: side effects! Discuss application with doctor prior to embarking on trip
Bepanthen® Bayer	Dexpanthenol	Nose ointment 2 x 5 g No info	Several times daily nasal	Dry, irritated, inflamed nasal mucosa	Highly effective, rapid action

* Take by mouth unless instructed otherwise.

Preparation	Active Ingredient	Form/Price	Dose*	Action/Indication	Notes
Betadine® Mundipharma	Iodine	10 ml bottle CHF 9.65	Generous local application Undiluted	Disinfectant	Iodine allergy, thyroid disease
Bioflorina™	live enterococci (intestinal flora)	35 cps CHF 21.60	2–3 cps daily	To prevent or treat attacks of diarrhoea	
Brufen® Abbot	Ibuprofen	20 x 400 mg foil-wrapped tablets CHF 9.15	400–600 mg Up to 4 x daily	Pains, joints, swellings of the joints	Allergic reactions Allergy to aspirin Gastrointestinal complaints Kidney failure
Carbolevure® Robapharm	Live yeast	20 cps Adults CHF 20.55	1 cps 3 x daily	Diarrhoea and for regulating and normalising intestinal flora	
Cialis® Lilly	Tadalafil	No info.	1 tbl 24 hrs prior to ascent	Prevention of HAPE, erectile dysfunction	Potential exacerbation of headaches contingent on altitude
Ciproxin® Bayer	Ciprofloxacin	6 x 250 g tablets CHF 18.70	2 x 250 to 2 x 500 mg for min. 3 days	Infections of gastrointestinal and urogenital tract	NB: Side-effects! Discuss application with doctor prior to embarking on trip
Comfeel Plus Coloplast	Polyurethane, Caroxymethyl cellulose, Pectin, Gelatine	No info.		Skin protection for open wounds featuring extensive weeping, abrasions, chronic wounds	
Dafalgan® Bristol-Myers Squibb	Paracetamol	16 x 1 g foil-wrapped tablets CHF 7.95	500 mg–1 g up to 4 x daily	Pain, fever, common cold	Liver toxicity in overdose
Decadron® Dexamethasone®	Dexamethasone	20 x 1 mg tablets approx. CHF 8.70	4 mg 4 x daily	Strong anti-inflammatories, Mountain sickness, HACE, severe allergic reactions	A number of side effects, including reduced stress tolerance, ability to make judgments, risk of overestimating one's abilities. Dosage related to problems contingent on altitude

Preparation	Active Ingredient	Form/Price	Dose*	Action/Indication	Notes
Diamox® Vifor Friburg	Acetazolamide	25 x 250 mg tablets CHF 15.15	250 mg 2 x daily depending on indication (see Chapter 17)	Stimulate respiration Prevention and treatment of altitude sickness	Tingling, impaired sense of taste, muscle spasms
Flamazine® Solvay Pharma	Silver sulfadiazine	Ointment 20 g CHF 10.20	1 x daily, apply directly to wound in layer of 2–3 mm	Minor burns, skin infections, infected wounds	
Floxal® BAUSCH & LOMB SWISS	Oflaxacin	Exe ointment 3 g CHF 9.10 UD eye-drops 30 x 0.5 ml CHF 16.95	4 x daily 1 drp. Inflammation: every 30 mins 1 drp. 48 h 3 x daily. One strand of 1 cm local application	Topical antibiotic Conjunctivitis Contact lens-related inflammation of the cornea	Stop wearing contact lenses
Fucithalmic® Leopharma	Fusidic acid	Monodose Liquid Gel 12 x 0.2 g CHF 16.35	1 drp. every 12 hrs Local application	Antibiotic for use with bacterial conjunctivitis snow blindness	Remove contact lenses
Hystoacryl® Braun	n-Butyl-2-Cyanoacrylate	5 Amp. € 148.27		Tissue adhesive small wounds (see Chapter 16)	Very expensive
Imodium® Janssen-Cilag Loperamide® MEPHA	Loperamide	No info.	1–2 x 2 mg cps, then 1 cps. for each subsequent attack of diarrhoea up to max. 8 mg daily	Acute and chronic diarrhoea	NB: fluid and electrolyte replacement. This is an emergency medication!
Itinerol® Vifor Friburg	Meclozini-2 HCl, Pyridoxini-HCl	No info.	1 supp. daily	Nausea and vomiting of whatsoever origin, travel sickness	For children 3 months–6 years, children 6–12 years as well as adults
Lacrycon® Thea Pharma	Hyaluron acid	Daily dose 20 x 0.65 ml CHF 21.15	4 x daily 1 drp. Local application	Crocodile tears syndrome Dryness of the eyes	
Lysopain® N Boehringer Ingelheim	Lysozyme, Bacitracin	24 Lozenges CHF 9.50	4–8 tbls. daily	Local analgesic, acute, inflammatory, painful disorders in the area of the mouth and pharynx	Not if patient unable to tolerate fructose. Consult a doctor if no improvement within 5 days

Preparation	Active Ingredient	Form/Price	Dose*	Action/Indication	Notes
Motilium lingual® Janssen-Cilag	Domperidone	30x 10mg tablets CHF 14.30	10mg up to 3x daily before meals sl	Promotes passage through gastro-intestinal tract, "gastric disorders" such as abdominal pain after meals, bloating, flatulence and heartburn	Not indicated where pituitary disease or severe gastro-intestinal disease is present, interactions with other medicines
Nasobol® Inhalo Sanofi	Cineol, Levomenthol, Oil of Rosemary, Oil of Thyme	30 tablets CHF 11.50	3–4 treatments per day Inhalations	Respiratory diseases	Hot water required Highly effective, low weight
Neocitran® Novartis	Phenylephrine Pheniramine Ascorbic acid, Paracetamol	No info.	3 pouches or effervescent tablets daily	Reduces swelling, pain killer, antipyretic, influenza	See Paracetamol
Neosporin® GlaxoSmithKline	Neomycin, Gramicidin, Polymyxin	Eye drops 5ml CHF 9.60	2–4x daily 1–2drps. Local application	Topical antibiotic Conjunctivitis	Allergy to individual substances
Nexium® Astra Zeneca Omeprazol® Mepha	Omeprazol	14x 20mg MUPS tablets CHF 47.70	40mg 1x daily	Inhibits formation of stomach acid, heartburn, acid regurgitation, stomach pain	Interactions with other medications Headaches Indigestion
Oculac® Novartis	Povidonum K 25	20 SDU 0.4ml eye drops CHF 11.80	4x daily 1drp. Local application	Crocodile tear syndrome Dryness of the eyes	
Buscopan® Boehringer Ingelheim	Scopolamine butylbromide	20x 10mg drgs. CHF 12.50	3–5x daily 1–2drgs.	Antispasmodic and analgesic action on the muscles of the gastrointestinal tract	Contra-indicated for certain muscles and disorders of the large bowel
Tramal® Grünenthal	Tramadol	50x 10mg cps CHF 6.90	1–2cps, max 8cps daily	Severe pain	Reduction in awareness, contra-indicated in the case of respiratory problems, can trigger dependency

Preparation	Active Ingredient	Form/Price	Dose*	Action/Indication	Notes
Tylenol® Children Jannsen Cilag	Paracetamol	No info.	Weight-related	See Dafalgan	Pay attention to instructions given by medical practitioner
Viagra® Pfizer	Sildenafil	No info.	25 mg 3 x daily	Treatment of HAPE, erectile dysfunction	As for Cialis®
Vibrocil® Novartis	Dimetidine	Nasal drops, Nasal spray, Nasal gel No info.	3–4 drps. 3–4 x daily local application	Decongestant for reducing inflammation in the nasal mucosa due to rhinitis	Not for long-term therapeutic use: damage to mucosa!
Vigamox® Alcon	Moxifloxacin	5 ml. Drp Opht, dropper CHF 16.95	3 x daily 1 drp. for 4 days local application	Topical antibiotic Inflammation of the cornea	Allergies. Stinging and burning when applying drops. Do not wear contact lenses during therapy
Viscotears® Novartis Vismed® TRB Chemedica SA	Carbomer 980 Hyaluron acid	Liquid gel 30 x 0.6 g CHF 15.65 eye gel UD 20 x 0.45 ml CHF 18.50	3–4 x daily local application	Crocodile tears syndrome Dryness of the eyes	
Zolpidem® Stillnox®		10 x 10 mg tablets approx. CHF 6.00	10 mg 1 x daily local application	Sleep disturbances	Not > 4 weeks. Paradox and psychiatric disturbances, amnesia, dependency
Zyrtec® UCB Pharma	Cetirizine	10 foil-wrapped tablets (separable) CHF 13.50	10 mg 1 x daily	Allergic reactions, hay fever	Rarely fatigue. Interactions with other medications. Does not work immediately

The above is a nonbinding selection of medications covering all the drugs mentioned in the various chapters. The selection has been compiled by the authors independently of one another. There are no agreements in existence with the pharmaceutical companies cited. Details of medications originate from the Swiss Medicines Compendium (www.kompendium.ch) dated 19.01.2010. The only side effects mentioned are those that occur in and are relevant to the outdoor environment and which could be dangerous. No all side effects have been mentioned by far! Please ensure that you read the enclosed slip carefully or ask specialists in the field. Copyright by Documed AG, Basel, Switzerland 2010. The pharmaceutical company, if it is the main manufacturer of the medication, is mentioned along with the nonbinding recommended retail price (in the case of SL -specialty list- preparations maximum price to the public incl. VAT; for non-SL preparations in accordance with manufacturer's information incl. VAT). The publishers accept no liability for any claims that may be derived on the basis of the above information.

22.2 Lake Louise Score

22.2.1 Lake Louise Score for Small Children up to 3 Years of Age

The level of the score is calculated from the total of the fussiness score (FS) and the child-specific symptom score (= pediatric symptom score, PSS). Fussiness is defined as a state of irritability without any clearly recognizable cause which lasts for at least two hours. The diagnosis of altitude sickness designates it as probable in the event of a fussiness score of at least 4, a symptom score of at least 3 and consequently a total score of at least 7, naturally assuming an acute exposure to altitude at a height of >2500 m.

Fussiness score (total of extent and intensity)

Extent of inexplicable fussiness

0	1	2	3	4	5	6
None			Intermittent			Constant

Intensity of inexplicable fussiness

0	1	2	3	4	5	6
None			Moderate			Hard crying

Child-specific symptoms score (Total based on eating, playing and sleeping behaviors)

Rate how well your child has eaten today?
- 0 normal
- 1 slightly less than normal
- 2 much less than normal
- 3 vomiting or not eating

Rate how playful your child is today?
- 0 normal
- 1 slightly less than normal
- 2 much less than normal
- 3 has not played at all

Rate ability of child to sleep today?
- 0 normal
- 1 slightly less or more than normal
- 2 much less or more than normal
- 3 not able to sleep

22.2.2 Lake Louise Score for Primary School Children

The first question gives a general impression of the overall condition of the child and provides clues as to whether the symptoms listed in the following agree with their overall condition.

A diagnosis of AMS is probable if:

- A gain in altitude of more than 2500 m has been registered during the past three days
- Headaches and one additional symptom listed are a feature
- A total score of at least 3 (excluding Point 1) is achieved

1. How do you feel at the moment?

I'm feeling very well	0
I'm feeling well	1
I'm not feeling so good	2
I'm feeling very poorly	3

2. Have you got a headache/pains in your head?

I haven't got a headache	0
I've got a little headache	1
I've got more than just a little headache	2
I've got a bad headache	3

3. Are you hungry?

I'm hungry/I'm not feeling off-color	0
I'm not really hungry/I'm feeling a little bit off-color	1
I feel poorly/I've been sick	2
I feel very poorly/I've been really sick	3

4. Are you tired?

I'm not tired	0
I'm a little bit tired	1
I'm more than a little bit tired	2
I'm very tired	3

5. Do you feel dizzy?

I'm not feeling dizzy	0
I'm feeling a little bit dizzy	1
I'm feeling more than a little bit dizzy	2
I'm feeling very dizzy (everything's going around)	3

6. How did you sleep last night?

As well as I always do	0
Not so well as usual	1
I woke up very often in the night	2
I could not sleep	3

Now add up all the points in 2.—6. to obtain the total score for the child.

Mild AMS = Score of 3—5 (corresponding global assessment based on 1st of 0 or 1)
Severe AMS = Score of > 5 (corresponding global assessment based on 1st of 2 or 3)

22.2.3 Lake Louise Score for Young Persons and Adults

A diagnosis of AMS is probable if:

- A gain in altitude of more than 2500 m has been registered during the past three days
- Headaches and one additional symptom listed are a feature
- A total score of at least 3 is achieved

Please assess your current condition and tick off the relevant symptoms:

1. Headaches

0 No headaches
1 Mild headaches
2 Moderate headaches
3 Severe headaches rendering me incapable of functioning

2. Gastrointestinal Complaints

0 None/normal appetite
1 No appetite/nausea
2 Moderate nausea and/or vomiting
3 Severe nausea and/or vomiting rendering me incapable of functioning

3. Fatigue–Weakness

0 None at all
1 Slight fatigue and/or weakness
2 Moderate fatigue and/or weakness
3 Severe fatigue and/or weakness rendering me incapable of functioning

4. Dizziness – Drowsiness

0 None at all
1 Slight dizziness/drowsiness
2 Moderate dizziness/drowsiness
3 Severe dizziness/drowsiness rendering me incapable of functioning

5. Difficulties in sleeping

0 I have been sleeping as well as ever
1 I haven't been sleeping as well as I normally do
2 I have been waked up repeatedly, have been sleeping badly
3 I haven't been able to sleep at all

Now add all the points together to get the total score

Mild AMS = Score of 3—5 (corresponding global assessment based on 0 or 1)
Severe AMS = Score of >5 (corresponding global assessment based on 2 or 3)

Global Assessment

If you have any of these symptoms, in what way do they affect your ability to function?

0 Not at all
1 Slightly reduced
2 I find it difficult to continue to function
3 I am practically incapable of functioning and can only lie about

22.3 Links

Swiss Alpine Club (SAC):	**www.sac-cas.ch**
Swiss Mountain Medicine Society:	**www.sggm.ch**
Alpine Rescue Switzerland:	www.alpinerettung.ch
German Society for Mountain and Expedition Medicine:	www.bexmed.de
German Alpine Club:	www.alpenverein.de
French Alpine Club:	www.ffcam.fr
Mountain Medical Intervention Group:	www.grimm-vs.ch
High-Altitude Medicine and Biology:	www.liebertpub.com
Himalayan Rescue Association of Nepal HRA:	www.himalayanrescue.org
Himalayan Rescue Association:	www.everester.org
Hypoxia Symposia:	www.hypoxia.net
Institute of Mountain Medicine Studies:	www.iemm.org
International Society for Mountain Medicine:	www.ismmed.org
International Society of Travel Medicine:	www.istm.org
International Commission for Alpine Rescue:	www.ikar-cisa.org
International Porter Protection Group:	www.ippg.net
Istituto nazionale per la ricerca scientifica e tecnologia sulla montagna:	www.inrm.it
Italian Alpine Club:	www.cai.it
Italian Alpine Rescue:	www.alpinia.net/soccorso.php www.soccorsoalpino.org (South Tyroll)
Medex – Medical Expeditions:	www.medex.org.uk
Food Guide Pyramid:	www.sge-ssn.ch
Austrian Alpine Club:	www.alpenverein.at
Austrian Society for Alpine and Mountain Medicine:	www.alpinmedizin.org
Travel Medicine Information:	www.safetravel.ch
Argentine Society for Mountain Medicine:	www.samm.org.ar
Italian Society for Mountain Medicine:	www.medicinadimontagna.it
Swiss Forum for Sport Nutrition:	www.sfsn.ethz.ch
International Union of Alpinist Associations:	www.theuiaa.org
Wilderness Medical Society:	www.wms.org
WSL-Institute for Snow and Avalanche Research SLF:	www.slf.ch

22.4 Lexicon*

Achilles tendon reflex: A slight tap on the Achilles tendon generates a stretching movement in the ankle joint. When this movement is reduced or if it is totally absent by comparison to the opposite side, compression of the nerve root may be present.

Acid–Base Balance: The human body is able, by exercising different mechanisms, to maintain its acid base balance and hence the pH value in the blood at a constant level within restricted limits.

Acidosis: The pH level in the human body is too low (acid).

After Drop (Post-Rescue Death Syndrome): Circulatory arrest that occurs in conjunction with the rescue of an injured person is known as After Drop. The same term is used in a range of different situations.
In the case of persons suffering from hypothermia (e.g. victims of avalanches) the flow of blood to the surface of the body is reduced and the warm blood is concentrated on the organs essential for survival, or the body core. A big difference in temperature occurs between the core and the skin. When the patient is moved or warmed up again, mixing of warm blood (core) and cold blood (skin, extremities) takes place. As a consequence of sensitivity to temperature, which is a feature of the dromotropic system of the heart, it is possible that fatal disturbances to heart rhythm may ensue with cardiac arrest. More recent research, however, tends to indicate heart overload as a result of the sudden backflow of a large quantity of blood.
In a mountain rescue context, post-rescue death syndrome is often attributable to suspension trauma. In this a person may be suspended for a long period of time which leads to the blood pooling in the lower extremities. If the blood suddenly streams back into the organism on rescue this may also lead to overloading of the heart and circulatory failure. Toxic substances as lactate and potassium may also be present in high concentrations.
Where persons who are buried or trapped are concerned, post-rescue death syndrome is frequently due to the fact that, following relief of pressure, the blood supply to crushed limbs is restored and therefore injured structures start to bleed again. In the case of these victims, there is also a danger that the hormonal stress reaction may be suspended. Before rescue persons who are not unconscious find themselves in an extreme stress situation. At the same time stress hormones (adrenaline and cortisol) ensure that organ functions essential to life are maintained. Once the rescue has taken place this stress mechanism is reduced and the blood circulation maintained by the stress hormones collapses.

* A number of medical terms are explained in the original text and are not listed below.

Alkalosis: The pH level in the human body is too high (basic).

Allergen: A substance which, through the agency of the immune system, triggers hypersensitive reactions. An allergen is an antigen; the reaction caused by it is an allergic reaction. The immune system of allergic patients reacts to contact with the allergens by forming specific antibodies.

Alveoli: Air sacs in which the exchange of gases is effected between inhaled and exhaled air and the blood.

Autonomic nerve system (vegetative nerve system, VNS): It is by way of the VNS that biologically fixed, automatic sequence regulatory processes are transmitted which monitor the functions essential to life such as heartbeat, respiration, blood pressure, digestion and metabolism so as to maintain inner homeostasis. It is not possible for a human being to consciously control these functions. The autonomic nerve system is subdivided on the basis of functional and anatomical factors into a sympathetic and a parasympathetic system. These are antagonistic in terms of their effect. Activating, action-promoting stimuli are conveyed via the sympathetic nervous system whilst the opposite e.g. rest-promoting impulses are transferred via the parasympathetic system.

Bladder dysfunction: The inability to release urine or uncontrollable discharge of urine.

Cerebral arteries: The cerebral arteries are the blood vessels that supply the brain with oxygen. Starting at the base of the skull they branch out into a number of arteries that are connected with one another in annular format and penetrate as far as the individual sections of the brain by way of small branches.

Cerebral (O)edema: A disturbance in the regulation of the supply of blood to the brain caused by a lack of oxygen from 400 up to 4500 m which leads to (blood) fluid accumulation in the connective tissue of the brain. The lead clinical symptom is severe disturbance to balance associated with extreme headaches resistant to pain killers. Added to this may be vomiting, disturbances of consciousness or even coma.

Chemoreceptors: These are specialized sensory cells that are geared to chemical substances transported in the air or dissolved in fluids. They play a major role in the sense of smell and taste.

Convection: The transfer of heat from one place to another.

Cyanosis: In medicine the term **cyanosis** (from the Greek *kuaneos* "blue") is used to describe a violet to bluish discoloration of the skin, the mucous membranes, lips and finger nails. The particular hue does not necessarily have to occur at the same time or to the same extent in all specified areas. The cause of cyanosis is, as a rule, a deficient supply of oxygen to the blood, which may be due to an insufficient concentration of oxygen in the respiratory air (long-term stay at high altitude) or in the event of pathological changes to the lung or the heart.

Cystic Fibrosis: A congenital genetic metabolic disorder where the composition of the secretions from various glands is changed. The secretion becomes viscous. This results in disturbances in function of different kinds in the affected organs, especially the increasing development of chronic coughing and pneumonia.

Dehydration: Lack of water in the body due to excessive loss of fluid (sweating, respiration, urine and bowel movements) or too little intake of fluid.

Euler-Liljestrand Reflex: Describes the relationship between ventilation and the supply of blood to the lungs. If part of the lung ceases to be ventilated, the blood vessels will automatically be constricted so that the flow of blood is reduced.

Fracture: Breaking of a bone.

Free Radicals: Atoms or molecules with at least one unpaired electron are described as radicals and these are in most cases particularly reactive. As a result free radicals play an important role in relation to a series of biological cell processes because they are capable, as a result of cell damage, of contributing to the aging process. Thus illnesses such as cancer or diabetes etc. may occur.

Glycogen: Is a polysaccharide. It assists in the short to medium term storage and provision of glucose as a source of energy.

Hematoma: Effusion of blood, bruise or colored stains.

Hem iron: The trivalent iron present as a binding compound in the red blood pigment (hemoglobin) or in muscle cells (myoglobin). Iron can also occur in the form of free iron in the diet. In animal products such as lean meat, liver or fish iron occurs in both forms and the proportion of hem iron is around 50 up to 80 %. Hem iron is present in the largest proportions predominantly in red meat. In foods derived from plant matter (such as vegetables and cereals) iron occurs only in its free form.

Hyperventilation: Rapid deep breathing. It is possible to distinguish between pathological and physiological hyperventilation. In pathological hyperventilation, caused by stress or anxiety, the patient breathes out too much CO_2 (carbon dioxide) so that a change in the acid base balance occurs. As a result dizziness, pins and needles in the hands and spasms may occur. Physiological hyperventilation is a normal adaptation phenomenon during exposure to altitude.

Hypoxia Normobaric/Hypobaric: Hypoxia is defined as a lack of oxygen in the tissue. Normobaic hypoxia occurs when the concentration of oxygen in the respiratory air is reduced (e.g. due to the introduction of nitrogen or carbon dioxide) with no change to air pressure (change of gas mixture in an enclosed chamber or with a stationary mask system). Hypobaric hypoxia is the reduction in the oxygen content of the respiratory air due to a reduction in air pressure (natural altitude conditions or in a vacuum chamber).

Inverted Lasègue's Sign: This is a nerve stretching test (root L2—L4), in which the leg (patient lies on his stomach) is bent at the knee. If this causes shooting pains along the front of the thigh, then a positive inverted Lasègue's is present and hence possible nerve compression.

Kelty Camp Chair® or Crazy Creek® Chair: This is a type of camping stool with an upholstered seat and upholstered backrest without metal legs.

Lasègue Sign: This is a nerve stretching test (roots L5 and S1), where the outstretched leg (patient lies on his back) is raised in the passive state. If pain is experienced along the length of the leg, then a positive Lasègue and hence possible nerve compression is present.

Lateral Foot: Outside edge of foot.

Long-Line Rescue (Helicopter): The Long Line System is used in the rescue of injured mountaineers from vertical and overhanging rock faces. A rope up to 200 meters long is latched up underneath the helicopter. The user will be able to use this to reach the accident victim even on high steep rock faces. If the victim of the accident is located under an overhanging rock the rescuer will be able to get to him using a telescopic rod.

Luxation, Dislocation (Latin luxare = dislocate, sprain): A complete or incomplete (subluxation) loss of contact of the ends of bones that form the joints. It is always the bone on the distal side of the body that is designated as the dislocated bone. Any dislocation represents a serious injury to a joint.

Macronutrients: The macronutrients include fats, carbohydrates and proteins.

Medial Foot: Inside of the foot.

Median nerve: The median nerve is a branch arising from the brachial plexus which is in part responsible for bending the fingers and for the nerve supply to the muscles in the ball of the thumb. In addition, the sensitivity (response to touch) of the thumb, index and middle finger tips on the back of the hand and almost the whole of the palm of the hand (apart from the little finger, half of the ring finger and the outside of the thumb) is taken care of by this nerve.

Micronutrients: The micronutrients include vitamins, minerals and trace elements. These need to be absorbed together with food and do not supply energy. Part of their function, for example, is to help build up macromolecules.

Mixed venous blood: This means blood that originates in the upper and lower vena cava and is "mixed" in the right atrium of the heart before passing through the right ventricle into the pulmonary artery. Sampling the blood is a highly complex affair and can only be carried out using a special catheter. The mixed venous blood provides information on the oxygen consumption of the peripheral organs.

Muscle Relaxants: Muscle-relaxing drugs.

Night Sweats: Night sweats result in dripping wet hair and nightwear that is wet through over a large area.

Oxidative Processes: Chemical reactions at cell level assisted by oxygen. So-called free radicals may emerge from oxidative processes. Oxidation in itself can destroy biochemical processes and important substances. Well-known anti-oxidative substances include vitamins C, E, beta-carotene and trace elements such as zinc, copper, manganese and selenium.

Paraplegia: Complete paralysis of both legs.

Patellar Tendon Reflex: A light tap on the patellar tendon will cause the lower leg to jerk upwards. If, in a comparison with the opposite limb, this happens to a lesser extent or not at all this is a possible indication of the presence of a compression of the nerve root.

Phasic Muscles: The muscles are composed of red and white muscle fibers. The red muscle fibers are also called "tonic muscles" and are fibers that demonstrate a high myoglobin content. The red muscle fibers are required for endurance sports. "Phasic muscles" means the white muscle fibers which, by contrast to the red fibers, contain only a small amount of myoglobin and correspondingly not long-term endurance components. However, they have a high contraction capability. The white fibers are needed, for example, in activities such as weight lifting where heavy weights need to be handled within a short period.

Polyglobulia: Polyglobulia means enhanced regeneration of the blood. This can happen, e.g. at high altitude, where the body forms an increased quantity of red blood corpuscles so as to raise the number of oxygen carriers.

Polytrauma: Polytrauma is the term used to designate several injuries to different regions of the body which have occurred at the same time, of which a minimum of one injury or the combination of several injuries represent a threat to health.

Pulmonary Hypertonia: Pulmonary hypertonic is the term used to describe an increase in blood pressure in the pulmonary circulation. This may be caused by disorders affecting the valves of the heart, the vessels of the lung or a fall in oxygen partial pressure such as occurs at high altitude.

Pulmonary (O)edema: Pulmonary (o)edema is a nonspecific accumulation of fluid in the connective tissue of the lung. Causes include changes in pressure in the blood vessels such as (e.g.) in the case of High Altitude Pulmonary (O)edema, or due to infections or drowning. In High Altitude Pulmonary (O)edema caused by drowning it is possible to distinguish between drowning due to ingesting fresh water as opposed to salt water. A feature of drowning in salt water is that the high salt concentration leads to an influx of fluid from the blood vessels into the connective tissue, in the case of fresh water it is damage to the surface lining of the alveoli of the lung. The outcome of any type of pulmonary (o)edema is that the person affected is no longer able to absorb sufficient oxygen into the **circulatory system.**

Radicular Pains: These are pains which emanate from the nerve roots and which can be assigned to a pain pathway along the leg and extending into the area of the foot. Often simultaneous discomfort occurs in the relevant area of the skin.

Rectal Disorder: Spontaneous, involuntary bowel movement.

RICE Rule/PECH-Regel: Basic rule that can be applied for all acute injuries. **RICE (PECH** in German) is an acronym that stands for **R**est (**P**ause), **I**ce (**E**is), **C**ompression, **E**levate (**H**ochlagern).

Saddle Anesthesia: Reduced sensitivity **(Hypesthesia** up to **Anesthesia)** with its typical spread, the form of which corresponds to jodhpurs. The feeling of numbness comprises the area of the **genitalia,** the region around the sphincter muscle and the insides of the thighs. Acute occurrence saddle anesthesia is associated with a problem at the level of the spinal cord. Frequently urinary and/or stool incontinence and impotence with a lack of sphincter muscle contraction are features. Should these symptoms occur it is essential to get to a medical center without delay.

Sensorimotor System: Interplay of sensory and motor skills, i.e. perception of stimulus by one sensory organ and subsequent motor behavior.

Shock: A life-threatening condition in which the circulation of blood in the organs is reduced. As a result a deficiency of oxygen in the tissues and, by way of a final consequence, metabolic disturbances occur. The cause is an absolute or relative reduction in the amount of blood circulating.
Accompanying bleeding = **hemorrhagic shock**
Accompanying blood poisoning = **septic shock**
Accompanying an allergic attack= **anaphylactic shock**
Accompanying failure of neural regulation (spinal cord injuries) = **neurogenic shock**

Slackline: Type of trend sport involving balancing on a wide band and thus training balance, coordination and concentration. Training for climbers etc.

Stagnation: Means that a particular variable is lacking in growth.

Tetraplegia: A form of paraplegia where all four limbs, i.e. both legs and arms, are affected.

Thromboses, Embolisms: Thrombosis is a disorder of the vascular system in which a blood clot **(thrombus)** in a **blood vessel,** mostly venous, forms. Causes include changes in the composition of the blood, damage to the vessel wall or instances where no further transport of the blood takes place. Flushing a thrombus away may present a further complication and this can lead to a (pulmonary) embolism. This is an acute blockage of the arteries of the lung which can lead to a disturbance to the exchange of gases and to cardiac stress. A sizable pulmonary embolism can be fatal.

Trisomy 21: (Down's Syndrome, Mongolism), genome mutation in humans in which Chromosome 21 (or part of it) is triplicated. This results in babies being born mentally handicapped.

Vasoconstriction: Narrowing of the blood vessel (this results in a worsening of performance in terms of blood flow in the affected organ and a reduction in heat output/loss of heat).

Vasodilation: Widening of the blood vessels (this gives a better flow of blood within the affected organ and increased heat output/loss of heat).

Ventricular Fibrillation: A life-threatening disturbance of the cardiac rhythm where there is no pulse and accompanied by a procession of disordered stimuli in the ventricles of the heart and where the heart muscle no longer contracts properly. Untreated, ventricular fibrillation will lead directly to death due to the lack of pumping action of the heart.

VO_2max: The maximum oxygen uptake (VO_2max) indicates the maximum number of milliliters of oxygen that can be utilized by the body in a state of physical exertion. It may be used to assess endurance capacity.

Wind Chill Factor: The **wind chill** describes the difference between the measured air temperature and the temperature felt as a function of wind speed. The wind chill factor is caused by the dissipation of warm air close to the skin as well as the associated increase in the rate of evaporation.

23. Authors

Dr. med. **Anna G. Brunello,** Swiss Medical Society (FMH) Critical Care Medicine, Anaesthesia and Emergency Medicine SGNOR (Schweizerische Gesellschaft für Notfall- und Rettungsmedizin - Swiss Society for Emergency and Rescue Medicine) is employed as an intensivist and anaesthesiologist at the Canton Hospital Graubünden and assists the Swiss Air Rescue Service Rega as an emergency medical practitioner. She is a member of the Board of the SGGM (Schweizerische Gesellschaft für Gebirgsmedizin – Swiss Mountain Medicine Society) and has been active for many years in training lay people (Swiss Alpine Club) and professionals (ERC, International Master in Mountain Medicine). She is an active mountaineer and has taken part in several expeditions to the Peruvian Andes, the Himalayas and Greenland.
Contact Address: brunelloa@hotmail.com

Dr. med. **Martin Walliser** is general surgeon and Head of Accident Surgery at the Cantonal Hospital of Glarus. In his function as Vice-Chairman, he is an active Member of the Board of the Swiss Mountain Medicine Society (SGGM) as well as being involved in the medical training of laypersons (mountain guide courses of the Swiss Association of Mountain Guides SBV, SAC, SOA etc.) and further in professional medical training programs (ATLS, SGGM etc.).
He has been a mountain guide since 1993 and regularly participates in projects that take him not only to the Alps but also to South and North America, Asia and Africa.
Contact Address: walli@spin.ch

Dr. med. **Urs Hefti** is the Head of the Swiss Sport Clinic Bern. He is a trauma surgeon and orthopaedic and sports medicine specialist. In addition, he is a clinical emergency physician as well as being an emergency doctor with REGA. In his capacity as member of the Swiss Mountain Medicine Society (SGGM) he has been active on various committees, including the Medical Committee of the International Mountaineering and Climbing Federation (UIAA) and the SAC. In addition, he has set up courses in sport climbing and medicine as well as the Altitude Medicine course in Zermatt, which has been certified by the UIAA/ICAR/ISMM as the primary specialist course worldwide for «Expedition and Wilderness Medicine». In 1998 he worked with the Himalayan Rescue Association (HRA) in Pheriche, Nepal.
He has led four major scientific research expeditions (Shisha Pangma, Muztagh Ata, Pik Lenin, Himlung Himal) and has climbed a number of high mountains on several

continents, one of which was the 8046 m high Shisha Pangma. He is a founder member of www.swiss-exped.ch – the Association for the Promotion of Training, Education and Research into Mountain and High Altitude Medicine.
Contact Address: swissyeti@bluemail.ch

Dr. med. **Daniel Walter** is an FMH physician specialising in general medical practice with his own practice in Jenaz (GR). He has completed a range of additional training courses, including in sport medicine (SGSM), in emergency medicine (SGNOR), chiropractics (SGMM) as well as in mountain and high altitude medicine (International Diploma of Mountain Medicine). Mountaineering in all its different aspects is his passion. Through participating in a range of different expeditions he has been able to gain experience in the care of expedition members as well as the local residents. For some years he has been active in the presentation of training courses focussing on high altitude medicine at Kobler & Partner, Berne. In addition, he is involved in the training of senior tour guides, mountain guides and hut wardens (SAC).
Contact Address: daniel.walter@praxisjenaz.ch

Dr. med. **Urs Wiget,** (retired) FMH, emergency physician SGNOR. Still working as a trainer in emergency medical services, sports and mountain medicine attending to a wide diversity of patients. Active on the mountain scene for 50 years, he has been a participator/doctor/leader on 10 major expeditions in the Himalayas and in the Andes. Derives great satisfaction from leading treks (Ladakh/Zanskar) and accompanying adventure tours (Thailand, Cambodia, Oman, Zanskar) in his capacity as a physician. Was team doctor for Alinghi in Ras al Kaimah and Valencia. He has always spent (and is still spending) a lot of time with children (his own 6 and others) in the mountains, as well as with his wife Susi Kriemler in the Himalayan Rescue Organisation Dispensary in Pheriche/Khumbu/Nepal.
Contact Address: udw@uitikon.ch

Urs Hirsiger is a certified dietician trained at a professional college and a member of the Swiss Association of Certified Dieticians (SVDE). For the past 10 years he has been running an independent practice in Sursee and works alongside the regional family doctors. As a member of the specialist Sports Nutrition group (collaboration with ETH Zurich and BASPO in Magglingen) he works in close collaboration with representatives of a very wide range of sporting trends. With experience of mountaineering spanning over 30 years, including sport climbing and high Alpine tours, he is a very enthusiastic mountaineer familiar with the whole of the Alpine region and beyond as well as long-distance treks. Having worked his way up from a participant on J+S courses to course leader, he is routinely to be found on the SAC basic training course.
Contact Address: urs-hirsiger@bluewin.ch.

PD Dr. med. **Susi Kriemler,** FMH (Swiss Medical Society) Paediatrics and Sport Medicine SGSM, is a lecturer and research associate at the Institute for Sport and Sports Sciences and at the Swiss Tropical and Public Health Institute of the University of Basle where she has been involved with movement in childhood for a number of years and in so doing endeavours to bring motherhood, mountaineering and high altitude medicine under a single umbrella. She is the author of a range of alpine medicine publications with the focus on children.
Contact Address: susi.kriemler@unibas.ch

Alexandre Kottmann, M.D., is an anesthetist and emergency Physician. He is completing his training as an intensivist at the University Hospital of Bern. Alongside this he works regularly in the pre-clinic at Rega. He is a member of the Medical Commission of ICAR (International Commission for Alpine Rescue) and represents Rega and the Swiss Alpine Rescue service. He is a member of GRIMM and Board member of the Swiss Society of Mountain Medicine. Since 2009 he has been Course Leader on the SSMM Courses for Doctors in Mountain Medicine and spends a great deal of time himself in the mountains.
Contact Address: alex.kottmann@me.com

Dr. med. **Christophe Marti,** FMH Internal Medicine. Works as a consultant at the Canton Hospital, Geneva, in the intensive care unit, emergency and internal medicine. He is active in training laypersons for the SAC, youth and sport and the Swiss Mountain Guides Association. An active mountaineer, he is frequently to be found in the Alps and has also taken part in climbs in South America and the Karakorum.

Dr. med. **Thomas Szeless,** FMH Internal Medicine. «From my childhood days I have been an enthusiastic explorer of the mountains that define and replicate themselves across our land and of Nature who transports us with every step on a journey through time.»

Dr. med. **Roland Albrecht,** FMH specialist in intensive medicine and anaesthesia, SGNOR emergency doctor as well as member of the Board of SGNOR und EUSEM (European Society for Emergency Medicine). Since1.7.2008 consultant and member of the Management Committee of the Swiss Air Rescue Service (REGA). He acts as a representative on the Foundation Board of the Alpine Rescue Service Switzerland and sits on various other committees. Address: Swiss Air Rescue Service (REGA), REGA Center, PO Box 1414, 8058 Zurich Airport.
Contact Address: roland.albrecht@rega.ch

Andres Bardill has been active either on a part- or full-time basis as a mountain guide since 1989. Since 2006 he has, in his capacity as Managing Director of Alpine Rescue Services (ARS), been responsible for deployment and training within the organisation and for ensuring that it is ready for operation and has made a significant contribution to building it up. As a trainer with J+S, on the SGGM doctors' courses, IKAR, and internally within the ARS he maintains permanent contact with mountain rescuers and partner organisations at a national and international level.

Dr. med. **Eckehart Schöll,** FMH Anaesthesiology and Clinical Emergency Medicine SGNOR, Emergency Doctor SGNOR. Since 2002 he has been Editor of the specialist journal of the Swiss Mountain Medicine Society (SGGM), the Forum Alpinum, Course Leader SGGM courses «Sport Climbing and Medicine» as well as «High Altitude Medicine », as well as being a passionate mountaineer and climber.
Contact Address: schoell@forum-alpinum.ch

Dr. med. **Christian Schlegel,** FMH for Physical Medicine and Rehabilitation, Sport Medicine SGSM and Manual Medicine SAMT. Has been based at the Swiss Olympic Medical Center in the Medical Health Center of the Grand Resort Bad Ragaz since 1998. For 18 years he has been a trainer in ski and mountain skills at the ETH Zurich, for 17 years he has been Federation Physician to the Sport and Ice-climbing National Team. Chief Medical Officer to the Swiss Olympia Delegation in Vancouver 2010.
Contact Address: Christian.Schlegel@resortragaz.ch

PD Dr. med. **Andreas Schweizer,** Orthopaedic and Hand Surgery FMH, is based at the University Hospital Balgrist in Zurich. Among other interests, he has been engaged in scientific research into climbing injuries to the hand and forearm and has for the past 20 years been an active sport climber and boulderer. Address: University Hospital Balgrist, Forchstrasse 340, 8008 Zurich.
Contact Address: andreas.schweizer@balgrist.ch

† Dr. med. **Hans Peter Bircher** died in a tragic climbing accident in Sardinia in Mai 2012. He was working as Orthopaedic Surgeon (FMH, EBOT) and Chief Medical Officer at the Zug Cantonal Hospital. Following his dissertation in Altitude Medicine at the Margheritahütte (the highest alpine hut in Europe), he has been on two expeditions in the Himalayas, consolidating his knowledge of Altitude Medicine. Sport climbing in a number of amazing locations worldwide, including in Bolivia and Madagascar, was his favourite hobby.
We not only lost a competent Orthopaedic Surgeon and caring doctor but also a good friend and mountain pal. Always positive and enthusiastic for all kinds of alpine adventures – we are missing him!

PD Dr. med. **Yann Villiger** is FMH in Anaesthesia and Intensive Care focussing on Cardiac Anaesthesia and Emergencies and is the Chief Medical Officer at the Hôpitaux universitaires de Genève. He is an ACLS Instructor and undertakes regular flights in his capacity as a REGA doctor in Geneva. His experience of the high mountains stretches back 25 years and he has held a Paragliding Pilot's Licence since 1991. His experience does not only extend to flying but also to the medical care of accident victims.
Contact Address: Yann.Villiger@hcuge.ch

Dr. med. **Tobias Merz** is a senior staff specialist in Internal Medicine and Intensive Care at the Department of Intensive Care Medicine of the University Hospital Berne, Switzerland. As a passionate mountaineer, he often visits the Andes and the Himalayas. He is the author of a range of scientific publications on the subject of Altitude Medicine compiled on the basis of experience acquired through participation in research expeditions.
Contact Address: Tobias.Merz@insel.ch

Prof. **Marco Maggiorini,** Chief Medical Officer at the University Hospital Zurich Dept. for Medical Intensive Care Unit. Having obtained the title of Consultant for Internal Medicine, Cardiology and Intensive Medicine, his current activities relate to the practice of Intensive Medicine. Involved in research into Altitude Medicine for more than 25 years, he is the author of several studies on the epidemiology and pathophysiology of Altitude Sickness, in particular High Altitude Pulmonary Edema as well as prophylaxis and therapy in relation to these complaints.
Contact Address: marco.maggiorini@usz.ch

Dr. med. **Bruno Durrer** is a mountain guide, General Medicine FMH, Emergency Doctor SGNOR, Sports Medicine SGSM and Medical Director of the Rescue Helicopter Station Air Glaciers and the Ambulance Service, Lauterbrunnen. He has his own General Practice in Lauterbrunnen and Mürren with the focus on Emergency Medicine, Sport Traumatology and Mountain and Sport Medicine. Since 1980 he has been on approx. 3000 helicopter rescue missions. He has taken part in a range of expeditions to Nepal, Tibet, Pakistan, South America and Africa. Bruno Durrer is a Member of the Board and a Foundation Member of various national and international Mountain Medicine Commissions and Societies (UIAA, ISMM, SGGM, ICAR) and has published a range of papers on accidents involving the effects of cold, avalanches and lightening as well as relating to mountain rescue medicine. He is a co-founder and was the responsible Head of the Swiss Courses for Medical Practitioners in Mountain Medicine from 1990 to 2004 and, in his capacity as a racing doctor, has offered his services at various major sporting events (Lauberhorn Abfahrt Ski Race, Inferno Abfahrt and Triathlon, Jungfrau Stafette).

Dr. med. Dr. phil. **Daniel Barthelmes** (FMH Ophthalmology) works at the Department of Ophthalmology at the University Hospital Zurich. Participating in the research expedition to Mt. Muztagh Ata, together with his colleagues Dr. med. Martina Bösch (Ophthalmology Clinic Zurich), Dr. med. Tobias Merz, Dr. med. Urs Hefti and others, he compiled and published several scientific studies related to changes of the eye at high altitude which are considered seminal in the field.

Dr. med. **René Meyrat,** specialist in dermatology and venerology, more specifically allergology FMH and clinical immunology, works in a group practice in Chur.

Dr. med. **Christian Giger** is a neurosurgeon focused on spine surgery. He is a member of the Swiss Society of Neurosurgery and mamber of the Swiss Society of Interventional Pain Management. A passionate mountaineer, ice climber and skier, when not in the hospital he can usually be found on the best slopes.
Contact Address: giger.christian@gmail.com

Dr. med. dent. **Gian Andrea Hälg.** Following a period as an assistant in a private practice and 5 years of clinic and scientific activity with a lectureship in the area of reconstructive dental medicine and implantology at the University of Zurich, he has been active since the summer of 2009 as an independent dentist in a joint practice in Samedan, near St. Moritz. «This means that I am back in the beautiful surroundings of the mountain valley Engadin, which is where I grew up and where, through the medium of ski and mountain bike, I am consistently finding new nooks and crannies which have lost none of their ability to bewitch»."

Dr. med. **Katharina Schenk-Jäger,** senior consultant at the Swiss Toxicological Information Centre (STIC) specialising in mushroom poisoning, certified mushroom controller, Association toxicologist for the Association of Swiss Mycology Societies VSVP.
Contact Address: katharina.schenk@usz.ch

Dr. med. vet. **Jacqueline Kupper,** Expert in poisonous plants and adviser in animal toxicology at the Toxicological Information Information Centre Zurich (STIZ) and at the Vetsuisse Faculty of the University of Zurich, Institute for Veterinary Pharmacology and Toxicology. ***Contact Address:*** jacqueline.kupper@usz.ch

Dr. med. **Stefanie Meusel,** FMH Internal Medicine Branch working as a family doctor in the «Praxis Feldmühle» group practice in Kriens. For many years member of the Board of the SGGM where she worked as a recorder. A number of trekking trips in Asia and South America, International Diploma of Mountain Medicine, basic experience in mountaineering and climbing. ***Contact Address:*** Stefanie Meusel, Praxis Feldmühle, Obernauerstrasse 40, 6010 Kriens.

24. Index of Illustrations

Sources of Illustrations, Drawings and Diagrams

Our sincere thanks to all who have contributed to the supply of illustrations.

Tommy Dätwyler (Cover photo: Patient evacuation on Pik Lenin, 7134 m, Pamir, Kyrgzstan), Willi Kuhn (among others, frontispieces Chapter 1 "Training Camp in Namibia" and Chapter 22 "Via Ferrata on Piz Trovat"), Anna Brunello (among others, frontispieces Chapter 2 "[Too] Much Weight on the Arctic Circle Trail, Greenland"), Urs Hirsiger (among others, frontispiece Chapter 3 "Halt by the Cross at the Summit"), Urs Wiget (among others, frontispieces Chapter 16 "Kala Patar, Khumbu, Nepal," Chapter 4 "Kids at Everest Base Camp," Chapter 5 "Girlish Euphoria at High Altitude," Chapter 6 "Oswald in Oman" – with the kind permission of Oswald Oelz and Chapter 16 "The Mother and Necklace:" Ama Dablam 6856, Khumbu Nepal"), Alex Kottmann (frontispiece Chapter 7 "The Long and the Short of it – Grand Jorasses, Mont Blanc"), Urs Hefti (frontispieces Chapter 8 "Happy Wandering post-Hip Replacement" and Chapter 12 "Bike Fun in the Engadine National Park"), Thomas Bärfuss (frontispiece Chapter 9 "Primary Care on Gemsfreiheit, Piz Palü"), Dominik Hunziker (among others, frontispieces Chapter 10 "Look, No Ropes: Next to the Accident Site, Sella Glacier, Bernina," Chapter 14 "Preventive Intervention in the Gorge, Bergell," Chapter 20 "Training in Suspension on a Rope" and Chapter 21 "Route Impassable – Evacuation in Bernina Region"), Rainer Eder (frontispiece Chapter 11 "Andi Schweizer in Speibl, Telli"), Remy Wenger, Speleo-Secours Switzerland (frontispiece Chapter 15 "Standard Equipment for a Cave Rescue"), Tobias Merz (among others, frontispiece Chapter 17 "High-Altitude Camping on Muztagh Ata, 7509 m Pamir, Kyrgzstan"), Christian Giger (frontispiece Chapter 19 "Arctic Midday Sun, Norway" and "Arctic Sun" Ski Tours in Norway). For all other illustrations our thanks go to Dani Walter (Chapter 1), Eckehart Schöll (Chapter 9.2), Martin Walliser (Chapter 9.3), Bruno Durrer (Chapter 10, 18, 20), Patrik Koster (Chapter 14), Martina Bösch (Chapter 17), Matthias Gutmann (frontispiece Chapter 18 "High Altitude Camping in the Early Morning – Pik Lenin, 7134 m, Pamir, Kyrgzstan"), Daniel Barthelmes (Chapter 19), René Meyrat (Chapter 19), Franco Brunello (Chapter 19), Gianni Haelg (Chapter 21.2), Jacqueline Kupper (Chapter 21.3) and Katharina Schenk (Chapter 21.3).

The majority of drawings originate from "Basic Education in Medical Services" from the Swiss Army, valid as of 1st January 1987, Part II, Instruction Sheet 59.11/IId. For permission to use this we extend our thanks to Niklaus Hofer (High Command, Swiss Army). Thanks are also due to Andréas Meyer (Coordination Unit for the Protection of Amphibians and Reptiles in Switzerland [Karch]), Urs Klemmer (Swiss Resuscitation Council), Stephan Harvey (Institute for Snow and Avalanche Research SLF) and Prof. Robert Steffen for kindly providing numerous items of additional teaching materials and information.

25. Index

E. Landolt/K. M. Urbanska

Our Alpine Flora

The glorious colours and the diversity of shapes of Alpine plants delight every alpinist and hiker! Those who take time to look closer at the plants and their dwellings will be rewarded with discovery of many interesting relationships between plants and their environment, and will enjoy their ever varying appearance and the multitude of forms. The SAC guidebook helps the reader to know diverse aspects of the plant life in the Alps. It also points out some problems: which faraway lands the Alpine plants come from? Why is the plant cover near Zermatt village different from that high up at the foot of the Eiger? How do some Alpine plants still manage to grow above 12 000 ft, whereas the others do not even reach the timberline. To make easier the recognition of species, the booklet is equipped with colour photographs, mostly taken in natural sites. In addition, about 75 species are presented in ink drawings! A practical fieldguide for amateur botanists, it is also an important reference work for all those with an interest in alpine plants.

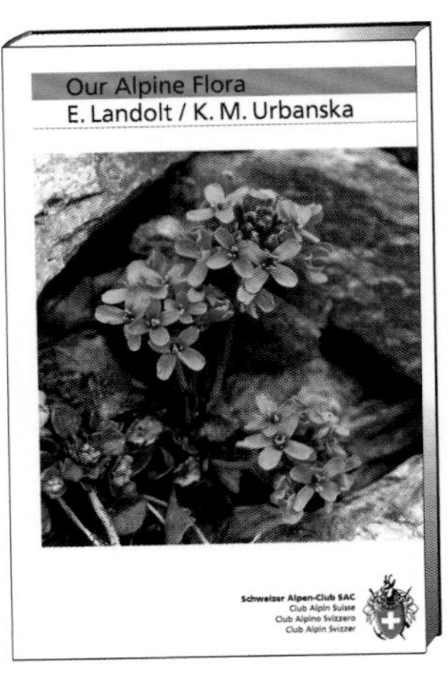

480 pages
136 color photos
140 drawings

3rd edition

ISBN 978-3-85902-219-5

Eric Pointner/Egon Feller

Oberwallis

Goms/Aletsch-Brig/Simplon/Visp/ Saastal/Mattertal/Raron-Siders

2000 routes in 99 climbing areas: presented here is an incredibly diverse climbing landscape situated in the middle of the highest mountains of Switzerland. More than 250 multi-pitch routes up to 800 m in length are to found in this guide!

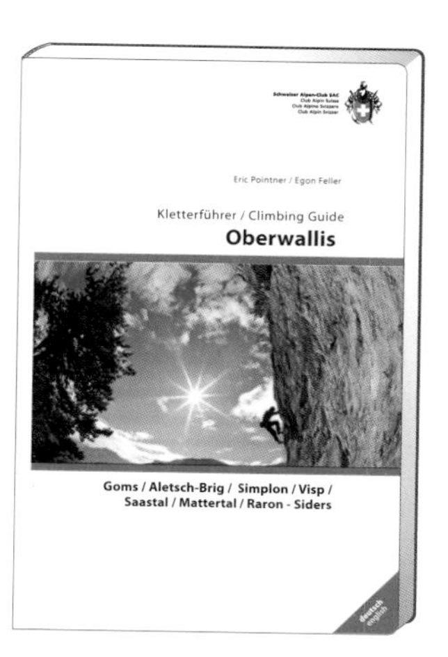

D/E
352 pages
81 color photos
18 photos black-white
159 pictures
of climbing routes
70 topographies

ISBN 978-3-85902-310-9

Remo Kundert/Marco Volken

Huts in the Swiss Alps

The "Hüttenbuch" (Hut Book) describes around 330 huts and bivouacs in the Swiss Alps, including all of the accommodation provided by the Swiss Alpine Club as well as numerous other huts and mountain guesthouses. It also contains the following, detailed information: coloured pictures of the huts, map extract with marked ascent routes (summer/winter), information about arrival via public transport, addresses and telephone numbers for information and reservations, staffing times and catering options, information about climbing crags, information about mobile phone signal, paths to other mountain huts and villages.

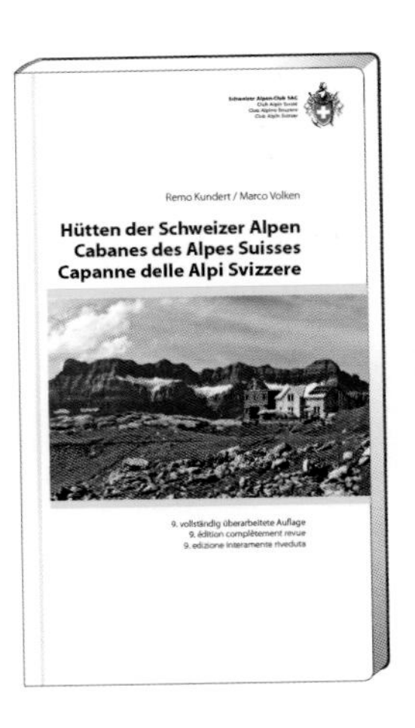

D/F/I
416 pages
346 color photos
345 maps

9th fully revised edition

ISBN 978-3-85902-346-8